INDEPENDENT LIFEBOATS

IN THE BRITISH ISLES

serving England, Wales and Scotland station by station

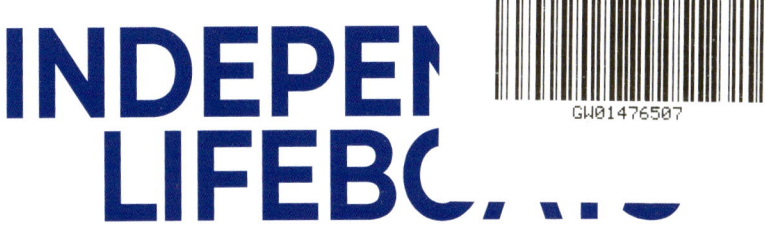

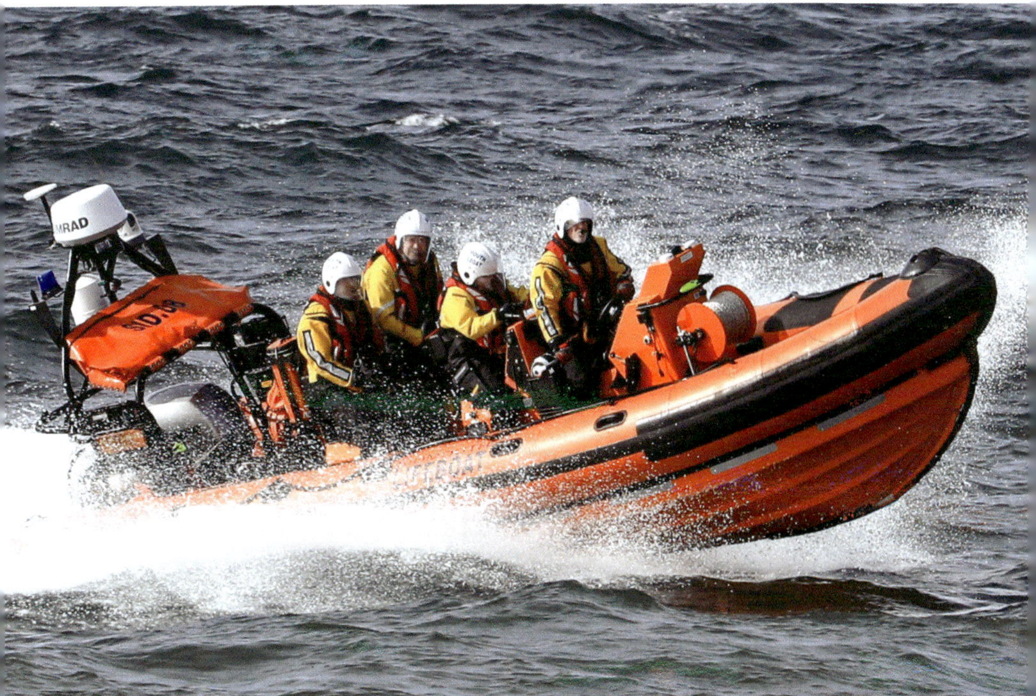

Martin Fish and Nicholas Leach

FOXGLOVE PUBLISHING

First published 2022

Published by Foxglove Publishing Ltd
Foxglove House, Shute Hill,
Lichfield WS13 8DB
United Kingdom
Tel 07940 905046

© Nicholas Leach and Martin Fish 2022

The right of the authors to be identified as the Authors of this work has been asserted in accordance with the Copyrights, Designs and Patents Act 1988.

All rights reserved. No part of this book may be reprinted or reproduced or utilised in any form or by any electronic, mechanical or other means, now known or hereafter invented, including photocopying and recording, or in any information storage or retrieval system, without the permission in writing from the Publishers. British Library Cataloguing in Publication Data.

ISBN 978-1-909540262

Typesetting and layout by
Nicholas Leach/Foxglove Publishing

The scope of this book

This volume covers the independent lifeboat stations of England, Wales and Scotland, and is arranged in geographical order, starting in north-east England and going south and clockwise round the coast, ending at St Abbs in the Scottish Borders. Trying to determine which independent lifeboat operators to include and which ones to omit was a little difficult. The authors have covered what they believe to be all the major coastal independent lifeboat organisations around the three nations, and the inland operations which have significant rescue craft. The stations and boats of Ireland have not been included, partly because it has proved difficult to travel round them and partly because there are so many. The individual entries for each station include photographs of the lifeboats past and present where possible, as well as details of the organisations' histories, and its current assets. Flood and water rescue boats operated by fire services, beach lifeguard units, mountain rescue and lowland search teams rescue boats have not been included.

CONTENTS

HISTORY OF INDEPENDENT LIFEBOATS   4

ENGLAND – EAST COAST   11
    Boulmer, Runswick, Hornsea, Hessle, Humber

ENGLAND – EAST ANGLIA   25
    Mundesley, Sea Palling, Hemsby, Caister, Felixstowe

ENGLAND – SOUTH COAST   43
    Pett Level, Southsea (Portsea), Hamble, Gosport, Solent, Sidmouth, Hope Cove

ISLE OF WIGHT AND CHANNEL ISLANDS   67
    Ryde, Sandown, Freshwater, Jersey, St Helier

BRISTOL CHANNEL AND SOUTH WALES   85
    Burnham-on-Sea, SARA (Tewkesbury, Upton-upon-Severn, Sharpness, Beachley, Newport), Loughor, Ferryside

ENGLAND – NORTH WEST   105
    Liverpool, Southport, Flookburgh, Ulverston, Askam (Duddon), Haverigg, Maryport

SCOTLAND   129
    Glencaple (Nith), Mossyard, Port William, Glasgow, Loch Lomond, Dornoch, Findhorn, St Abbs

INLAND LIFEBOATS   148
    York, Ratcliffe-on-Soar, Nottingham, Watersafe UK

CLOSED STATIONS   150
    Blyth, Cleethorpes, Birling Gap, Guernsey, Portishead, Clovelly, Stonehaven

SUMMARY OF INDEPENDENT LIFEBOAT STATIONS   158

MAP OF INDEPENDENT LIFEBOAT STATIONS   160

HISTORY OF INDEPENDENT LIFEBOATS

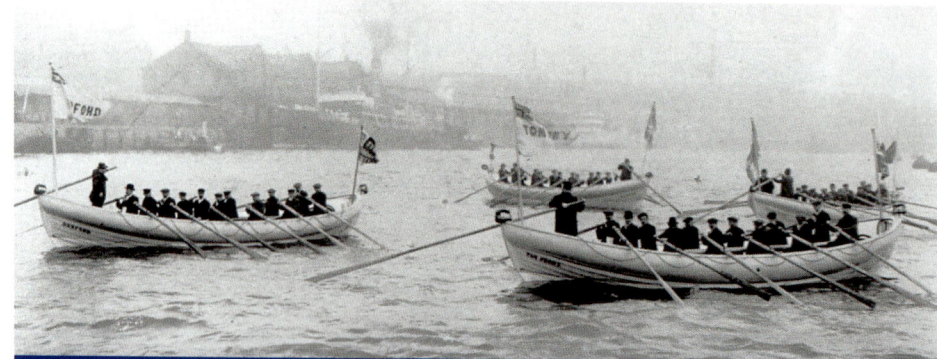

The Tyne Lifeboat Society's lifeboats in the early 1900s. The Society operated lifeboats from the 1770s to the 1930s. The lifeboats pictured here are, from left to right, Bedford, Willie Wouldhave (in background), Tom Perry and James Young, all of which were of the North Country type favoured in the north-east. (Supplied by Stephen Landells)

Around the coasts of the United Kingdom and Ireland is a network of lifeboat stations which operate independently of the Royal National Lifeboat Institution (RNLI). The 'independents' are funded privately and most are registered charities, relying on donations to remain operational. They operate lifeboats and water rescue services twenty-four hours a day, year-round, with crews made up entirely of volunteers. Their continued successful operation is a tribute to the enthusiasm and selfless dedication of those volunteers, who often undertake multiple roles to ensure the service is maintained.

Although the independent lifeboat stations are usually well-known in their locality, they can sometimes be overshadowed by the RNLI when it comes to publicity and fundraising. The national body has a multi-million pound budget to maintain its lifeboat stations around the UK and Ireland (238 in 2022). The management of such a complex and important service is undertaken from a large purpose-built headquarters site in Poole, where full-time staff provide the support needed to keep the RNLI's stations fully operational, from organising fund-raising campaigns to building state-of-the-art lifeboats. Operating alongside this national body, the independents play as vital a role when it comes to saving lives at sea.

Although the independent lifeboat organisations described in this book were mostly established during the late 20th and early 21st centuries, the oldest locally-operated lifeboats were in operation more than two centuries ago, before the RNLI had been founded (it was known as the National Institution for the Preservation of Life from Shipwreck when established in 1824, with the current title being adopted in 1854). The first lifeboat station, established in 1776 at Formby at

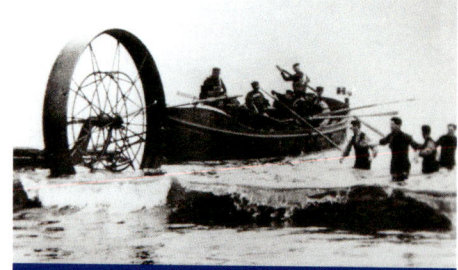

The Aberdeen lifeboat Bon Accord No.1 being launched off the beach. This boat, built by Forrestt & Son at Limehouse in 1853, was operated by the Aberdeen Harbour Commissioners independently of the RNLI until 1925, when the RNLI took over.

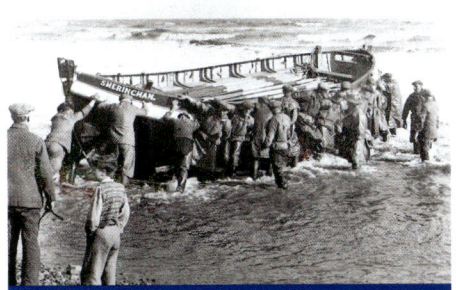

Henry Ramey Upcher being launched off the beach at Sheringham in the late 1920s. The lifeboat, 34ft 9in in length, was the second of two lifeboats operated by a Beachmen's Committee and funded by the local Upcher family. Built in the town in which she served, Henry Ramey Upcher was used as a lifeboat and crewed by local fishermen from 1894 to 1935.

the entrance to the Mersey, was a locally-funded and -managed affair, operating one of several lifeboats built for the Liverpool Dock Trustees (later Mersey Docks & Harbours Board). In 1790 the Glasgow Humane Society was founded and has provided a lifesaving service on the waterways of Greater Glasgow ever since.

Over the course of the next half century or so, many other lifeboats were provided, and all were funded and managed locally. On the north-east coast of England lifeboats were established at South Shields (in 1789) and at North Shields (in 1798) by local people, while at Sunderland the Humane Society provided a lifeboat. Early lifeboats covering Dublin Bay were financed by the port's Dock Trust, while elsewhere other lifeboats were funded and built through the initiatives of shipowners' groups at major ports such as Montrose, Aberdeen and Hartlepool.

During the first half of the 19th century, county and district associations sprang up in many places with the aim of providing a lifeboat. In 1806 a Humane Society was formed in Suffolk which financed local lifeboat activities at Pakefield, Lowestoft and Aldeburgh. Indeed, the coastal towns in Norfolk and Suffolk were home to many independent lifeboat operations during the 19th century, and the four non-RNLI lifeboat operations now thriving in Norfolk continue a long tradition of life-saving in the county.

But as the 19th century progressed, most of the independent lifeboat stations gradually came under the auspices of the RNLI. Then, as now, finance was a challenge for lifeboat operators, but the RNLI, by the second half of the century, was devising new and innovative ways to raise the funds needed to maintain a national lifeboat service, and was thus in a better position to take over all sea rescue operations. The great majority of independent bodies ceased their lifeboat operations before 1900, with one of the last to

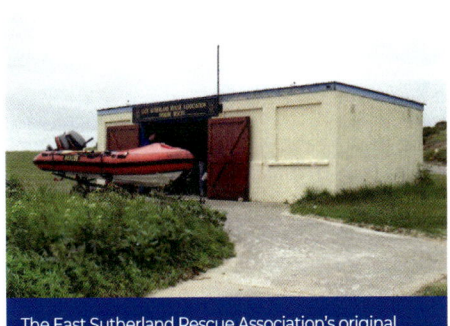

The East Sutherland Rescue Association's original lifeboat house on Dornoch Beach, with the inshore lifeboat Laura Sinclair II outside. The Association, whose boats cover the Dornoch Firth, opened a large brand-new purpose-built station in 2022.

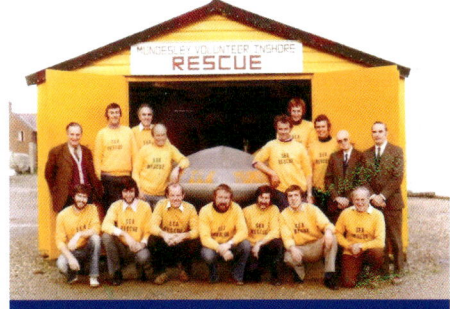

The early days at Mundesley Volunteer Inshore Rescue, with the crew and lifeboat outside their somewhat rudimentary boathouse. Mundesley, as with all independent lifeboat services, has come a long way since it was first established.

Independent lifeboats of Britain

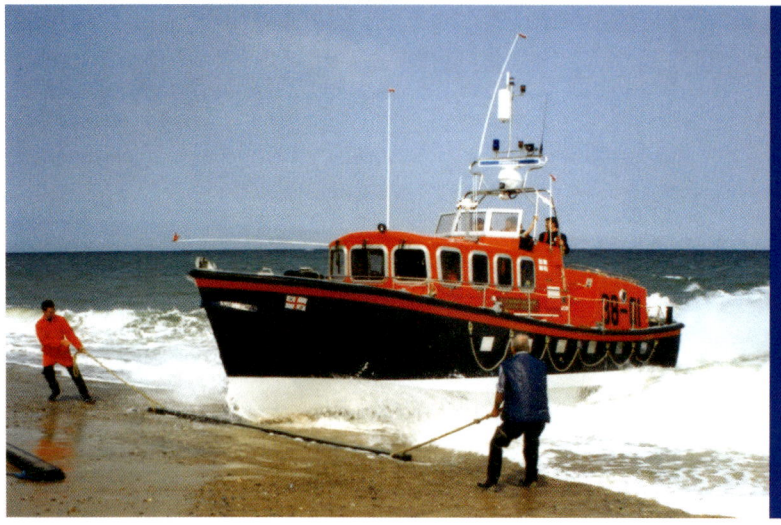

Caister lifeboat Bernard Matthews being recovered onto the beach, July 1995. Caister was the first independent lifeboat service to operate an offshore lifeboat. (Nicholas Leach)

maintain a lifeboat being the Aberdeen Harbour Commissioners, who passed responsibility for the port's lifeboats to the RNLI in 1925.

From the 1960s, new independent lifeboat operations began to be founded. The two main factors contributing to this were: (a) more people using the coast for leisure purposes, taking to the water, often in small boats, on sailboards or other craft, and needing help, and (b) suitable rescue craft being readily available and reasonably affordable. From the 1960s small, fast inflatables and rigid inflatables proved to be suitable rescue craft, and the RNLI began employing the inflatable inshore lifeboat in large numbers. Such craft,

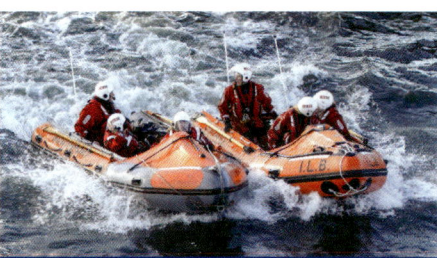

Two D class inflatable ILBs operated by the Southport Offshore Rescue Trust pictured on exercise in 2017. The Trust became the first Rescue Boat Organisation to be recognised by the MCA as a Probationary Declared Facility following a review of recognition for independents in 2019. (Martin Fish)

relatively cheap to acquire and maintain, could be feasibly operated as rescue boats by local coastal communities whose resources were limited.

Areas where boating activity was most intense, such as the Solent and around the Isle of Wight, saw some of the first independent lifeboats established, such as at Hamble (in 1968), Gosport and Ryde (both in 1969). Elsewhere, independent organisations were founded when the RNLI had closed a station against the wishes of the local communities, with Caister in Norfolk being probably the best-known example. When the RNLI withdrew in 1969, locals immediately got together to provide a rescue craft, and the service has since gone from strength to strength. Caister Volunteer Lifeboat Service, as it is now known, operates an offshore as well as an inshore lifeboat, has a modern purpose-built boathouse, and a lifeboat museum.

The Rescue Boat Code

Independent lifeboat organisations may be funded and managed locally, but they have to comply with various rules and regulations to gain Declared Facility status with the Maritime and Coastguard Agency (MCA). The MCA is the UK executive agency working to prevent the loss of lives at

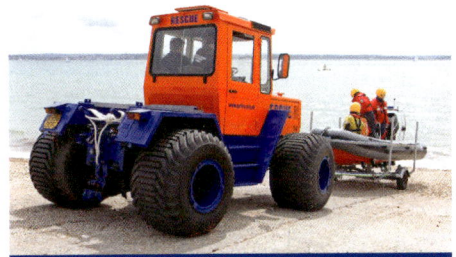

A wide variety of launching vehicles play a crucial role at independent stations, such as this Mercedes launching tractor used at Gosport. (Nicholas Leach)

sea and is responsible for implementing British and international maritime law and safety policy, which includes overseeing search and rescue (SAR) operations. The agency has a wide-ranging remit, but one of its primary responsibilities is coordinating SAR on the coastline and at sea through His Majesty's Coastguard (HMCG).

There are two levels of SAR facilities under the jurisdiction of the MCA: a Declared Facility and an Additional Facility. The Coastguard is able to call upon and co-ordinate the activities of both, but the Additional Facilities are usually used as a back up to Declared Facilities, which include the RNLI's lifeboat stations. A Declared Facility is available for civilian maritime SAR operations under the direction of HM Coastguard and must meet specific standards.

These standards were determined by the MCA through the Rescue Boat Code, under which all UK lifeboat stations, including independent organisations, operate. The Code was first drafted in 2005 by several organisations, including the RNLI, Royal Lifesaving Society UK (RLSS UK), Royal Yachting Association (RYA), Surf Life Saving Great Britain (SLSGB) and the Independent Rescue Boat Organisations. The role of Rescue Boat Organisations had hitherto not been specifically covered by any formally recognised national standard, as the MCA's existing safety codes of practice for small (up to 24m) vessels were not applicable because the rescue boats did not operate on a commercial basis.

The MCA reworked the small craft codes in 2011, taking into account updates to technical standards, and clarifying the requirements and responsibilities of Rescue Boat Organisations. The latest version of the document was published in March 2013 under the title Rescue Boat Code, The Code of Practice for Open Rescue Boats of Less than 15 Metres in Length.

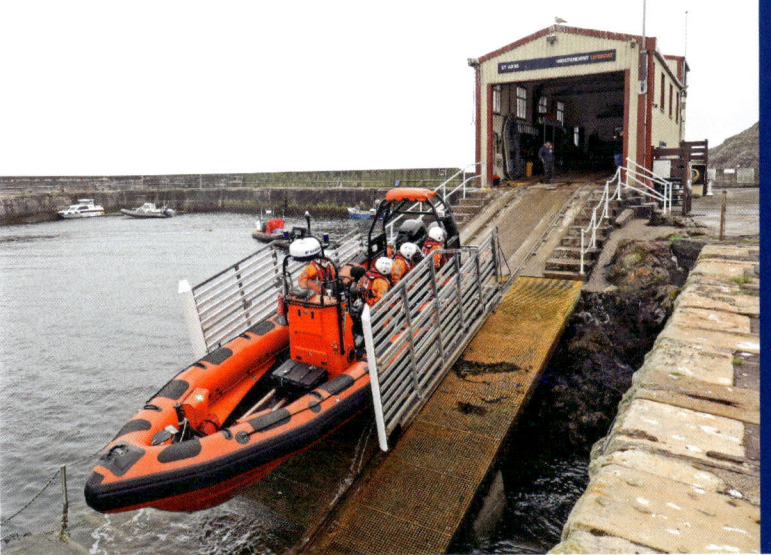

At St Abbs, the lifeboat house built by the RNLI just before the First World War was taken over by the independent St Abbs Lifeboat operation when that organisation was founded to reinstate an SAR service after the RNLI had closed its station. (Nicholas Leach)

Independent lifeboats of Britain

The safety of Rescue Boat Organisations and those they assist is dependent upon the successful integration of many factors, not simply the design of the boats and equipment. Therefore the Code includes sections on equipment, safety procedures, training and maintenance, and every Rescue Boat Organisation needs to demonstrate compliance with each section of the Code.

The Code presented a number of challenges for many of the Rescue Boat Organisations both in relation to technical compliance for rescue boats and wider requirements to produce documentation and systems to demonstrate that they complied with the Code. A review of the Declared Facility status was undertaken by the MCA which resulted in the re-assessment of all independent lifeboats. This process started in 2019 when Southport Offshore Rescue Trust became the first Rescue Boat Organisation to be recognised by the MCA as a Probationary Declared Facility for Provision of Inshore Search and Rescue. Over the next 12 months the MCA monitored the activities of the Trust, from call-outs to training exercises, to ensure the required standards were met, and this resulted in Southport becoming the UK's first independent lifeboat organisation to be a recognised Declared Facility under the new Code. A UK wide re-assessment then commenced for the rest of the independent declared lifeboats.

Funding challenges

Financing a lifeboat operation is expensive and raising the necessary money is often the biggest challenge faced by independent lifeboat operators as the acquisition and maintenance of lifeboats, equipment and shore facilities is dependent on a steady income stream. Fundraising takes place throughout the year, with annual lifeboat days in the summer being among the more high profile events at many independent stations. Although local fundraising is the most common way for raising the necessary finance, significant individual donations and bequests are not uncommon. Among those stations to benefit from individual generosity are St Abbs and Caister, where Boyd Tunnock and Bernard Matthews respectively have funded brand new lifeboats.

The 'independents' were given a financial boost in 2014 when the Conservative and Liberal Democrat coalition government announced that £5 million in grant funding would be made available over a five-year period to charities operating inland waterway safety boats, with awards being

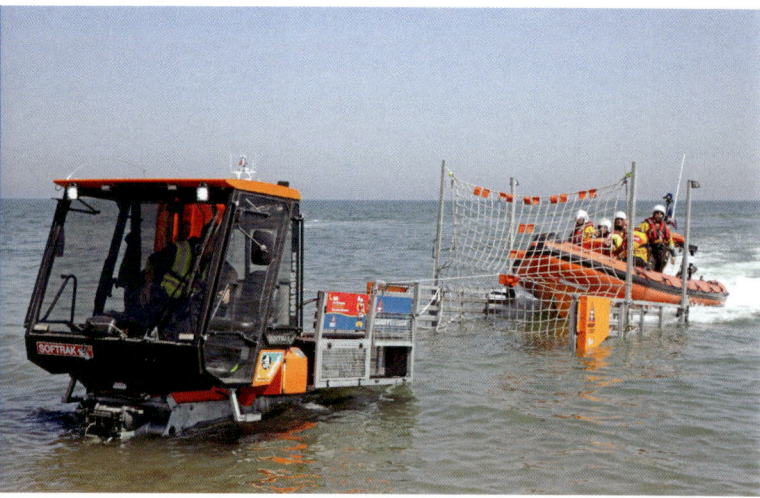

The Atlantic 75 B-762 was built by the RNLI in 2000 and was acquired by Hemsby Inshore Rescue in 2018. Pictured being recovered at Hemsby, the boat was renamed Sea Weaver for service with the Norfolk organisation. (Nicholas Leach)

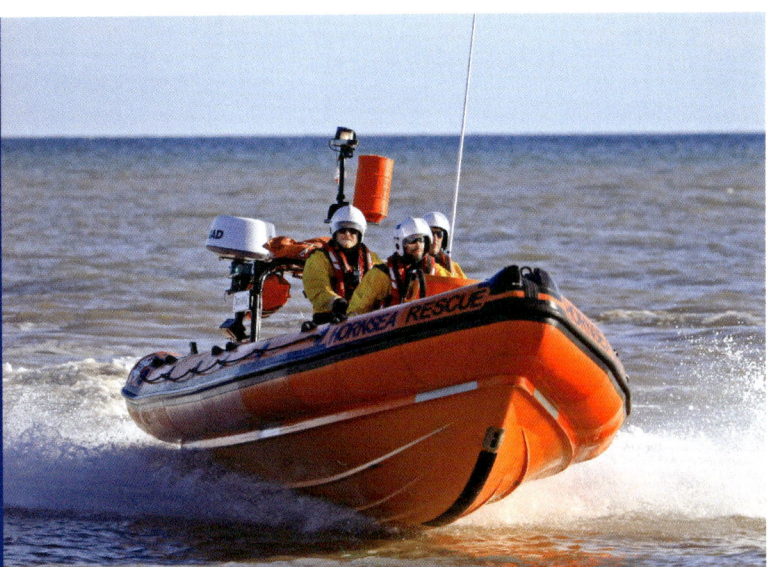

The former RNLI Atlantic 75 Duckhams 2001 (B-773) served the RNLI for 16 years before being sold out of service. She became the second former RNLI Atlantic 75 to serve at Hornsea when the independent station acquired her in 2019. (Nicholas Leach)

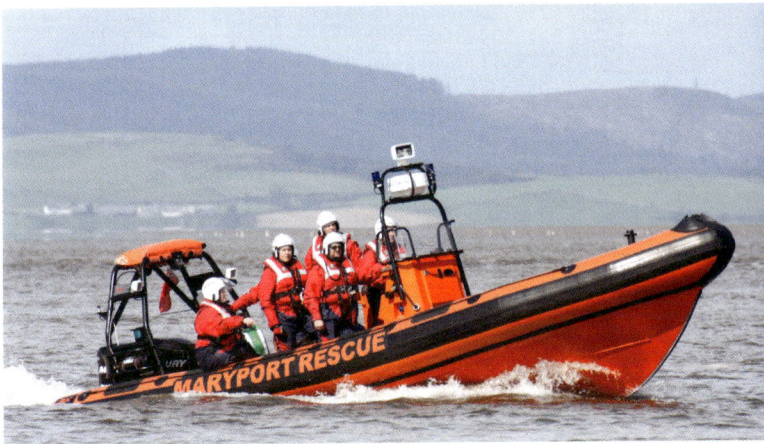

The MST Rescue 900 lifeboat E.ON Spirit of Maryport was purpose-built for the Cumbrian operator in 2009. (Martin Fish)

made annually. Transport Minister John Hayes formally launched the scheme in November 2014 to support the work of the life-saving charities that operate rescue boats on inshore waters, rivers, lakes and other inland waterways.

Independent lifeboat organisations were invited to bid for grants to fund equipment and associated items needed for rescue operations, including flood rescue. Funding was available only for specific projects, which did not include infrastructure, buildings or other structures, or vehicles not used to launch, recover or transport rescue craft. Training costs were supported in the first years of the Fund, but were later removed.

Eligible applications were considered by a panel with representatives from the DFT, the MCA, the RYA, the RNLI, the Department for Environment, Food and Rural Affairs (DEFRA), and the devolved administrations. Between 2014, when the scheme was launched, and 2020 the Rescue Boat Grant Fund provided £5.7 million to 104 charities around the UK. The last grant under the scheme was made in February 2020.

Independent lifeboats of Britain

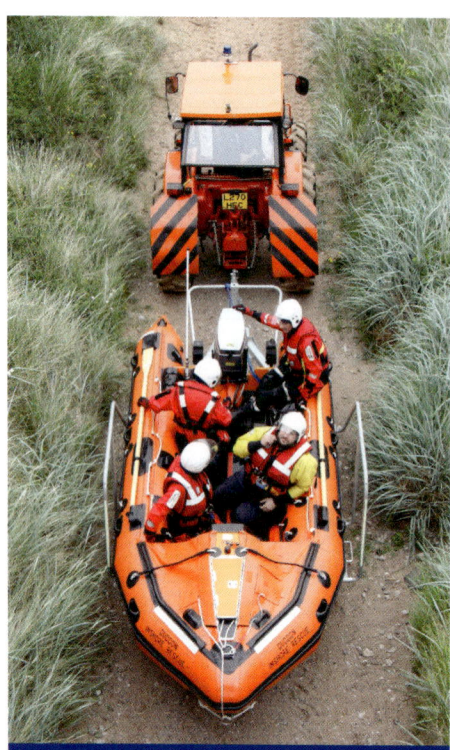

The IB1 type inshore lifeboat operated by Duddon Inshore Rescue, Cumbria, pictured in June 2016. The IB1 is designed and built by the RNLI. (Martin Fish)

Some of the more significant awards in 2020 went to Maryport Inshore Rescue, which received £77,000 to fund a new D class inflatable, a new communication system for the 9m MST lifeboat and new dry suits; Nith Inshore Rescue received £69,083 for a new outboard engine for the main rescue lifeboat, new PPE and personal floatation devices for volunteers, as well a new auxiliary boat road trailer; and Freshwater Independent Lifeboat was awarded £62,609 for power plant renewal, new PPE for crew, and an Automated External Defibrillator for the IB1 lifeboat.

A national organisation

A significant development in independent lifeboat operations took place in 2022 with the formation of the National Independent Lifeboat Association (NILA). Set up as a charity, the NILA was formed with the aim of promoting and supporting independent lifeboat organisations around the UK.

The NILA was founded by MP Anthony Mangnall after he visited an independent lifeboat in his constituency of Totnes and South Devon. This visit highlighted both the essential work undertaken by the UK's independent lifeboats and the many challenges they face, notably funding, public awareness and long-term support. As a result, Mangnall worked with colleagues in Parliament, as well as industry experts, to form the charity, which offers independent lifeboats support and raise their profile.

The NILA's stated mission is 'to give a voice, assistance and advice to the growing community of independent lifeboats across the United Kingdom, creating a valued, professional and recognised resource for water-based search and rescue.'

The NILA initially accepted members from all nations of the UK, and was officially launched at the Emergency Services Show at the National Exhibition Centre in Birmingham in September 2022. Members of the NILA remain independent but benefit from belonging to a larger organisation, such as gaining greater representation in Parliament, national promotion, and access to working groups where data and best practice is shared.

The association also aims to achieve recognition by the UK SAR Operators Group, joining the likes of the RNLI, Lowland Rescue (ALSAR), Mountain Rescue England and Wales, and the Royal Life Saving Society UK (RLSS). The Department for Transport has confirmed it is supportive of the NILA while the Maritime and Coastguard Agency has also welcomed the new Association too.

ENGLAND EAST COAST

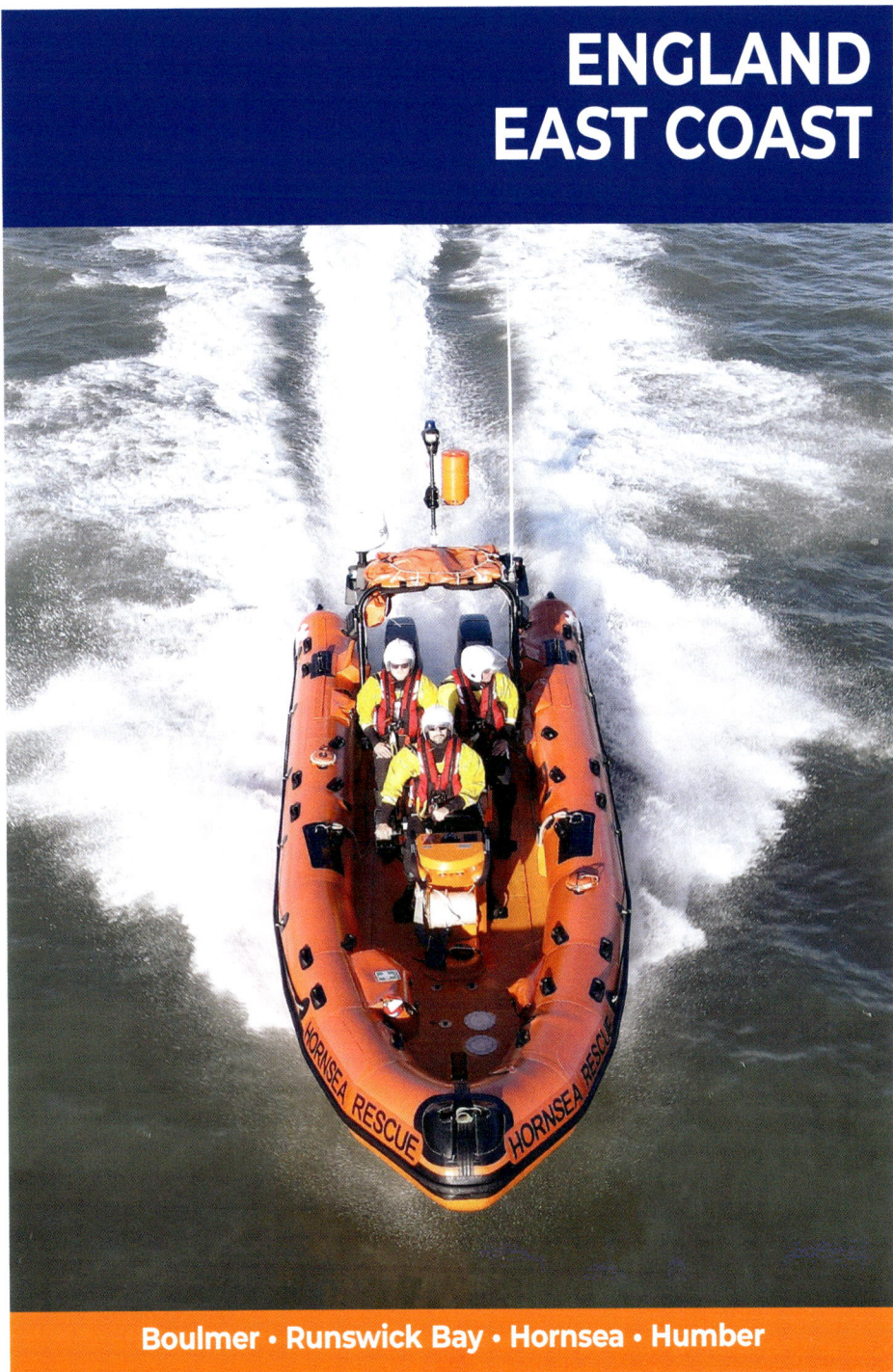

Boulmer • Runswick Bay • Hornsea • Humber

Independent lifeboats of Britain

BOULMER
Northumberland

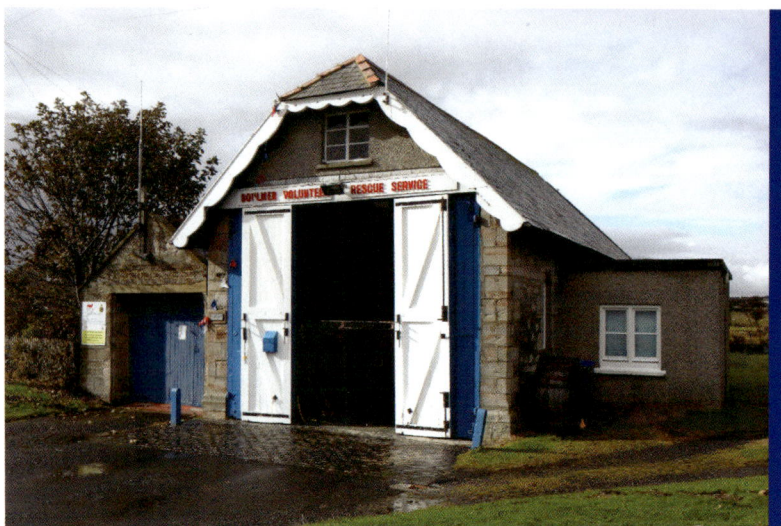

The lifeboat house built at Boulmer in 1872 by the RNLI, and used by the Institution until 1968. Since 1969 it has been home to the Boulmer Volunteer Rescue Service. The original RNLI service boards are on display inside. (Nicholas Leach)

LOCATION Northumberland
ORGANISATION Boulmer Volunteer Rescue Service
ESTABLISHED 1969
HISTORY Following a coastal review in 1967 the RNLI closed its station at Boulmer and withdrew the 37ft Oakley lifeboat on 1 March 1968, sending an inshore lifeboat the following day. However, at the end of summer 1968 this was withdrawn and the station closed. Local feeling was in favour of retaining a lifeboat, so in 1969 the Boulmer Volunteer Rescue Service was founded, with the RNLI offering the now empty lifeboat house to the service. After a considerable amount of local fund-raising, a boat was acquired and the station opened.

PREVIOUS ASSETS
1969 A Norwegian-built GRP-hulled Ancus

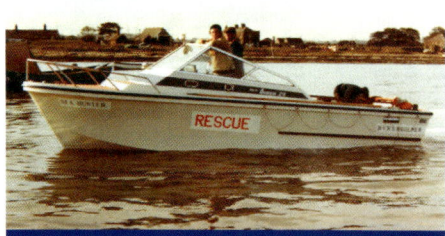

The first lifeboat to serve the Boulmer Volunteer Rescue Service was Sea Hunter, which was powered by twin 110hp Volvo petrol engines driving propellers through retractable outboard sterndrives. She was officially named Sea Hunter and launched by Her Grace the Duchess of Northumberland in September 1970. She served the station from 1969 to 1997.

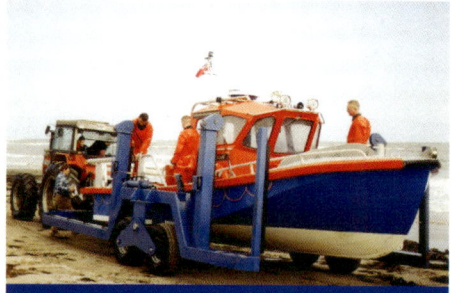

The second independent lifeboat at Boulmer, Duchess Elizabeth, served for nine years up to 2006. The purpose-built launching trailer featured four hydraulic lifting rams to which the lifeboat was attached by cables. After the whole unit had reached the water, the rams would lower the boat into the sea and the crew would release the cables. (Martin Fish)

Queen type boat was delivered, being available for service from early 1970. Named Sea Hunter, the boat was launched across the beach from a trailer drawn by a tractor.

1997 A new Wave Rescuer type boat, built by Alnmaritec, was acquired. The 9.35m by 3.3m aluminium-hulled boat was driven by two Castoldi waterjets powered by Volvo TA MD 200bhp engines, and was launched across the beach by a tractor from a purpose-built trailer. She was formally named Duchess Elizabeth by Her Grace, The Duchess of Northumberland at a ceremony on 16 August 1997. Capable of speeds up to 35 knots, Duchess Elizabeth was one of the fastest lifeboats in the UK when introduced in 1997. The design featured an enclosed wheelhouse with helmsman and navigator positions, a self-draining well deck with self-draining scuppers and a working deck aft over the engine covers .

2006 A new 30ft Tornado rigid inflatable, powered by twin 150hp outboard engines, was acquired. Named Pentland Knight, it cost £35,000 with the funds being raised locally.

RESCUES On 27 October 1972 Sea Hunter performed a notable service in association with the Rocket Apparatus Team, the rescue helicopter and the Amble lifeboat. They rescued the crew of the fishing vessel Nordboen in storm-force conditions. For this service, the crew were rewarded for their gallantry at a presentation in London where they were presented with silver plates by Secretary of State Peter Walker.

CURRENT ASSETS Tornado 5.5m rigid inflatable, named Boulmer Haven, on station 2013; Leyland 38TD tractor and trailer.

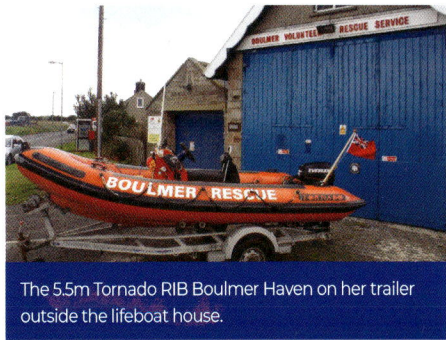

The 5.5m Tornado RIB Boulmer Haven on her trailer outside the lifeboat house.

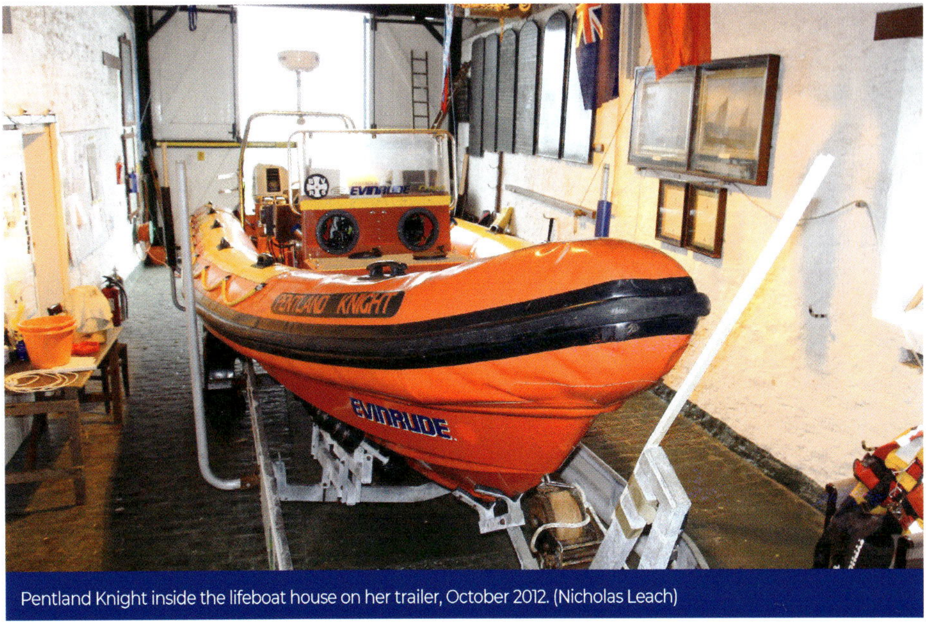

Pentland Knight inside the lifeboat house on her trailer, October 2012. (Nicholas Leach)

Independent lifeboats of Britain

RUNSWICK
North Yorkshire

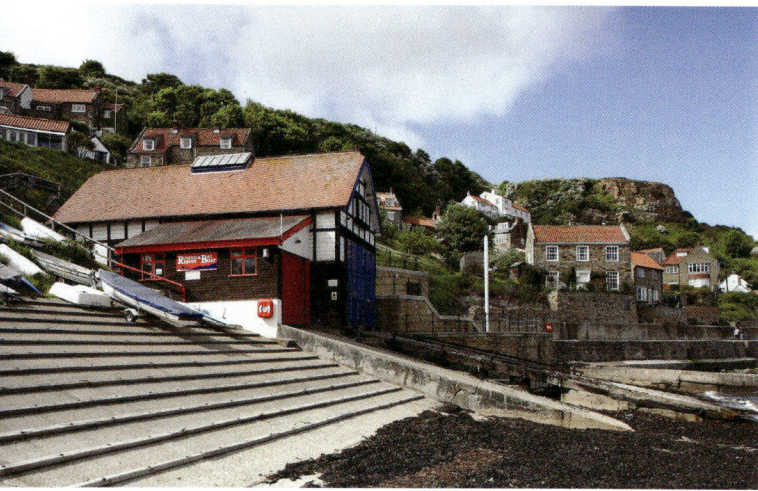

The former RNLI lifeboat house at Runswick Bay, built in 1910 and used until 1978,. The small tractor house, built in 1970, housed the Runswick Bay Rescue Boat. A powered winch is used to help with launch and recovery. (Nicholas Leach)

LOCATION Runswick Bay, Yorkshire
ORGANISATION Runswick Bay Rescue Boat
ESTABLISHED 1982
HISTORY The RNLI operated a lifeboat at Runswick Bay from 1866 until 1978, when the station was transferred to Staithes. However, local people felt a lifeboat was still needed so, at a meeting in the village in 1980, it was agreed to privately fund a fully equipped inshore rescue boat to work within the Bay. Funds were raised, a boat was found, and crew were trained as the Runswick Bay Rescue Boat was established.
PREVIOUS ASSETS
1982 The first rescue boat, named Claymoor, entered service. This 16ft inflatable boat was bought from Humber Boats in Hull and was powered by a 40hp Mariner outboard motor. Claymoor was launched 35 times in four years.
1986 A new rescue boat was purchased. Also built by Humber Boats, the 17ft rigid inflatable was powered by a 40hp Mariner engine and was faster and more manoeuvrable than her predecessor, as well as giving an improved ride for the crew. Named Christine Appleton after the late wife of the organisation's secretary, she launched 30 times on service.
1992 At ten years of operations, the RBRB obtained its next rescue boat, Lady Normanby,

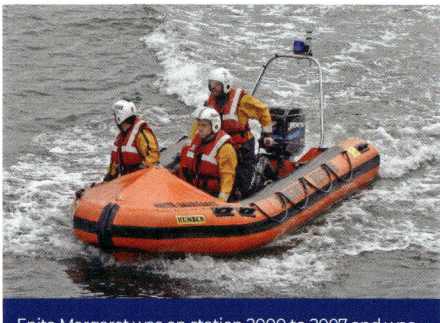

Enita Margaret was on station 2000 to 2007 and was launched on service 33 times. (Martin Fish)

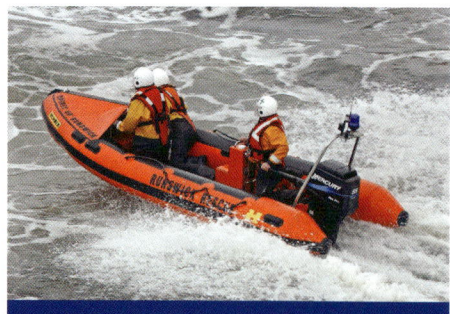

The Humber type rigid inflatable Spirit of Runswick at Whitby in 2008. She served from 2007 to 2010.

Independent lifeboats of Britain

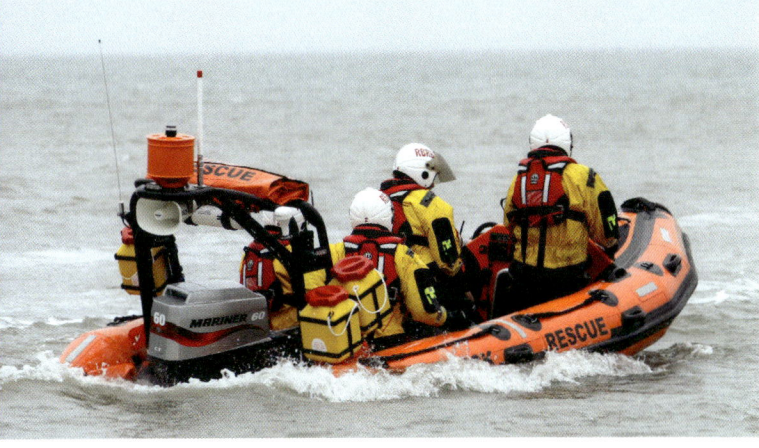

Runswick Bay Rescue Boat's current lifeboat, Spirit of Nagar, on exercise in April 2022. She entered service in 2020. (Martin Fish)

a 17ft rigid inflatable built by Humber Boats with a single 55hp Mercury outboard.

2000 A new lifeboat arrived in June. Named Enita Margaret, she was similar to her predecessor but a foot longer. She carried electronic aids including a GPS navigator and plotter.

2007 Another new lifeboat, Spirit of Runswick, entered service in April. The 5m Humber Assault rigid inflatable was driven by a 50hp Mariner engine. She had a top speed of 26 knots and was manned by three crew.

2010 The sixth rescue boat to serve RBRB, Spirit II, entered service. The Gemini GRX420 catamaran-hulled inflatable was powered by a 50hp Mariner two-stroke engine and had a draught of less than a foot. She was light, fast and manoeuvrable and was ideally suited to work close inshore along the rocky coast on either side of Runswick Bay's beach.

2015 A new lifeboat, named Freebird Fojt and identical to Spirit II, was placed on service. The lighter and more manoeuvrable Gemini type was well suited to operations in Runswick Bay. The new boat was fitted out to the exact design and specification internally as her predecessor by RBRB volunteers. Spirit II was retained for both training and as a replacement if any damage or maintenance issues took Freebird Fojt out of service.

2020 A new Ribcraft lifeboat entered service. She was formally named Spirit of Nagar on 18 July. Built in Yeovil, the boat was funded by a grant of £75,000 from the Department for Transport's Inshore and Inland Rescue Boat Fund.

CURRENT ASSETS 4.8m Ribcraft Professional, named Spirit of Nagar, on station 2020.

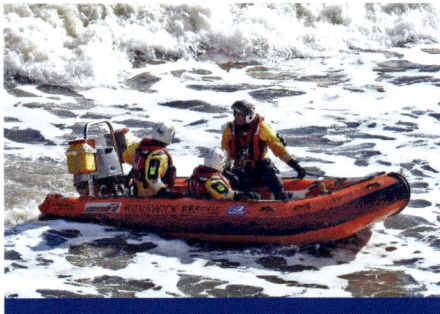

RBRB's sixth lifeboat, Spirit II, being launched; she was on station from 2010 to 2015. (Martin Fish)

Freebird Fojt in the surf off Runswick Bay; she was on station from 2015 to 2020. (By courtesy of RBRB)

Independent lifeboats of Britain

HORNSEA
East Riding of Yorkshire

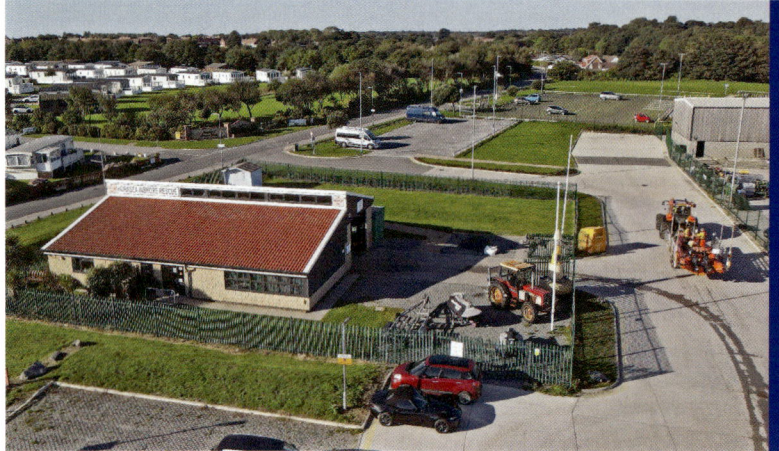

The lifeboat station at Hornsea, completed in 2010, is situated at the southern end of the South Promenade, close to Longbeach Leisure Park. (Nicholas Leach)

LOCATION Yorkshire
ORGANISATION Hornsea Rescue
ESTABLISHED 1993
HISTORY Hornsea Rescue was founded in the early 1990s following the withdrawal of the local Coastguard Patrol Boat. Auxiliary Coastguards had operated the boat throughout the year since the early 1970s. Although this was classed as a patrol boat, it was also used for rescues and saved numerous people. Following a Coastguard Review in the early 1990s, the policy on patrol boats changed and some Coastguard stations, including Hornsea, lost their boats. Hornsea' boat was transferred to the newly-formed Hull Coastguard Station.

Following the withdrawal, concern regarding the safety of bathers, fisherman and others was voiced and a public meeting supported the establishment of an independent rescue facility run by volunteers. In 1994 Hornsea Rescue was founded as a registered charity, which purchased an inshore rescue boat. Longbeach Leisure Park, at the southern end of South Promenade, near Hornsea Boat Launch, offered premises free of charge, and an old disused barn was converted into a boathouse.

While the service was grateful to the Leisure Park for the building, its location was not ideal from an operational point of view so

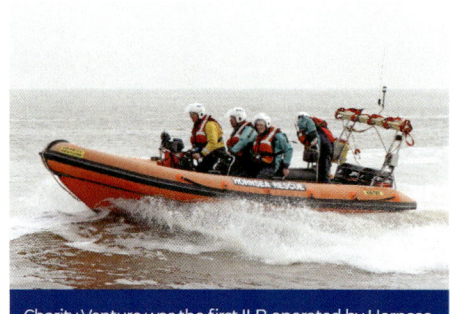

Charity Venture was the first ILB operated by Hornsea Rescue. (Nicholas Leach)

The Yamaha WaveRunner VX110 is powered by a four-stroke engine. (Nicholas Leach)

Independent lifeboats of Britain

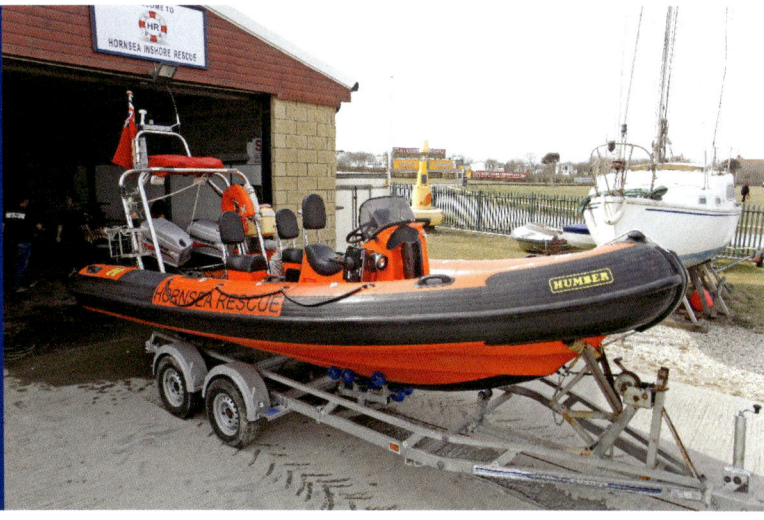

The 6m Humber Offshore Pro rigid inflatable Emily Laura, which was acquired in 2011, pictured in 2013. (Nicholas Leach)

a purpose-built rescue station on the seafront was built. Work started in August 2008 and it was completed two years later, being officially opened in December 2010 by HRH The Princess Royal. The new building has a boat hall for the rescue equipment, as well as a drying room, training and hospitality rooms, kitchen, toilets and operations room.

PREVIOUS ASSETS
1995 The first boat was a 5.85m rigid inflatable built by Ribtec of Southampton and delivered in December 1995. Named Charity Venture, it was powered by twin 60hp Mariner outboard engines giving a top speed of around thirty-five knots and was equipped with GPS navigation donated by Hornsea Lions. The boat has since undergone several upgrades, with new engines purchased in 2003 and fitted in the same year. The engines were replaced for a second time, in 2010, with twin Mercury 40hp two-stroke outboards.
2011 Following a generous anonymous gift, a new 6m Humber Offshore Pro rigid inflatable, powered by twin 60hp Mariner two-stroke outboard engines, was purchased. She was named Emily Laura at the request of the donors. The engines were modified with a post immersion restart system so that, in the

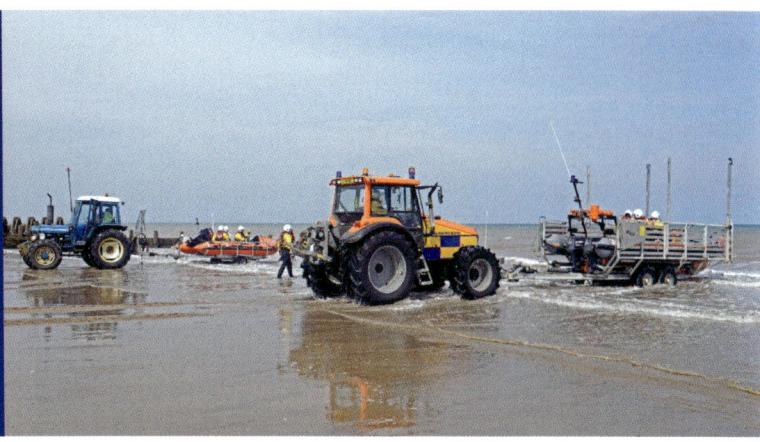

The Avon EA16 inflatable Pride of Hornsea and Atlantic 75 Charity Endeavour (ex-RNLI B-708) being launched on exercise, June 2019. (Nicholas Leach)

Independent lifeboats of Britain

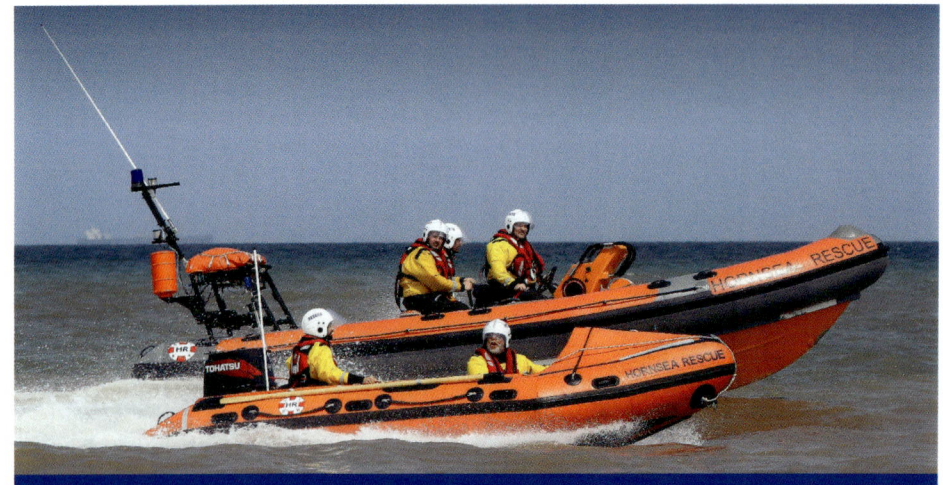

The Atlantic 75 Charity Endeavour (on station 2013-19) and inflatable Pride of Hornsea on exercise in June 2019. Both boats were taken out of service later that year. (Nicholas Leach)

event of a capsize, they can be restarted. Two tractors were available for launching, with the main vehicle, named Henry in honour of a former crew member, used most of the time.
2013 The former RNLI Atlantic 75 Bessie (ex-B-708) was acquired. Renamed Charity Endeavour, she served until 2019 and was launched using a standard ex-RNLI do-do carriage pulled by a Muir Hill launch tractor, which was specially adapted.
2019 An Avon EA16 inflatable was acquired from St John Ambulance service in Guernsey. Named Pride of Hornsea, she was launched by trailer using an International 1055 tractor, but was taken out of service and sold in 2021.
2019 The former RNLI Atlantic 75 Duckhams

The Atlantic 75 Spirit of Hornsea (ex-RNLI B-773) being launched on exercise. (Nicholas Leach)

2001 (ex-B-773) was acquired as a replacement for the first Atlantic 75; the boat, built in 2001, was seven years younger than the previous Atlantic, and was renamed Spirit of Hornsea.
2021 The D class inshore boat Pride of Hornsea was withdrawn and sold following a review of requirements, leaving the Atlantic 75 and jetski.
PWC The service has operated personal water craft (PWC) since 2005, when HSBC Bank, through its 'HSBC in the community' project, financed the purchase of a PWC, which was supplied by the local Jet Ski Centre at Fosse Hill. The Yamaha Wave Runner VX110 Deluxe watercraft, powered by a 110hp four-stroke engine, has a top speed of more than 50 knots. It can be operated by one person, and be launched in less time than larger vessels. A new Yamaha PWC was acquired in 2013.
RESCUES The most notable incident in which the station's volunteers have been involved came on 31 August 2011, when two people and their dogs were rescued. In very windy conditions, the young couple and their two dogs were cut off by the tide and in imminent danger as rough seas were rising up the cliffs. The PWC was launched at 3.30pm, followed by the inshore rescue boat, helmed by

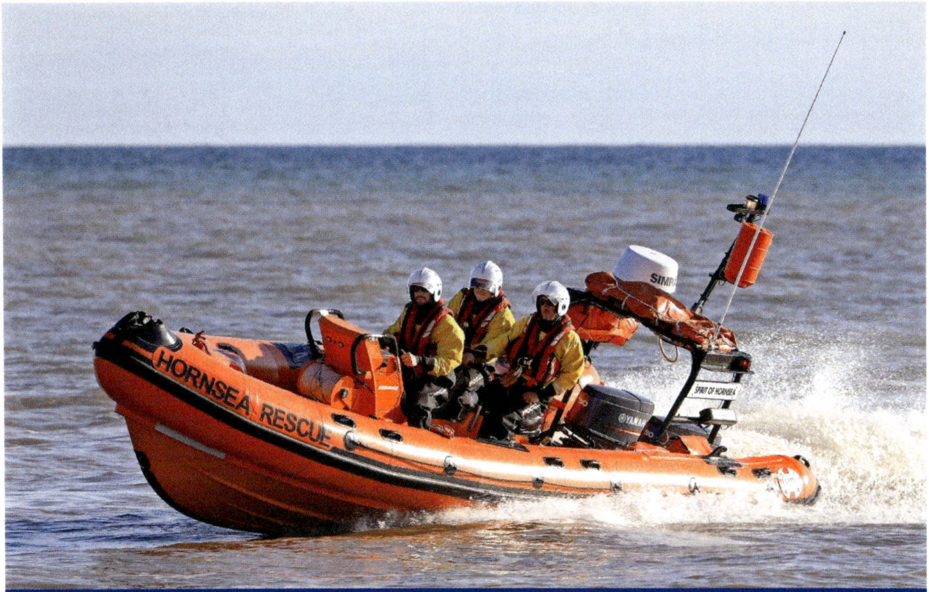

The Atlantic 75 Spirit of Hornsea (ex-RNLI B-773) on exercise off Hornsea, October 2021. (Nicholas Leach)

Coxswain Dave Pick, while Coxswain Neville Metcalfe was also on the boat and in charge of the operation. The couple were stranded at the base of the cliffs and were having to climb up the cliffs due to the incoming tide. Once on scene, the rescue craft were unable to get close in due to the shallow water and so crew members swam through the surf to effect a rescue. Rapidly deteriorating conditions made the situation hazardous, with the sea was rising up the cliffs, but the crew reached the casualties safely and managed to get them, and both their dogs, to the lifeboat.

CURRENT ASSETS Atlantic 75 Spirit of Hornsea (ex-RNLI B-773), acquired in 2019; launched by a Valmet /JAS P Wilson tractor and ex-RNLI do-do carriage. The Yamaha Rescue Water Craft is named Hornsea Jet.

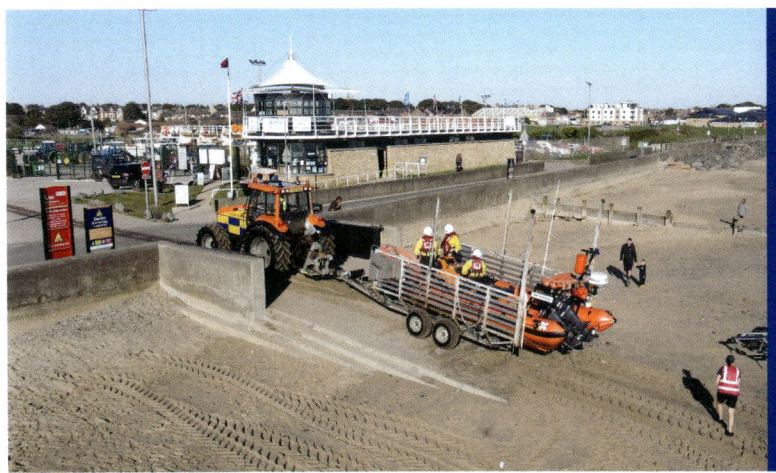

Atlantic 75 Spirit of Hornsea being recovered and taken back to the boathouse; launching and recovery involve taking the boat, on her carriage, across the South Promenade. (Nicholas Leach)

Independent lifeboats of Britain

HUMBER

East Riding of Yorkshire

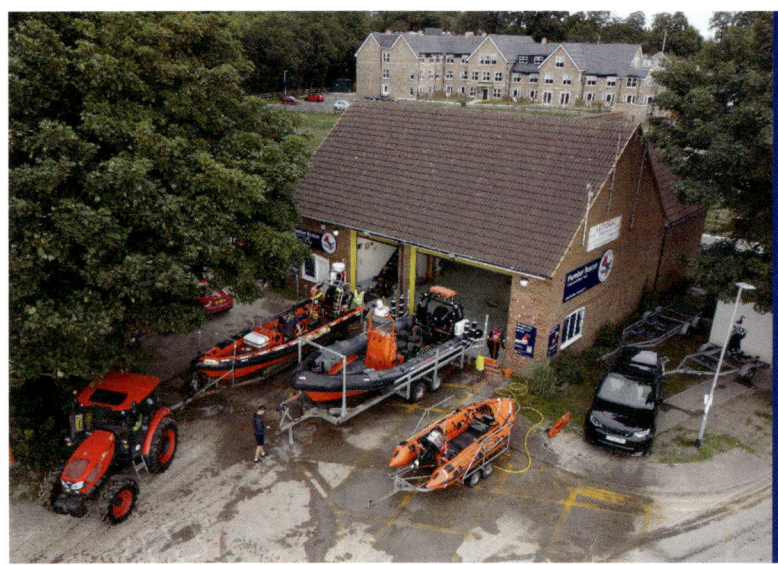

The boathouse on the Hessle Foreshore was opened in 1998 and houses two rigid inflatables, the launching tractor, Land Rover and a D class inflatable. (Martin Fish)

LOCATION Hessle Foreshore, northern bank of the River Humber
ORGANISATION Humber Rescue
ESTABLISHED 1990
HISTORY Humber Rescue is an independent charity responsible for the provision of a fast-response rescue boat on the rivers of the Humber Estuary. The area covered is approximately 540 square miles, and includes the rivers Trent, Ouse, Hull and Humber. Prior to Humber Rescue's founding, there was no dedicated rescue or safety vessel on the upper reaches of the Humber, one of the country's major rivers. The need for a rescue service on the river became apparent in the the late 1980s, particularly following the withdrawal of the pilot launch from Hull. An appeal organised by Radio Humberside and the Hull Daily Mail in 1989 raised sufficient funds to purchase a boat, trailer and launching vehicle, and Humber Rescue was launched in 1990.

PREVIOUS ASSETS
1990 When the service started, the boat was kept in a crew member's garden and towed to

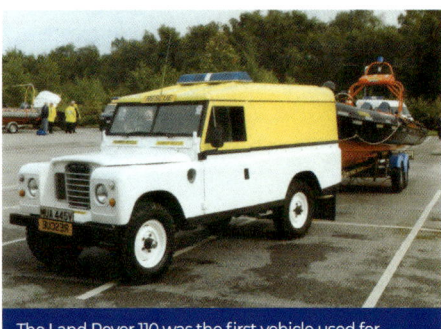

The Land Rover 110 was the first vehicle used for launching and recovering the lifeboat

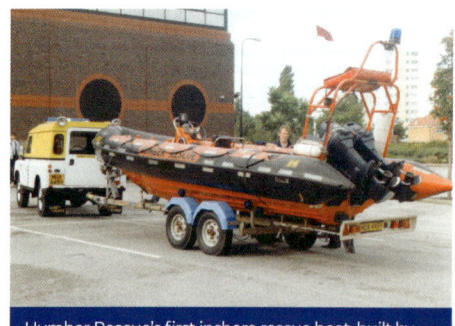

Humber Rescue's first inshore rescue boat, built by Humber Ribs and powered by twin outboard engines.

Independent lifeboats of Britain

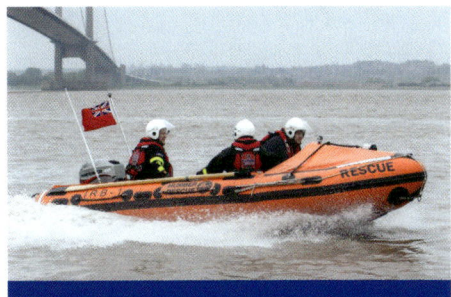

The Avon EA16 inflatable, named Sue Roberts, afloat for a training exercise in 2015. (Martin Fish)

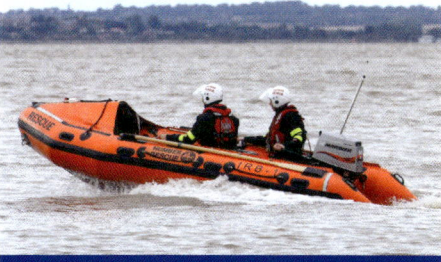

The ILB Sue Roberts, upgraded with a new 50hp Mariner outboard engine, training in 2022. (Martin Fish)

the river by Land Rover. The first lifeboat was a rigid inflatable manufactured by Humber Ribs in Hull, powered by twin Yamaha 60hp outboard engines. It was fitted with a centre steering console with seating for a helm and two crew members. A substantial roll bar was fitted over the engines at the stern supporting the airbag, radar reflector, aerials and lighting.

1995 A purpose-built lifeboat house was built close to the foot of the North Tower of the Humber Bridge. The boathouse, which was formally opened in 1998 by round-the-world yachtsman Tony Bullimore, was close to the slipway into the river enabling the boat to be launched within seven minutes of a call.

1998 The service's first large lifeboat was obtained to enhance operations. Built by Tornado International Boats in Hull, the rigid inflatable was powered by twin 130hp Honda outboard engines and carried GPS navigation and radar, which at the time was uncommon on rigid inflatable lifeboats. The lifeboat was named Olive Hunt after the founder of her namesake charity, which supports Humber Rescue. A Ford agricultural tractor was acquired for launching and recovery. When

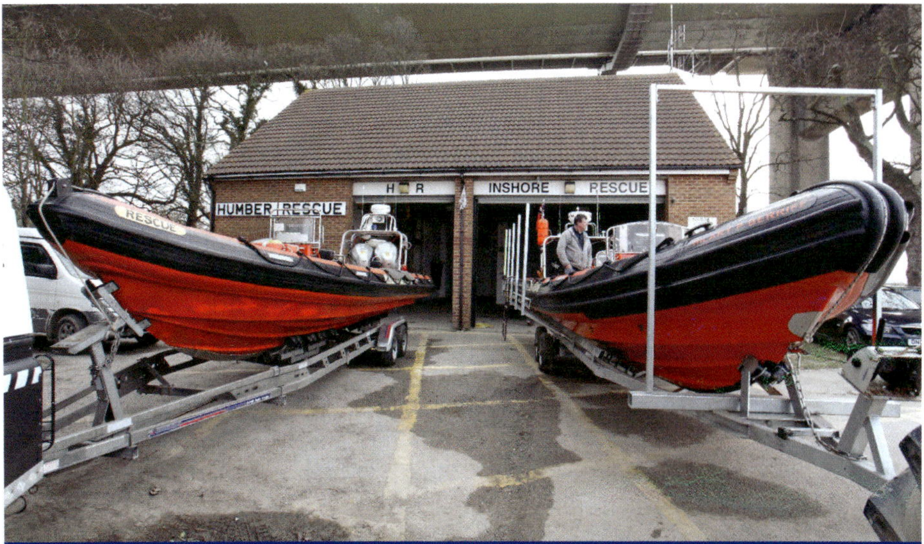

The 8.5m rigid inflatable Hilary P. Berriff (on right) on her launching trolley outside the boathouse, alongside the older boat, fully operational, which was used as a relief craft. (Nicholas Leach)

Independent lifeboats of Britain

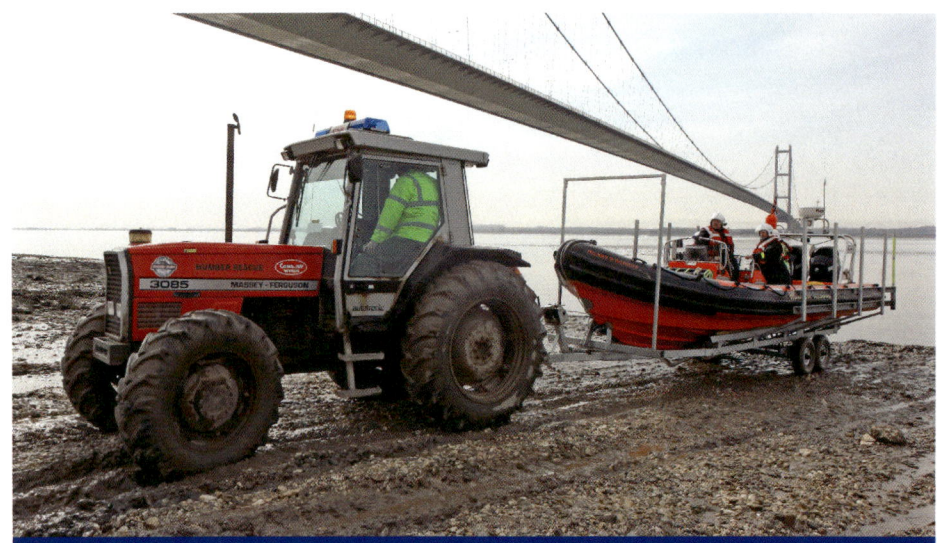

Launching the 8.5m rigid inflatable Hilary P. Berriff across the Hessle Foreshore in the shadow of the Humber Bridge. The station has a crew pool of approximately 18 and training is regularly undertaken. (Nicholas Leach)

this boat was replaced as the main lifeboat in 2011, it became the training craft and reserve boat if required. In 2021 during a major refit two 150hp Mercury Engines were fitted, as well as new communication and navigational equipment, and a new console.

2007 A new small Humber Ribs-built rigid inflatable, powered by a Honda outboard engine and named Rescue Junior, entered service. As the smallest rescue boat, it acts as a support vessel to assist with training, charity events such as the Humber swims, and can be deployed in response to flooding incidents.

2011 On 9 April a new lifeboat was officially launched on the Hessle Foreshore. It was named Hilary P. Berriff, after the wife of Humber Rescue founder Paul Berriff, by the Lord Mayor of Hull, David Gemmill OBE. Built by XS Ribs, the 8.5m by 2.9m rigid inflatable was powered by twin 200hp Mercury Verado engines giving a top speed in excess of 45 knots. She was equipped with two GPS chartplotters, two depth sounders and three VHF radios. Her high sheer bow and deep-V hull gave the craft a substantial internal freeboard. A Massey Ferguson 3125 tractor was used to get the boat afloat.

2014 A former RNLI D class inshore lifeboat (ex-D-546) was acquired and went into service in 2015. The EA16 type boat, built by Avon inflatables at Llanelli and fitted out by the RNLI in Cowes, was named Sue Roberts. Initially powered by a 40hp Mariner outboard, the boat was later upgraded with a 50hp Mariner outboard. The vessel is an ideal size for conditions on the Humber, being well suited to conducting searches close to the shore.

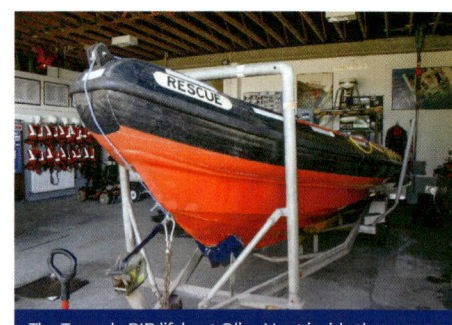

The Tornado RIB lifeboat Olive Hunt inside the lifeboat station in 2006 on the purpose-built stern-first launching trailer. (Martin Fish)

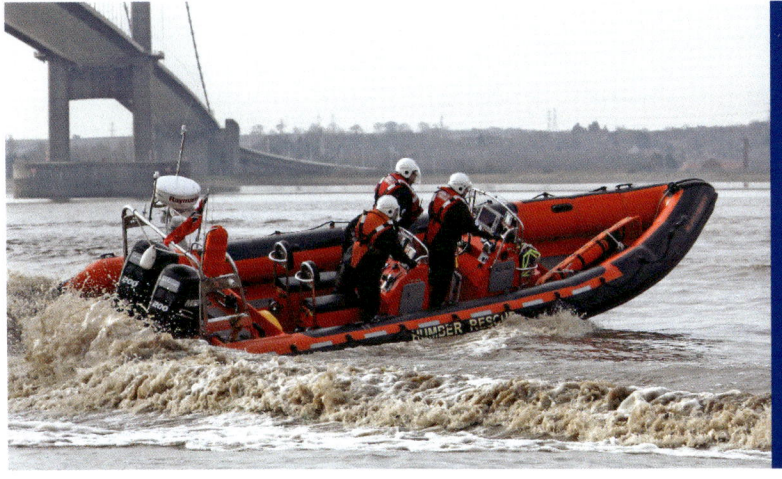

The 8.5m rigid inflatable Hilary P. Berriff in the river Humber. She was on station from 2011 to 2020. (Nicholas Leach)

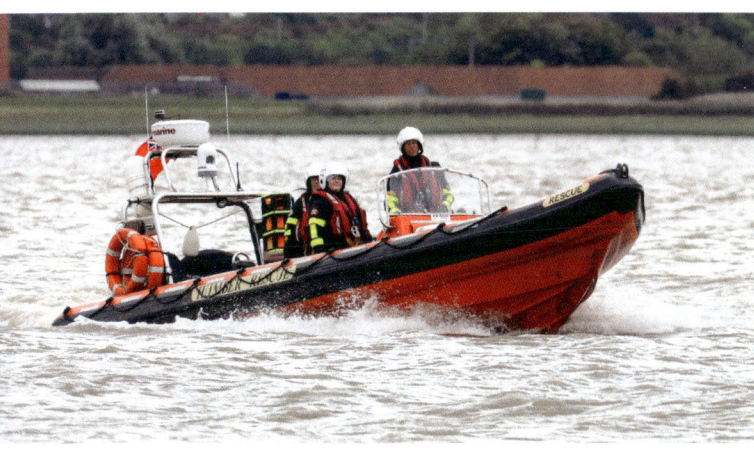

Humber Rescue's reserve and training lifeboat Olive Hunt on exercise in the river in 2022. Replaced as the main lifeboat in 2011, she underwent a significant refit and upgrade in 2021. (Martin Fish)

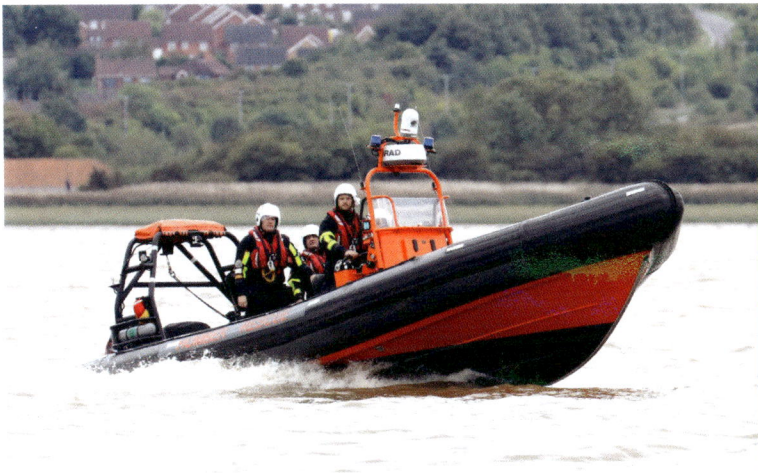

The MST 900W-SAR rigid inflatable, built in Liverpool, entered service with Humber Rescue in 2020; she is seen undertaking a training exercise on the Humber in September 2022. (Martin Fish)

Independent lifeboats of Britain

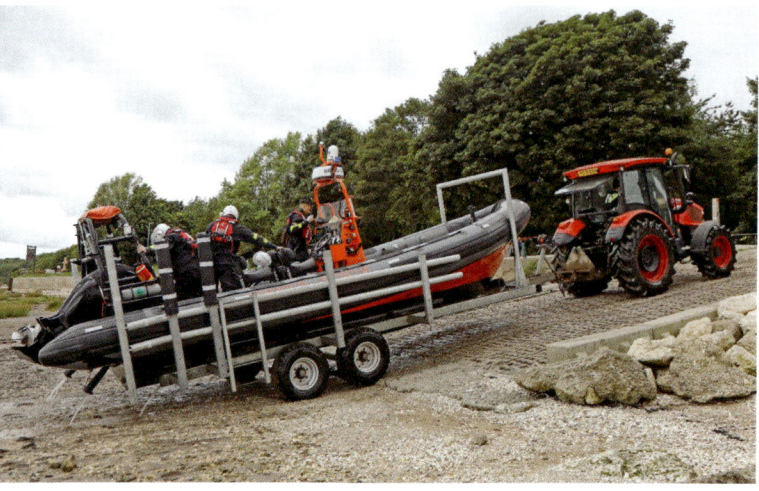

The MST 900W-SAR rigid inflatable being recovered using the Zetor tractor. (Martin Fish)

2020 In November a new MST 900W-SAR rescue boat came into service to replace the previous main lifeboat Hilary P. Beriff. The MST is powered by two 150hp Mercury engines giving a top speed of 42 knots, equipped with a range of communication and navigational equipment, including radar, a FLIR camera, and carries four crew with survivor capacity for 12. In the event of a capsize, a manually operated righting bag is fitted.

2021 A new Zetor Proxima CL 110 launching and recovery tractor arrived in October.

2022 The former RNLI IB1 D class inflatable D-704, purchased in 2020, became operational after a full refit and the installation of a new floor. Replacing the EA16 D class, the boat is powered by a 50hp Mariner outboard, and has a bow console containing navigation and communications equipment.

CURRENT ASSETS MST SAR-900W rigid inflatable, built by Marine Specialised Technology Group, on station in 2020; 8.5m Tornado Rigid Inflatable, named Olive Hunt, reserve lifeboat, on station 1998; Humber RIB, named Rescue Junior, on station 2011; IB1 D class inflatable (ex-RNLI D-704), on station 2022. All assets are launched into the River Humber from trailers, using either the Zetor Proxima launching tractor and a Land Rover Defender.

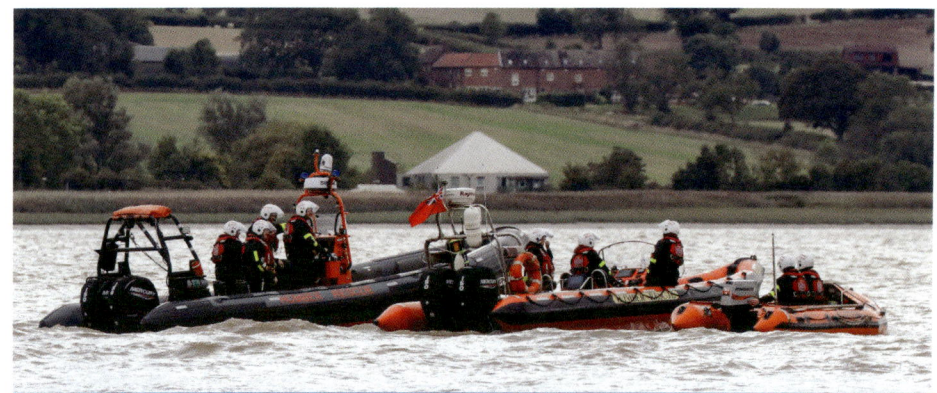

Humber Rescue's assets in the river while they were supporting a fundraising charity swim in 2022. (Martin Fish)

Independent lifeboats of Britain

ENGLAND
EAST ANGLIA

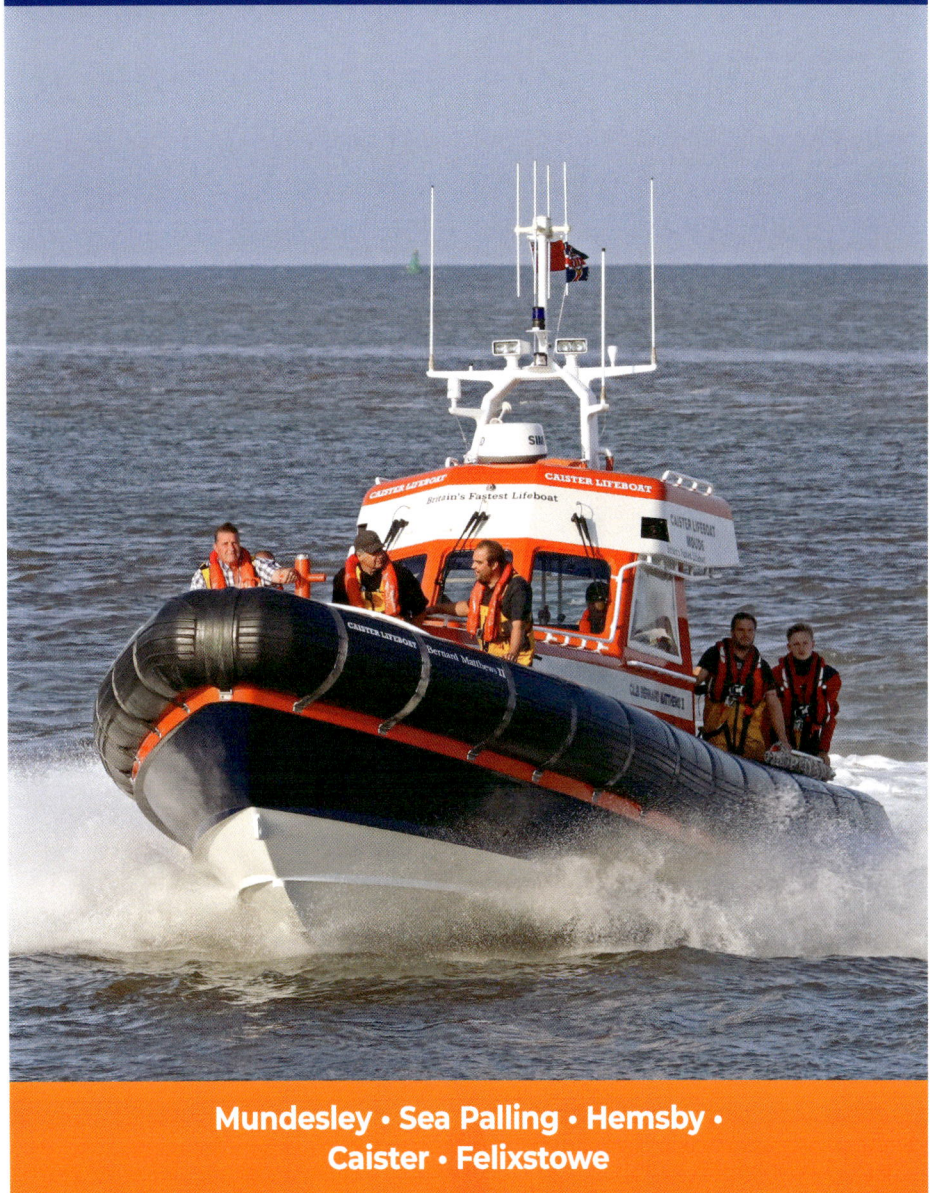

Mundesley • Sea Palling • Hemsby • Caister • Felixstowe

MUNDESLEY

Norfolk

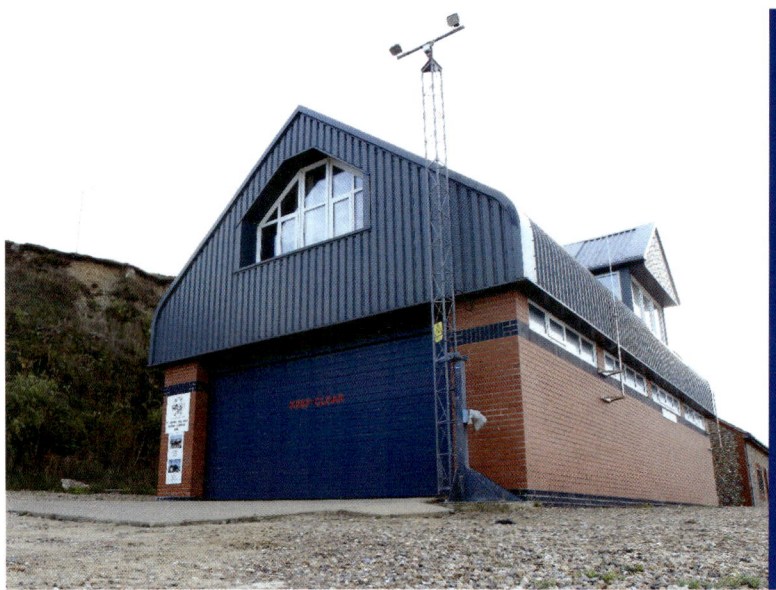

The lifeboat house built in 2006 for the ILB and launching vehicle, with a boathall on the ground floor and crew facilities and a lookout on the first floor. (Nicholas Leach)

LOCATION Norfolk
ORGANISATION Mundesley Volunteer Inshore Lifeboat Service
ESTABLISHED 1972
HISTORY Following an incident in 1971 when a drowning and near drowning of a man and his wife occurred while they were sailing half a mile off the beach at Mundesley, the Mundesley Parish Council called a meeting to discuss the feasibility of establishing an inshore lifeboat at Mundesley. The RNLI and Coastguard were approached but were unable to help. It was therefore decided to set up an independent rescue unit, funded and manned from within the village. Further meetings followed resulting in the formation of The Mundesley Volunteer Inshore Lifeboat Service Ltd, a limited company and registered charity. A board of directors was elected, with members chosen from the community

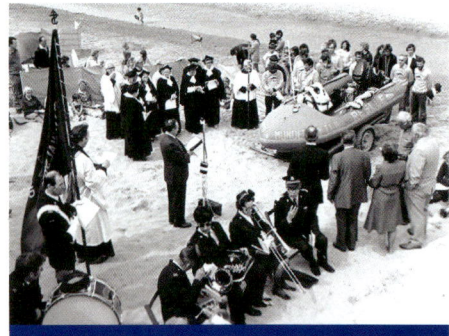

The scene during the dedication of the first Mundesley Volunteer inshore lifeboat.

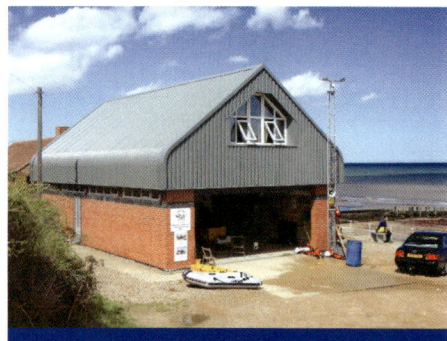

The lifeboat house built in 2006 is situated at the southern end of the small village. (Nicholas Leach)

Independent lifeboats of Britain

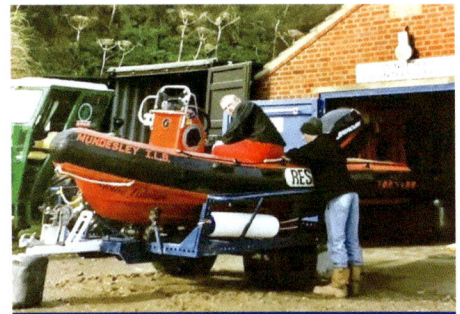

The 4.5m Tornado rigid inflatable lifeboat Mollie Tidman entered service in 1997.

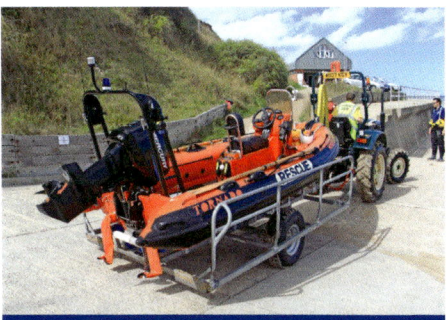

The 4.5m Tornado rigid inflatable lifeboat Footprints, built by Goodchild Marine, on her launching trailer.

and including crew members. The volunteer crew take care of the day-to-day running of the boat and the directors oversee the policy making and financial arrangements.

PREVIOUS ASSETS

1972 In spring a Zodiac inflatable was borrowed from a local businessman and was used to establish the station, operating from a temporary boathouse on the promenade at the east end of the village. Fundraising was undertaken and a 4m Avon Searider semi-rigid inflatable was purchased. A wooden hut was donated by a Bacton Gas Site contractor and converted into a boathouse.

1979-80 A new boathouse was constructed, with about £2,000 worth of materials being donated by local firms. The lifeboat crew undertook all of the building work, apart from the brickwork. The house, with a crew room and lookout on the first floor, was officially opened on 11 June 1980 by Cmdr P. Warrington RC, of HM Coastguard, and was dedicated by the Rev G. Norman.

1991 A new 4m Avon Searider was purchased, complete with a new 50hp Yamaha engine.

1997 A new Tornado rigid inflatable entered service and was dedicated in the spring, being named Mollie Tidman. She served until replaced with another Tornado craft, named Footprints, which was a 4.5m rigid inflatable fitted out by Goodchild Marine of Great Yarmouth using a Tornado hull, and was

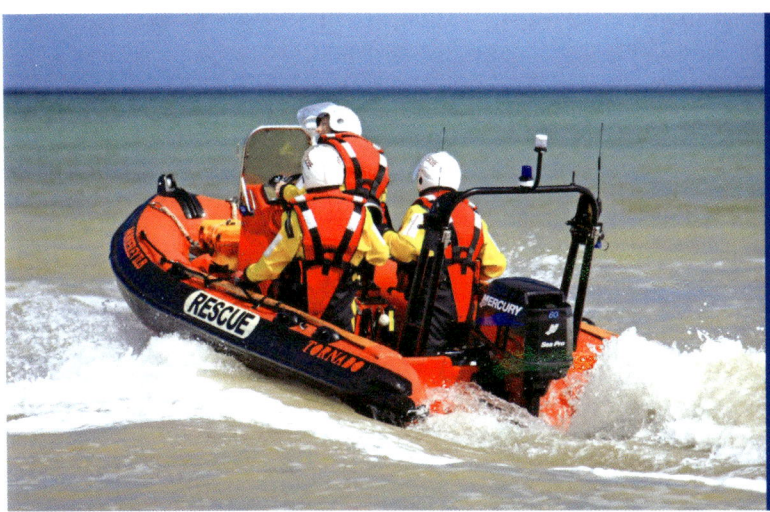

The Tornado inshore lifeboat Footprints on exercise off Mundesley, August 2010. She was powered by a 60hp Mercury outboard giving a top speed of 28 knots. (Nicholas Leach)

Independent lifeboats of Britain

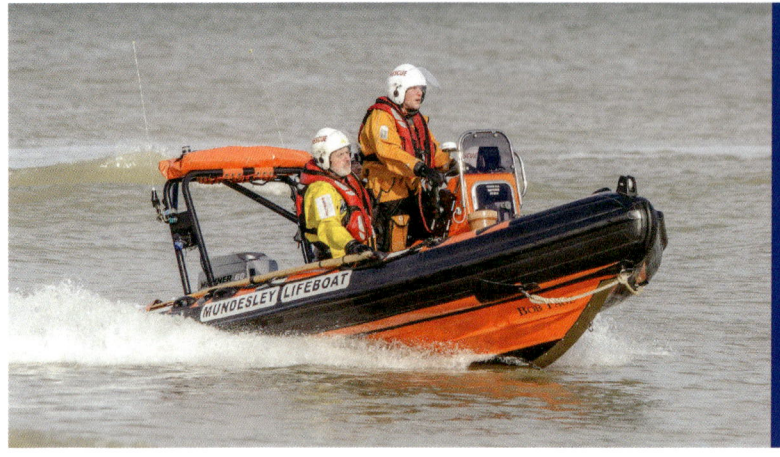

The 2012-built Ribcraft lifeboat Bob Page on exercise. She cost £30,000 and was funded from the legacy of Bob Page. (By courtesy of Mundesley Volunteer Inshore Lifeboat Service)

powered by a 60hp Mercury outboard engine.
2006 A new lifeboat station was built by Blyth and Sons, of Sheringham, funded by public donations, after a £100,000 appeal was launched in 2004. The new boathouse provided much improved crew facilities.
2012 A new lifeboat arrived in the spring. Built by Goodchild Marine, the 4.8m Ribcraft Professional hull was fitted with a 60hp Mariner outboard engine, had a centre console for the helm with VHF radio and GPS navigation equipment, and a roll bar at the stern with a righting airbag.
2018 An Arancia surf rescue boat, with a 30hp engine and launching trailer, was purchased to operated as a second lifeboat.
2021 A nearly new Loglogic Softrak launching vehicle was purchased from Caister Lifeboat and training in the use of a tracked launching vehicle began. Designs for a building to house the Softrak vehicle were also prepared.
2022 In 2021 the Service placed an order with Goodchild Marine Services who in turn ordered the base boat hull from Ribcraft in Yeovil. Powered by a 60hp Mariner outboard, a similar configuration to previous lifeboats was continued with a centre helm console and roll bar mounted righting airbag. On 10 July the volunteers marked the 50th anniversary of the Service's establishment with the dedication of the new boat, which was named Edna Claxton by North Norfolk MP Duncan Baker.
CURRENT ASSETS Ribcraft 4.8 Professional, on station in 2022, named Edna Claxton, launched by Shire 330 tractor and trailer; Arancia RIB with trailer.

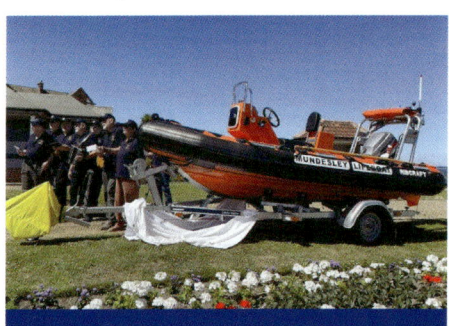

Naming and dedication ceremony for the new lifeboat Edna Claxton, July 2022.

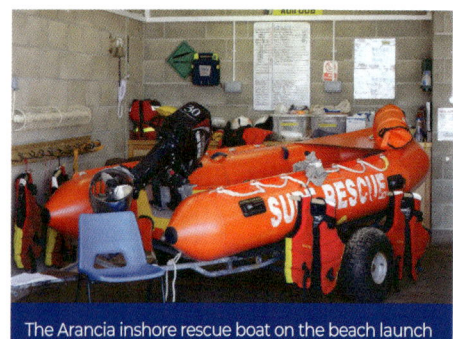

The Arancia inshore rescue boat on the beach launch trailer inside the boathouse, July 2021. (Martin Fish)

SEA PALLING
Norfolk

LOCATION North-east Norfolk
ORGANISATION Sea Palling Independent Lifeboat
ESTABLISHED 1972
HISTORY RNLI pulling and sailing lifeboats served at Palling from the 1850s until 1930, but no trace of the lifeboat house used by these boats remains. The life-saving tradition was re-established in 1972 when, with increasing numbers of tourists visiting Sea Palling, local residents thought it prudent to provide an inshore lifeboat and so formed the Palling Volunteer Rescue Service (PVRS). PVRS Ltd, administered by local volunteers, was formed as a registered charity to operate and finance an independent lifeboat service. Following much fundraising, the station's first inshore lifeboat, Hearts of Oak, entered service in 1974. The station covers the coast between Eccles-on-Sea and Winterton.

PREVIOUS ASSETS
1974 On 26 August the lifeboat Hearts of Oak entered service. The 16ft 6in inflatable inshore

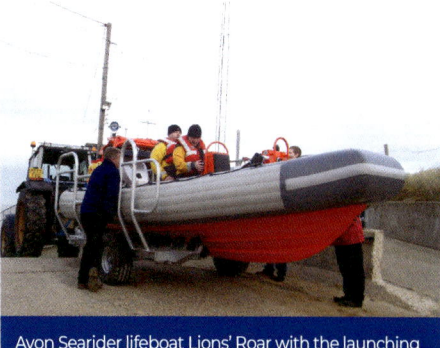

Avon Searider lifeboat Lions' Roar with the launching tractor on the access road to the beach.

rescue craft, named after one of the last RNLI lifeboats and powered by a 40hp outboard, was kept in a boathouse near the Village Gap.
1980 A new 5.4m Avon Searider rigid inflatable, named Leo, entered service. She was funded by local associations, including the Norwich Leo Club, which provided £1,500. Power came from a 75hp outboard, which gave the boat a top speed of 34 knots. This boat served for more 28 years.

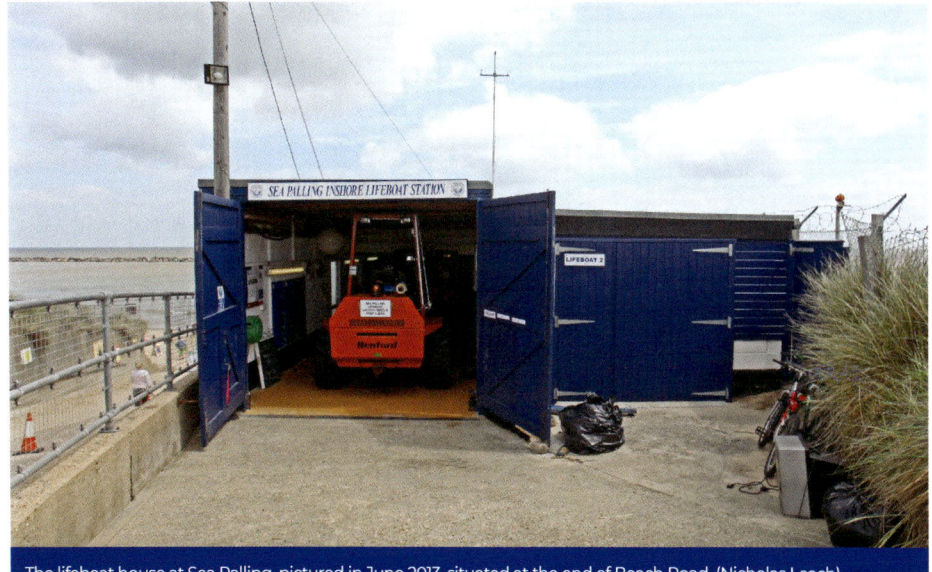

The lifeboat house at Sea Palling, pictured in June 2013, situated at the end of Beach Road. (Nicholas Leach)

Independent lifeboats of Britain

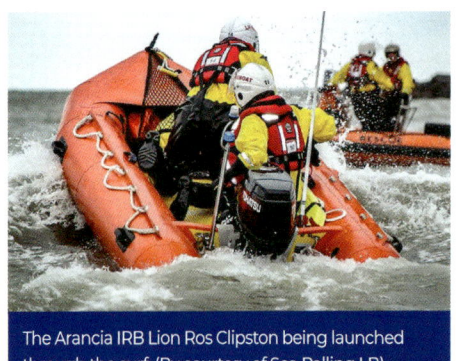
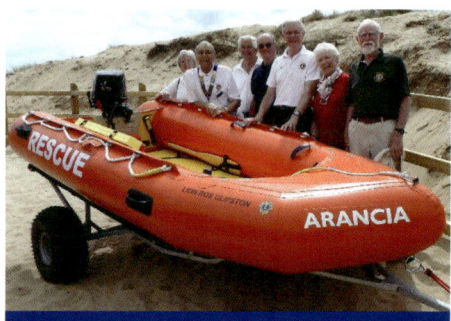

The Arancia IRB Lion Ros Clipston being launched through the surf. (By courtesy of Sea Palling LB)

The naming ceremony of the Arancia inshore rescue boat Lion Ros Clipston, July 2017.

2008 In April a new Avon Searider boat was acquired, named Lions' Roar in recognition of the continuing support of a major benefactor, the Hoveton and Wroxham Lions Club. Lions' Roar was formally blessed by the Bishop of Norwich on 4 May 2008 and provided a service 24 hours a day, all year round. She was a 5.6m Avon Adventurer rigid inflatable, powered by a 90hp outboard which gave her a top speed of 35 knots.

2011 On 1 September, while on a training exercise at night off Happisburgh, Lions' Roar hit an unidentified object and was severely damaged, which resulted in it being written off, so fund-raising began for a new boat, which was ordered in December from Hull boatbuilder Humber RIBs, with Norfolk-based Goodchild Marine contracted to fit it out.

2012 The new £22,000 boat came into service in May, and was formally named and dedicated on 4 June. The 5.7m Humber Sea Pro rigid inflatable was powered by a 90hp outboard engine, which gave a top speed of 36 knots. She was fitted with AIS, GPS, depth sounder, VHF, and other equipment.

2019 Lionheart underwent a major refit at

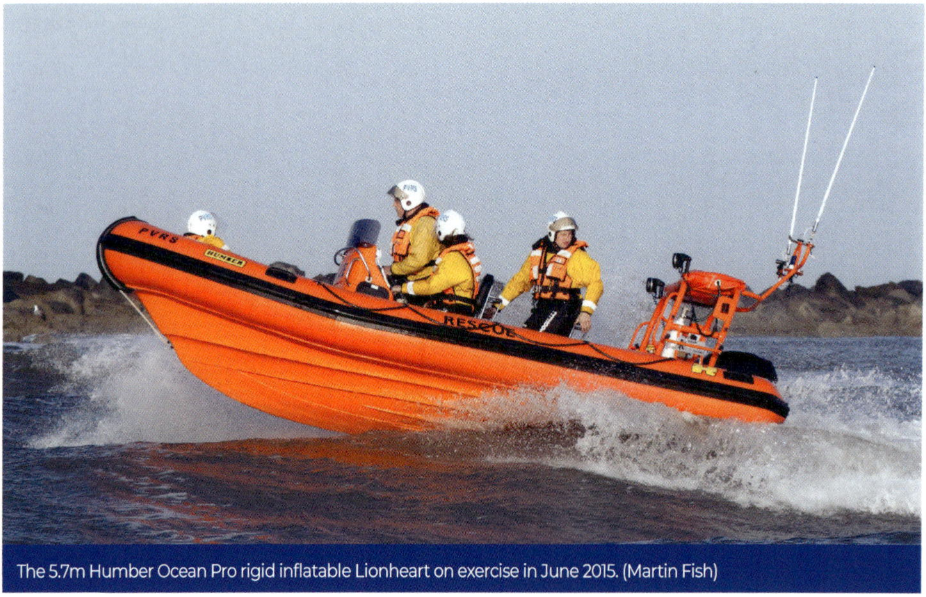

The 5.7m Humber Ocean Pro rigid inflatable Lionheart on exercise in June 2015. (Martin Fish)

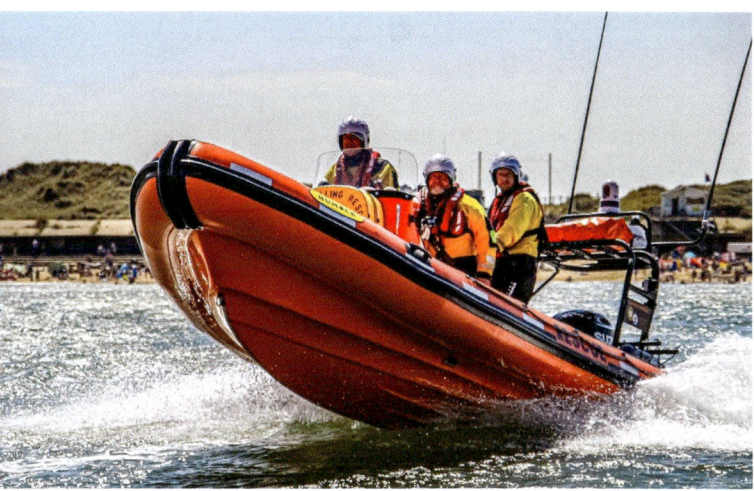

The 6.3m Humber Ocean Pro rigid inflatable, which entered service in 2022, off the beach at Sea Palling. (By courtesy of Sea Palling LB)

Norfolk Yacht Agency, which included being fitted with a new fuel tank and an upgrade to the electrical fit out. Radar was fitted, together with an forward looking infra-red camera.

2017 An Arancia IRB was obtained for operations around the reefs off the beach. Powered by a 30hp Tohatsu outboard, it was provided by the Wroxham and Hoveton Lions Club in memory of their Treasurer and was named Lion Ros Clipston in July. The IRB is launched by trailer with a Yamaha Grizzly Pro Quadbike. Previously a Rib-X Zapcat style craft had been used for inshore work.

2021 Additional facilities and toilets were installed next to the boathouse to improve welfare arrangements for the crew and remove reliance on local public toilets.

2022 Storage facilities were further extended, to improve housing for the Arancia IRB. In May a new 6.3m Humber Ocean Pro rigid inflatable entered service. Funded by the Norfolk Freemasons' Mark Benevolent Fund, the boat was powered by a 200hp Suzuki outboard. Slightly larger than the previous lifeboat, it arrived in May for crew training and sea trials, and was formally named Canon Portal at a ceremony on 24 July.

CURRENT ASSETS 6.3m Humber Ocean Pro rigid inflatable, named Canon Portal, on station 2022, equipped with Raymarine Radar, AIS and FLIR camera, launched by Benford 4x4 Launch Vehicle and Trailer; Arancia IRB Lion Ros Clipston, on station 2016, launched by Argo Responder vehicle and trailer.

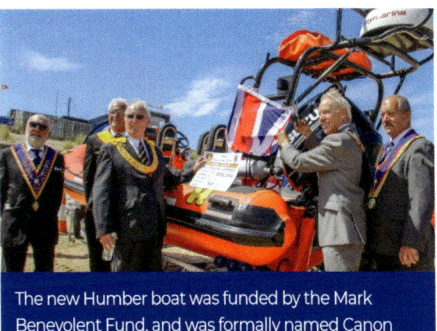

The new Humber boat was funded by the Mark Benevolent Fund, and was formally named Canon Portal at a ceremony on 24 July 2022.

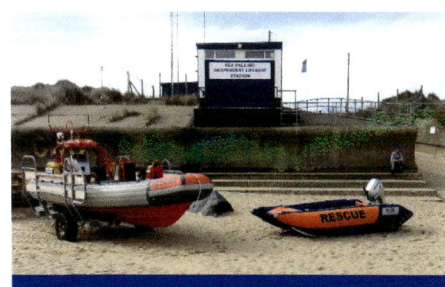

Avon Searider lifeboat Lions' Roar and the Rib-X Zapcat inshore rescue boat on the beach at Sea Palling in front of the lifeboat station.

Independent lifeboats of Britain

HEMSBY

Norfolk

LOCATION Norfolk
ORGANISATION Hemsby Inshore Rescue Service; known as Hemsby Lifeboat
ESTABLISHED 1975
HISTORY The Hemsby Inshore Rescue Service was formed in 1976 and became a charity by 1977. Its boats cover the seas off the Norfolk coast as well as the Norfolk Broads. Its foundation came about as the result of nine people drowning off the villages of Scratby, Hemsby and Winterton between 1973 and 1975. The Community Services Section of the Norfolk Broads Lions Club became concerned about the situation and decided to provide funds to purchase an inflatable craft with an outboard engine, a boat shed and all the other necessary equipment.

The new station was sited at Hemsby Gap, where the beach was most suitable for launching. At a meeting on 2 June 1976 it was decided that the organisation would be called Hemsby Volunteer Inshore Rescue Club. Peter Parsley, the village policeman, was appointed Chairman, and Andrew Fakes Secretary and Treasurer. The Lions Club donated the lifeboat and equipment to Great Yarmouth

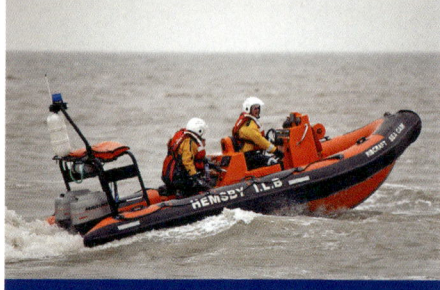

The 5.85m Ribcraft rigid inflatable Sea Cam was in service from 2001 to 2009.

Borough Council, which was responsible for the running costs and maintenance of the boat. The Service agreed to provide crew. Representatives from the Coast Guard, the RNLI, Caister and Sea Palling attended the preliminary meetings to provide advice.

The first year of the Club's existence proved difficult. From July to December 1976 an inflatable was loaned by the Sub-Aqua Club and fitted with a 10hp outboard for use by the Inshore Rescue Club. In December 1976 the Avon SR4M Searider rigid inflatable was delivered, and this boat entered service on 13 February 1977.

BOATHOUSE During 1986 the launching

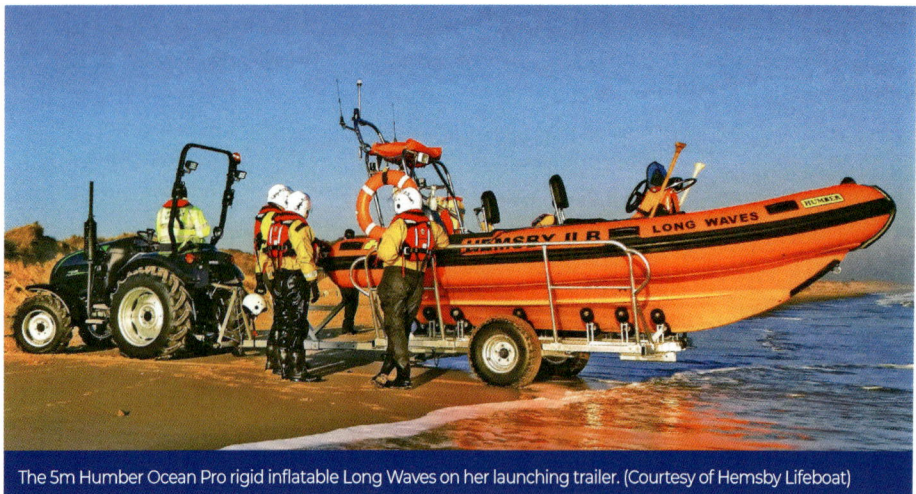

The 5m Humber Ocean Pro rigid inflatable Long Waves on her launching trailer. (Courtesy of Hemsby Lifeboat)

Independent lifeboats of Britain

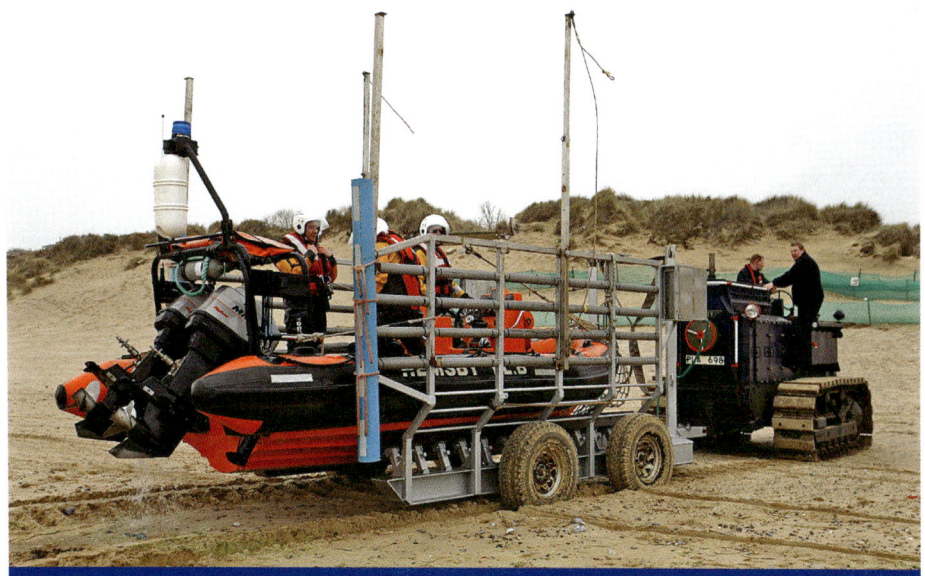

Recovery of the rigid inflatable Sea Cam at Hemsby following an exercise in March 2007. The Fowler tractor, built as T62 in 1954 for the RNLI, was acquired from the Caister Volunteer Rescue Service and used at Hemsby 2002 to 2009.

ramp from the lifeboat house was destroyed by the sea, making launch and recovery difficult. Continuing coastal erosion put the building at risk, so it was decided to construct a new boathouse, which was built and funded entirely by volunteers. Once a concrete base, capable of withstanding possible movement by sand, had been laid, a two-storey building was constructed to accommodate the boat and its equipment. The new boathouse was opened in 1989, having cost approximately £18,000 in total. During 2020-21 the existing station building was extended further to take a larger lifeboat and its launching vehicle.

PREVIOUS ASSETS

2009 Humber 5m Ocean Pro rigid inflatable Long Waves, launched by a Softrak vehicle and trailer, replaced 2021.

2021 On 12 December the Atlantic 75 lifeboat was named Sea Weaver in honour of a donor

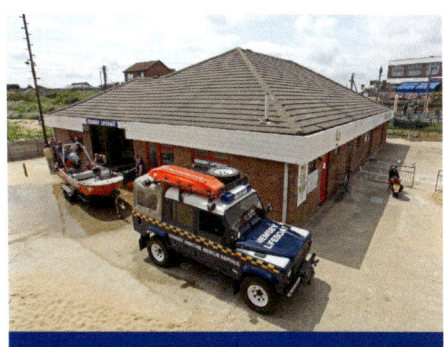

The lifeboat station near the beach, pictured in 2007, with the Land Rover and Broads boat outside.

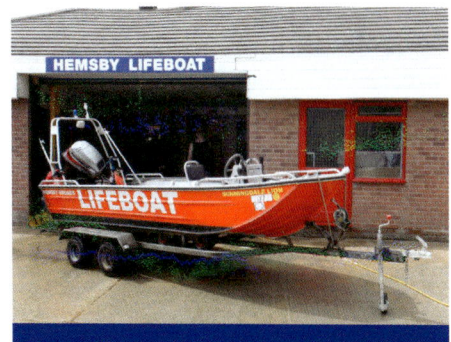

The semi-flat aluminium boat for use inland, with 125 miles of the Broads being covered.

Independent lifeboats of Britain   33

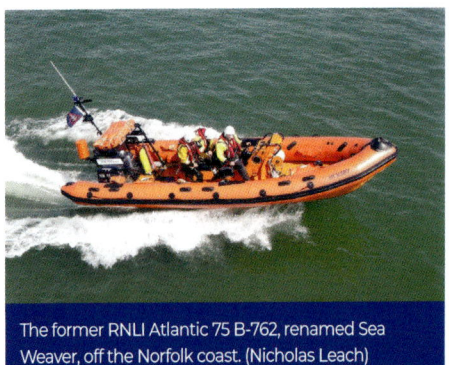

The former RNLI Atlantic 75 B-762, renamed Sea Weaver, off the Norfolk coast. (Nicholas Leach)

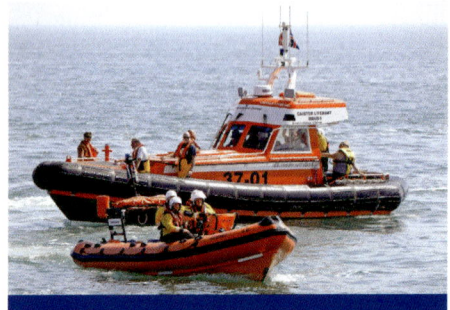

Atlantic 75 Sea Weaver with the Caister lifeboat Bernard Matthews II, August 2022. (Nicholas Leach)

who raised over £100,000 for the service. Sue was presented with a certificate signed by the crew on the day. During the ceremony, the Service also celebrated the fundraising efforts of East Anglia Working Newfoundlands, who have given many years of support to Hemsby, and the new Broads Rescue boathouse was named 'Newfoundlands' Boat House'. Sea Weaver was obtained by Hemsby in 2018 and work was carried out on the boat at Goodchild Marine prior to her becoming operational.

CURRENT ASSETS The former RNLI Atlantic 75 Jack and Joyce Burcombe (ex-RNLI B-762, built in 2000) was obtained from the RNLI in 2018, and entered service at Hemsby in 2021, being launched from a former RNLI drive on-drive off carriage; Loglogic Softrak vehicle used for launching and recovery, with plans to acquire a Talus MB-H tractor; Seastrike/Goodchild Marine semi-flat aluminium boat for use on the Broads, with Mitsubishi L20 4x4 vehicle and trailer, on station 2014.

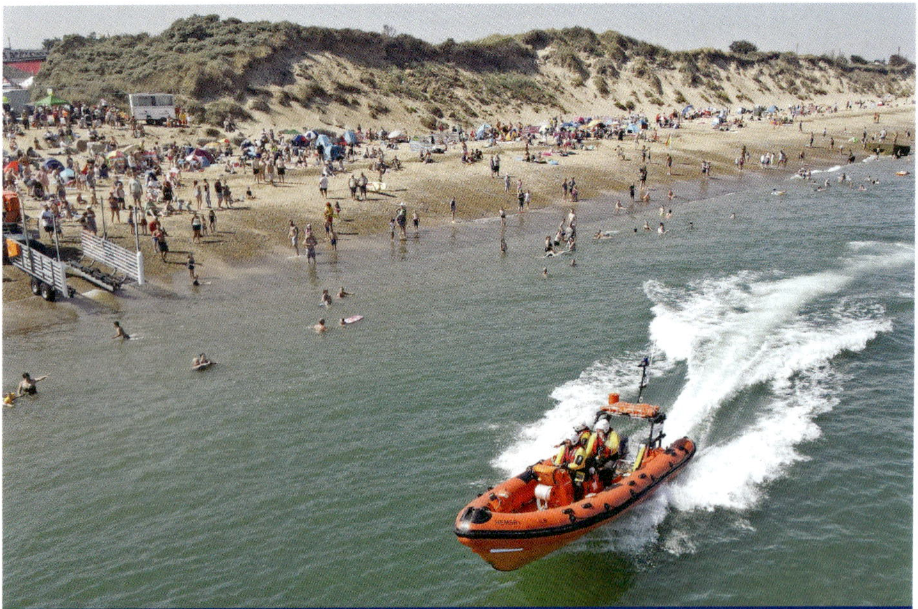

Atlantic 75 Sea Weaver on show during the station's annual lifeboat day, August 2022. (Nicholas Leach)

Independent lifeboats of Britain

CAISTER
Norfolk

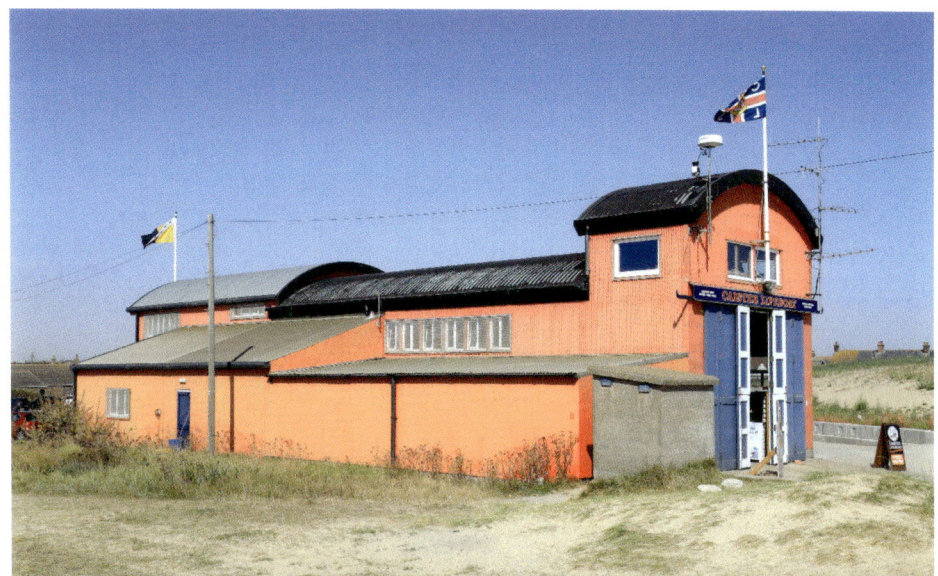

The lifeboat house built by the RNLI on the dunes in 1941. Caister Volunteer Lifeboat Service added extensions at the rear and on the south side to provide better facilities for the lifeboat and her crew. The building was used by the independent organisation until 2004, and was subsequently converted into an interactive museum, branded the Caister Lifeboat Experience, with former lifeboat Shirley Jean Adye as the centrepiece. (Nicholas Leach)

LOCATION Norfolk
ORGANISATION Caister Volunteer Lifeboat Service (since 1973)
ESTABLISHED 1969
HISTORY Caister independent lifeboat was established as Caister Volunteer Rescue Service, and is one of the best-known independent lifeboats in the country. The organisation was formed when, despite much local opposition, the RNLI withdrew their lifeboat from Caister in 1969. The ex-RNLI crew decided to form a rescue service and, as a temporary measure, 'Skipper' Woodhouse provided a 16ft fibreglass dinghy. A national appeal was launched to raise £50,000 to fund a boat. Although this did not generate enough funds, the children from Caister High School raised enough to fund an inflatable lifeboat, which saved four lives in 1971 and 1972 and was based in the old RNLI lifeboat house, which the service had taken over. In 1973, when the offshore lifeboat was acquired, the organisation was renamed Caister Volunteer Lifeboat Service and is a registered charity.

PREVIOUS ASSETS
1973 A former RNLI Liverpool class lifeboat,

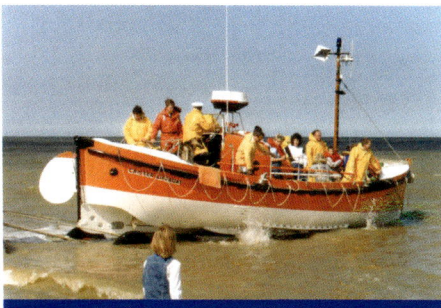

Launch of the 35ft 6in Liverpool class Shirley Jean Adye, the first Caister VRS lifeboat. (Paul Russell)

Independent lifeboats of Britain

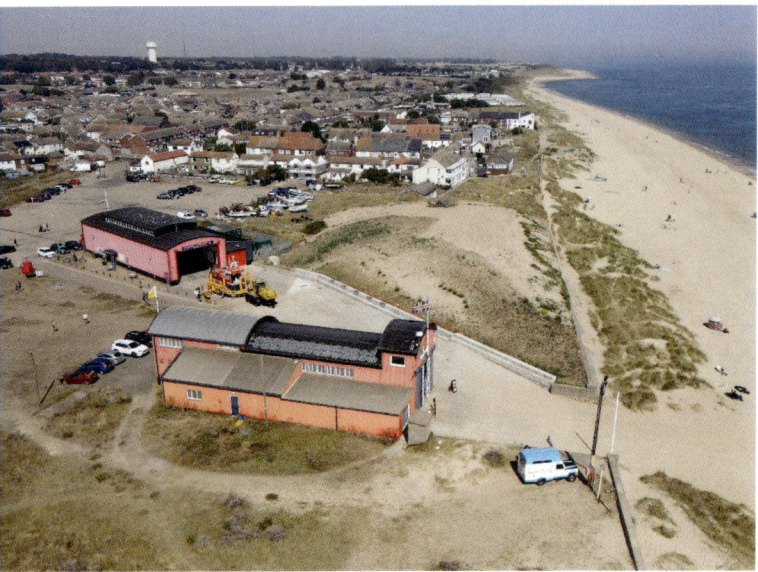

Overlooking Caister beach with the historic site from where Caister's lifeboats have been operated. The lifeboat house built in 1941 by the RNLI houses the Caister Lifeboat Experience, while the newer boathouse behind it in 2003-04 is used for the operational lifeboat.

W. Ross MacArthur of Glasgow (ex-ON-906), was bought for £4,300 from a Wells owner who had used her as fishing boat named Viking of Wells. Re-equipped to lifeboat standards, the boat was officially named Shirley Jean Adye and launched on 15 August 1973. A launching tractor was acquired for £3,850.

1991 On 18 June 1991 HRH Princess Alexandra officially named a new lifeboat which had been funded by a £400,000 appeal. It was named Bernard Matthews in recognition of the support and generosity of the well-known Norfolk turkey farmer. Based on an extended Brede class hull by Lochin Marine of Rye, the boat was fitted out at Goodchild Marine, Burgh Castle. She measured 38ft 6in by 8ft 10in and was powered by twin 240hp Ford Sabre diesels, giving a speed of 18 knots.

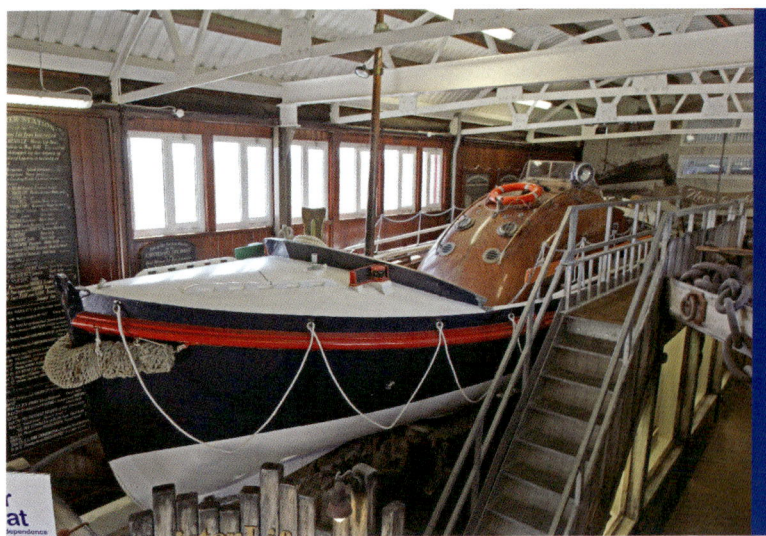

The former RNLI 35ft 6in Liverpool class lifeboat W. Ross MacArthur of Glasgow (ON.906), which was renamed Shirley Jean Adye for service at Caister, on display inside the old lifeboat house as the centrepiece of a museum telling the long history of the lifeboat service in Caister. (Nicholas Leach)

Independent lifeboats of Britain

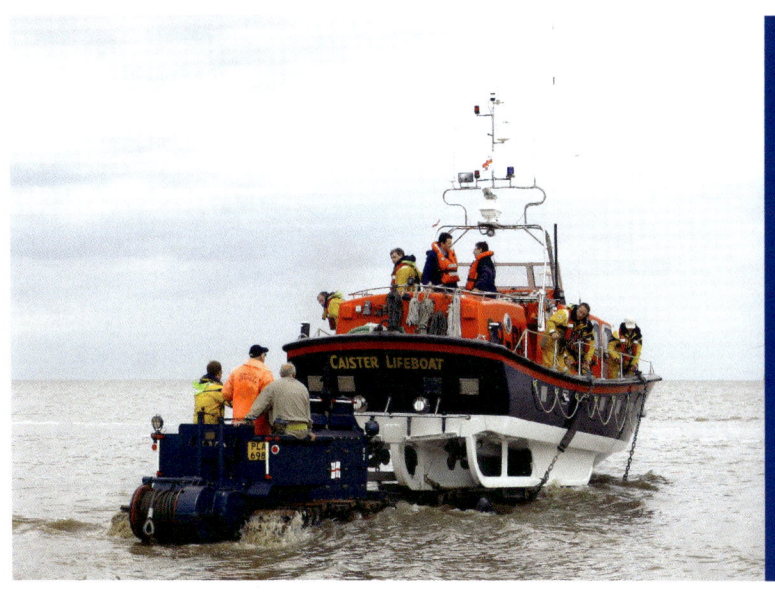

Launching the 38ft Lochin type lifeboat Bernard Matthews using the Fowler tractor (former RNLI T62). Bernard Matthews was on station from 1991 to 2004, and the tractor was in service from 1989 to 1997. (Nicholas Leach)

When replaced in August 2004, she was sold to Blyth Volunteer Lifeboat Service, but has since returned to Norfolk and is kept at Wells.
2001 An 4.5m Avon Searider rigid inflatable was funded by and named after Jim Davidson. The boat was formally christened on 9 September 2001 having been purchased with money raised by the donor at his charity show at the Wellington Pier during the 2000 season.
2004 The Caister VLS ordered a Valentijn type rigid inflatable lifeboat from Habbeké Shipyard, Volendam, in the Netherlands. Built at a cost of £450,000, the aluminium hulled Valentijn class boat measured 11m by 4.1m and was powered by twin Hamilton water jets driven by 250hp Volvo Penta engines giving a speed of 37 knots. Similar lifeboats are in widespread use along the Dutch coast. The new boat arrived at Caister on 29 August 2004 and was placed on service before the end of the year. She was formally named Bernard Matthews II, after the station's main benefactor, by HRH Prince Charles and the Duchess of Cornwall on 26 July 2005. The Caterpillar Challenger tractor was modified in the Netherlands and a new boathouse was built, adjacent to the old house, in Tan Lane.
2012 A new 5m Ribcraft ILB, named Fred Dyble, was placed on station in July. Bernard Matthews II had an extensive refit at

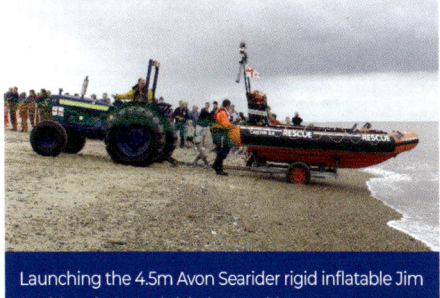

Launching the 4.5m Avon Searider rigid inflatable Jim Davidson in 2004. (Nicholas Leach)

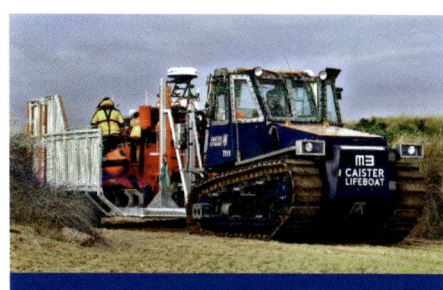

The former RNLI Talus MB-H tractor T111 launching the inshore lifeboat Fred Dyble II. (Keith Wood)

Independent lifeboats of Britain

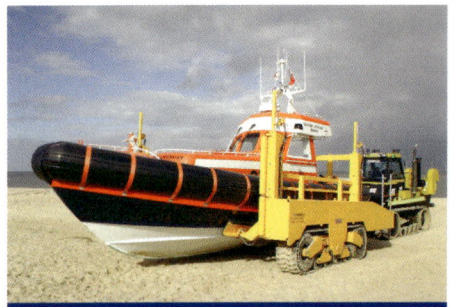

The Dutch-built rigid inflatable Bernard Matthews II arriving at Caister for the first time in August 2004.

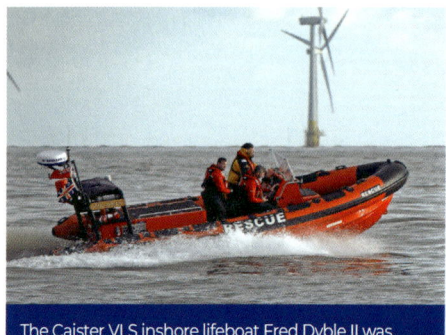

The Caister VLS inshore lifeboat Fred Dyble II was placed on station in 2019. (Keith Wood)

Goodchild Marine during October.
2014 An extension to the boathouse was completed to provide more space for the ILB.
2018-19 A new inshore lifeboat, built by Alicat Workboats in Great Yarmouth to an upgraded commercial specification, was commissioned; she entered service in March 2019. Named Fred Dyble II, she was powered by a 262hp Steyr inboard diesel engine and Hamilton waterjet, giving a speeds of 35 knots.
2019 The former RNLI Talus MB-H tractor T111 (ex-Peel) was purchased in December for launching the inshore lifeboat.
2022 Diverse Marine Ltd and Caister VLS signed an agreement in early February for construction of a first of class 14m lifeboat after a competitive tender process. The lifeboat was based on a design from Walker Marine Design, and built by Diverse Marine at Cowes. The 14m self-righting lifeboat has an aluminium hull, deck and coach roof, together with a resiliently mounted GRP wheelhouse to reduce noise and vibration. The air-conditioned wheelhouse has seats for six crew, with a central helm station forward. Power will come from twin Scania DI13-077M main propulsion engines driving twin Hamilton HJ364 waterjets for speeds in excess of 35

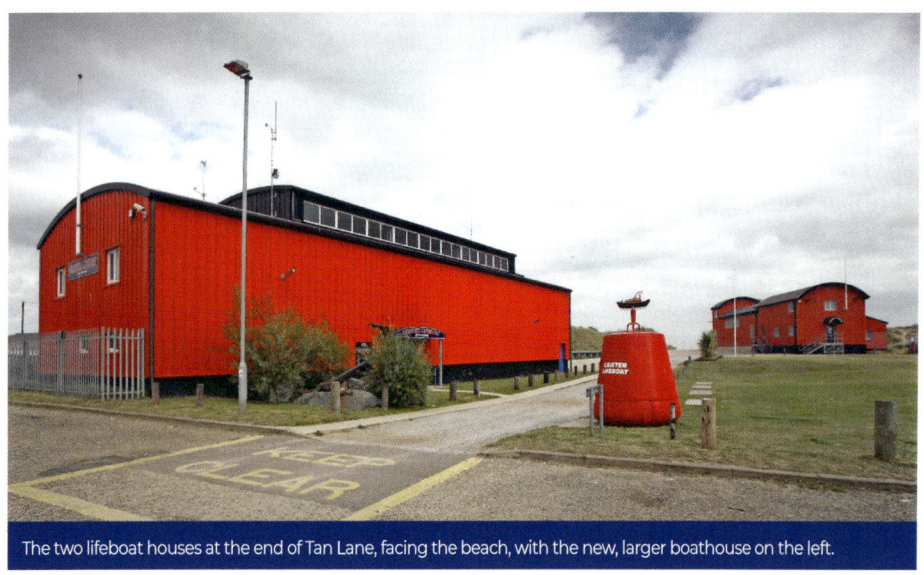

The two lifeboat houses at the end of Tan Lane, facing the beach, with the new, larger boathouse on the left.

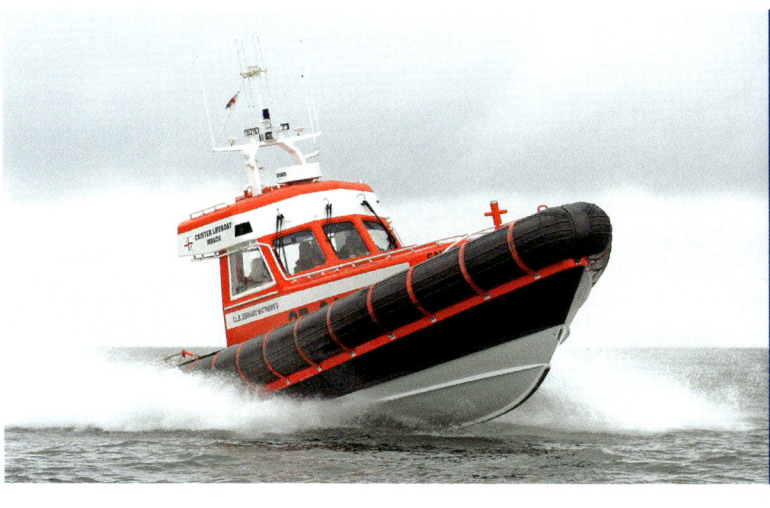

Bernard Matthews II makes an impressive sight as she arrives at Wells-next-the-Sea in August 2007 to take part in a gathering of lifeboats, past and present. (Nicholas Leach)

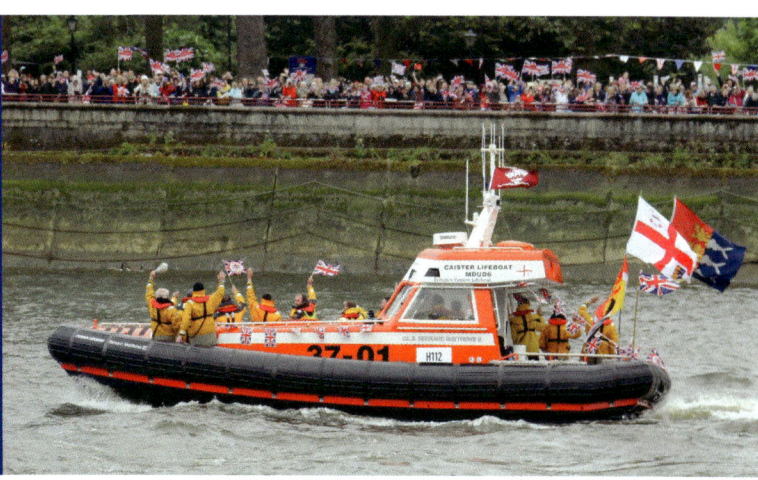

Bernard Matthews II in London participating in the Thames Diamond Jubilee Pageant parade on 3 June 2012. She joined the lifeboat contingent among the total of 670 boats that were involved. (Nicholas Leach)

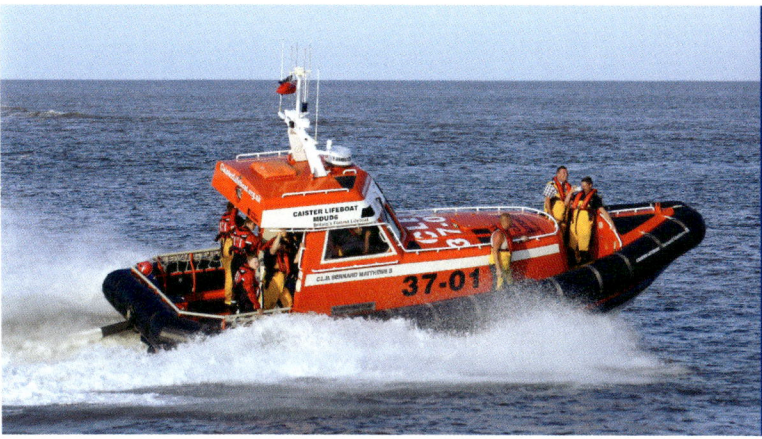

Bernard Matthews II at Gorleston for the RNLI station's annual lifeboat day in July 2018, during which she undertook demonstration rescues for the crowds on the pier. (Nicholas Leach)

Independent lifeboats of Britain

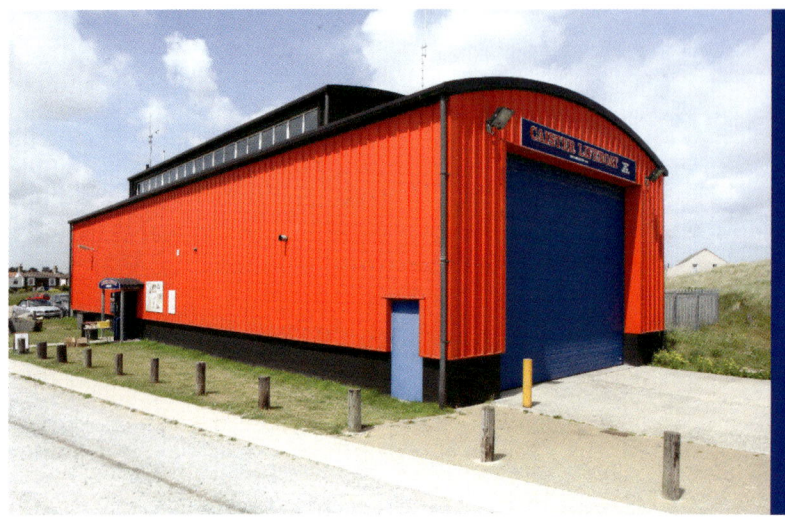

The lifeboat house built in 2003-04 for the Dutch-built lifeboat Bernard Matthews II and her launching rig. The building was altered in 2022 for a new British-built 14m lifeboat. (Nicholas Leach)

knots. The boat is to be in service in early 2023, with a new purpose-built launch vehicle. The main door of the lifeboat house was widened and access to the beach was enlarged in preparation for the new lifeboat.

CURRENT ASSETS Valentijn rigid inflatable Bernard Matthews II, launched by Caterpillar Challenger 65C tractor and hydraulic carriage, on station 2004; 7m Alicat inshore lifeboat Fred Dyble II, on station 2019, launched by Talus MBH Tractor (ex-RNLI T111) and carriage.

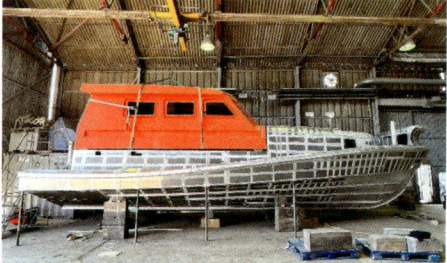

The new 45ft rigid inflatable lifeboat under construction at Diverse Marine, Cowes, July 2022.

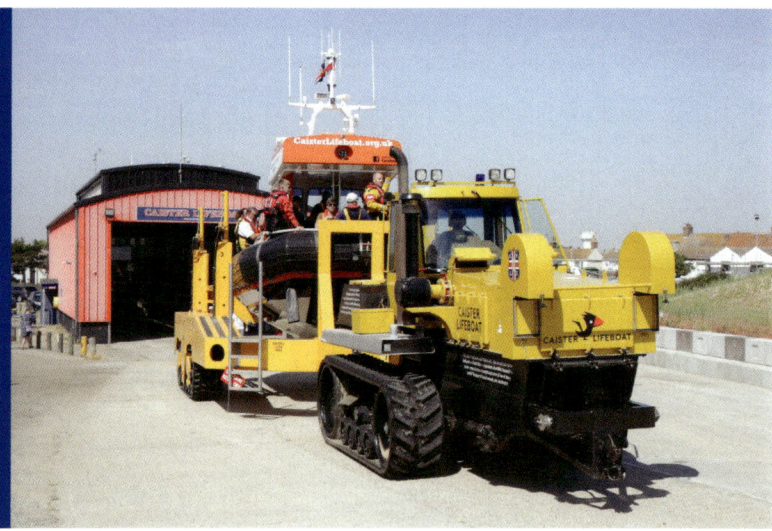

Bernard Matthews II being brought out of the lifeboat house for launching, August 2022. (Nicholas Leach)

Independent lifeboats of Britain

FELIXSTOWE Sussex

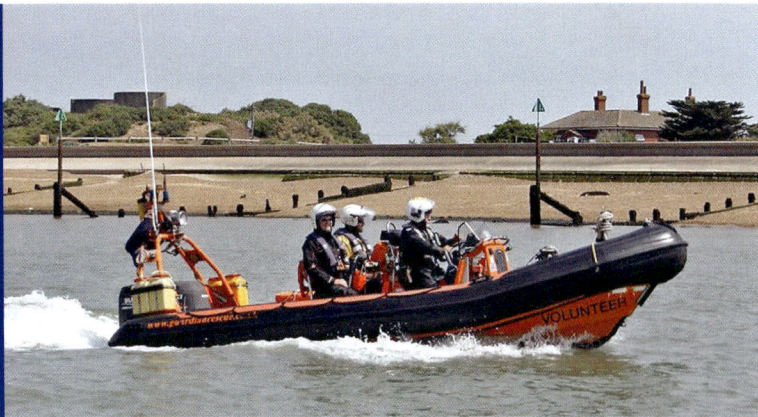

Felixstowe lifeboat Volunteer on patrol. The service offers Suffolk Resilience Cat 1-2 emergency response and is also a Suffolk Police Marine Support Unit. (By courtesy of FVCPR)

LOCATION Suffolk Yacht Harbour, Levington; shore facility at Railway Approach
ORGANISATION Felixstowe Volunteer Coast Patrol Rescue Service
ESTABLISHED 1997
HISTORY The Felixstowe Volunteer Coast Patrol Rescue Service (FVCPR) was formed in 1997 by two former Coastguards to fill the gap in marine safety cover left by the withdrawal of the Felixstowe Coastguard Patrol Boat. Its mission is to promote sea safety awareness, and to protect and preserve life at sea by the provision of a Volunteer Coast Patrol Rescue Service. The service maintains two lifeboats, which are based at Suffolk Yacht Harbour, Levington, which operate on a patrol basis.

Initially the service used a 4m Avon Searider rigid inflatable named Guardian, but, after this was overwhelmed working on the Deben Bar, and as the service was being tasked more frequently and further afield, a larger purpose-built rigid-hulled inflatable boat was deemed necessary in 1998. Named Volunteer, the new boat entered service in 2000 and was initially kept afloat at Levington. In 2011 Volunteer had a major refit, which saw her sponsons replaced and her electronics renewed.

In December 2013, when the Service was deployed by road to respond to the East Coast tidal surge flooding emergency, the lifeboat Volunteer and 4x4 support vehicle were involved in a serious road accident. A gust of wind turned the boat and the vehicle over, injuring the three crew. The Service was kept operational temporarily using a 24ft Halmatic Arctic rigid inflatable powered by twin 225hp engines, named Guardian. This was the former Essex Police boat Seaaxe, which was purchased through a grant form the Suffolk PCC. However,

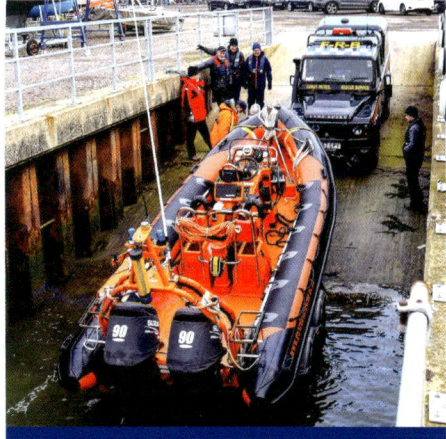

FVCPR lifeboat being launched at Suffolk Yacht Harbour, Levington. The boat patrols regularly during weekends. (By courtesy of FVCPR)

Independent lifeboats of Britain   41

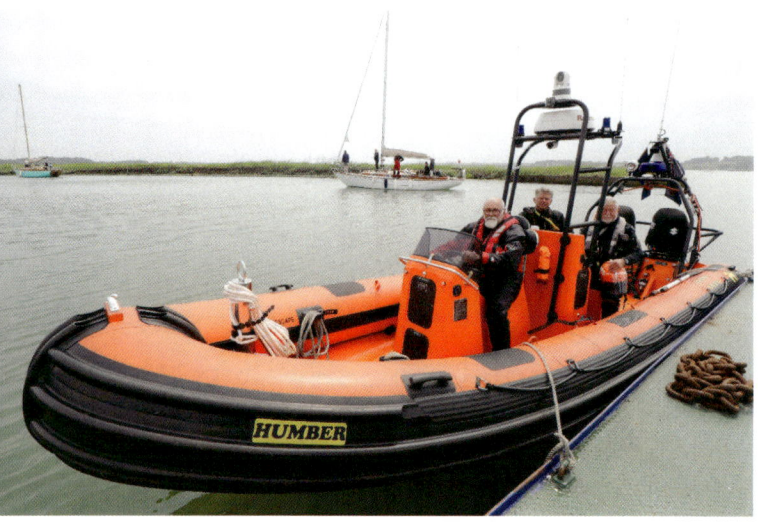

The Humber Ocean-Pro rigid inflatable at Suffolk Yacht Harbour, Levington, with her crew on board prior to heading out on patrol. (Nicholas Leach)

this boat was costly on fuel and unsuitable as a rescue platform, so was sold in 2015 to the UKBF, and the proceeds went towards a new boat.

In 2018 the East of England Co-op leased its old dairy site in Felixstowe to the FVCPR, part of a package of support for the independent charity. This was the FVCPR's first secure base, housing the lifeboats, and used as a training facility.

CURRENT ASSETS The service operates two boats, Volunteer and Last Orders, and both have trailers so that they can be moved from Felixstowe to Levington as necessary.

VOLUNTEER 6.3m x 2.34m Humber Ocean-Pro rigid inflatable; built by Humber Inflatables, Hull; crew three, displacement 1,700kg, range 70 miles, twin 90hp Suzuki outboards, speed 38 knots; named by Lady Eva English, Felixstowe Mayor Cllr Malcolm Minns; on station June 2000.

LAST ORDERS 7.5m x 2.54m Humber Ocean-Pro rigid inflatable, crew three, 100-mile radius, displacement 1,750kg, twin 115hp Suzuki outboards, speed 40 knots, named 14 July 2019 by the High Sheriff of Suffolk, Ros Eminson, and sponsor Mrs Jo Wenham; on station February 2020.

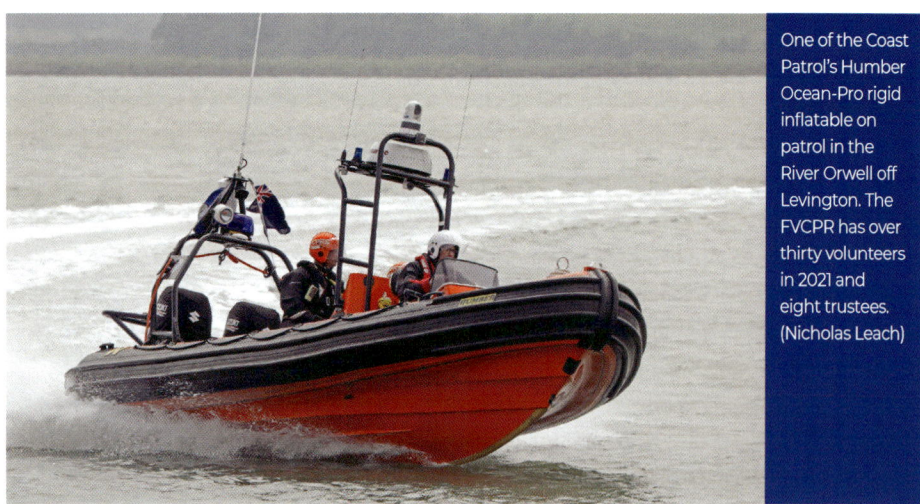

One of the Coast Patrol's Humber Ocean-Pro rigid inflatable on patrol in the River Orwell off Levington. The FVCPR has over thirty volunteers in 2021 and eight trustees. (Nicholas Leach)

ENGLAND SOUTH COAST

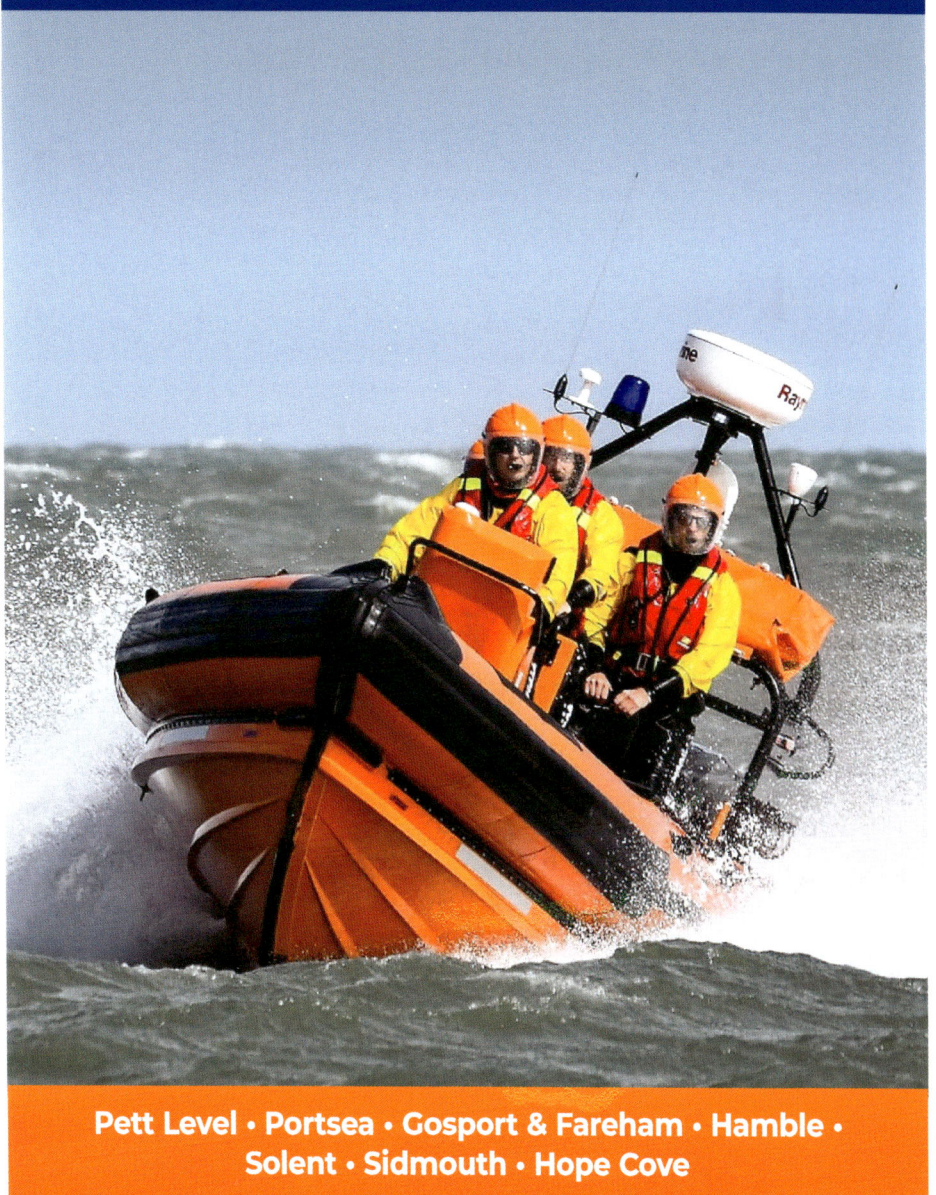

Pett Level • Portsea • Gosport & Fareham • Hamble • Solent • Sidmouth • Hope Cove

PETT LEVEL — Sussex

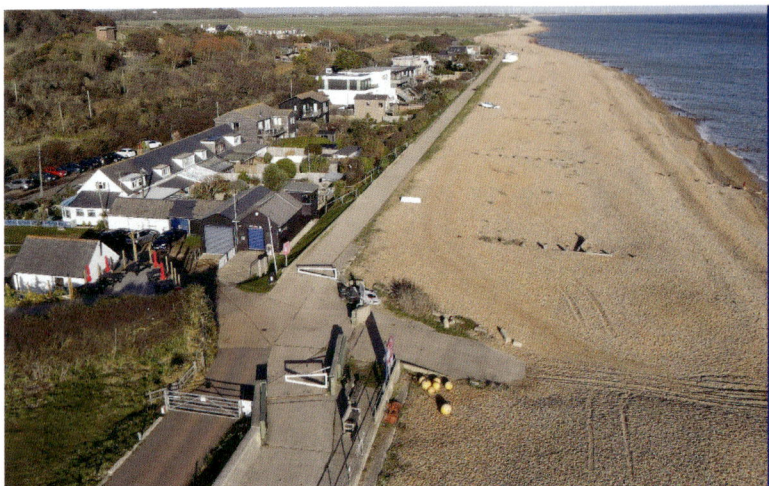

The Pett Level Rescue Boat operates from a small boathouse at the eastern edge of the village, with the boats being launched over the shingle beach. (Nicholas Leach)

LOCATION Pett Level, Sussex
ORGANISATION Pett Level Independent Rescue Boat
ESTABLISHED 1971
HISTORY The first rescue boat at Pett Level arrived in 1970 when it was based at the New Beach Club and was manned by local club members. The need for a rescue boat came about after two brothers, supported by club members, launched a rowing boat in a fierce gale to save the crew of a small fishing boat in trouble off Pett Level beach. The first lifeboat was an Avon Searider Deluxe rigid inflatable powered by a single outboard engine. The lifeboat was launched from a trailer over the steep shingle beach, and a small temporary boathouse was built on the seafront. The volunteers at Pett have been involved in

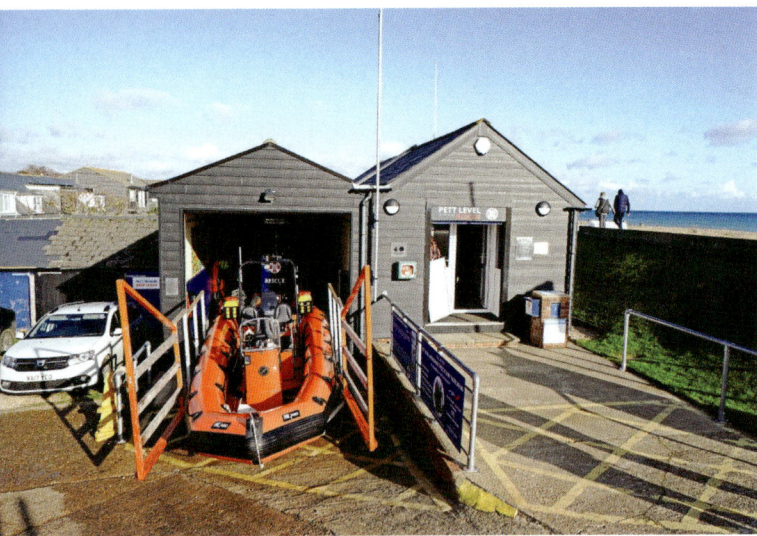

The Pett Level Rescue Boat is kept in one half of the double boathouse, with the other half providing crew and training facilities, and a small souvenir shop. The station was was rebuilt in 2012 to improved better facilities. (Nicholas Leach)

Independent lifeboats of Britain

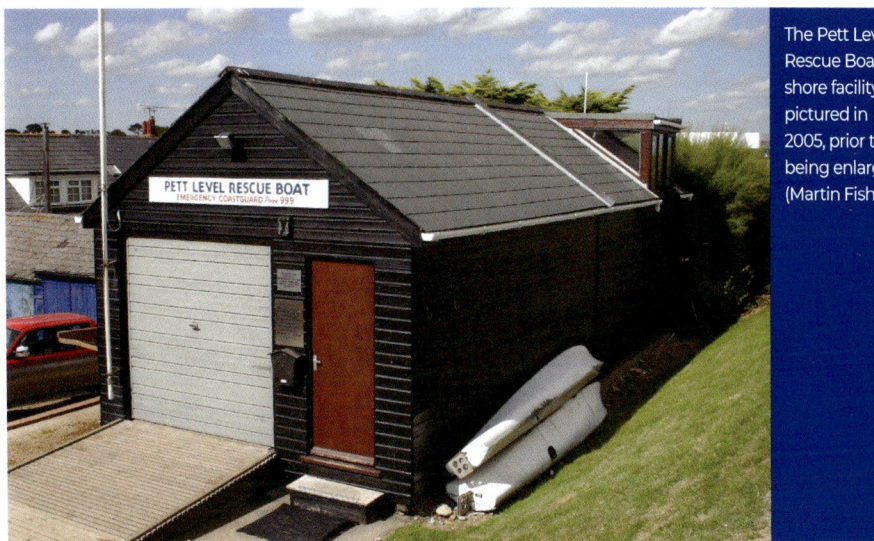

The Pett Level Rescue Boat shore facility, pictured in 2005, prior to being enlarged. (Martin Fish)

searches for missing vessels and people, rescues from stranded vessels, saving swimmers swept out to sea, assisting walkers cut off by the tide at Fairlight, and helping during flooding in Pett Level and Robertsbridge.

PREVIOUS ASSETS

2006 A new 4.7m Avon Searider rigid inflatable, named Lou Parsons and powered by a single 70hp Yamaha outboard, was acquired. It featured a central console for the helm and a crew member, and a basic roll bar over the engines for the VHF aerial and navigation lights. Launching and recovery were achieved using an all-terrain dumper truck, which was subsequently extensively rebuilt into a bespoke launching vehicle by Rye Recovery, who installed a winch which is used on the shingle areas of the beach. A bow launching trailer provided safe launching into surf.

2008 Rye Mayor Sam Souster attended the naming ceremony of the new lifeboat, an XS Ribs rigid inflatable with a tiller-steered 15hp Yamaha four-stroke engine. The boat, which cost around £5,000, was named Mary Newgate after benefactors Mary Marshall and the Newgate Club in London. Julie Marshall, Mary's daughter, and Robin Gosling-Smyth, representative of the Newgate Club, were present at the ceremony. The boat was used for inshore work and flood relief.

2012 Following the rebuilding of the lifeboat

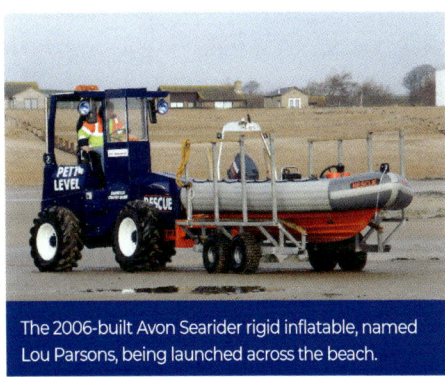

The 2006-built Avon Searider rigid inflatable, named Lou Parsons, being launched across the beach.

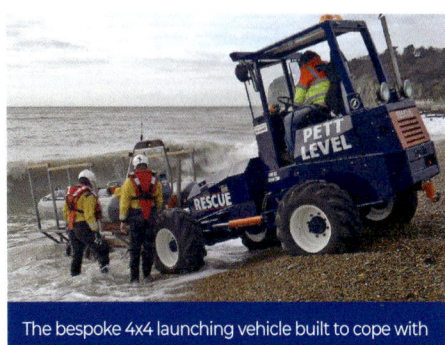

The bespoke 4x4 launching vehicle built to cope with challenging beach conditions at Pett.

Independent lifeboats of Britain

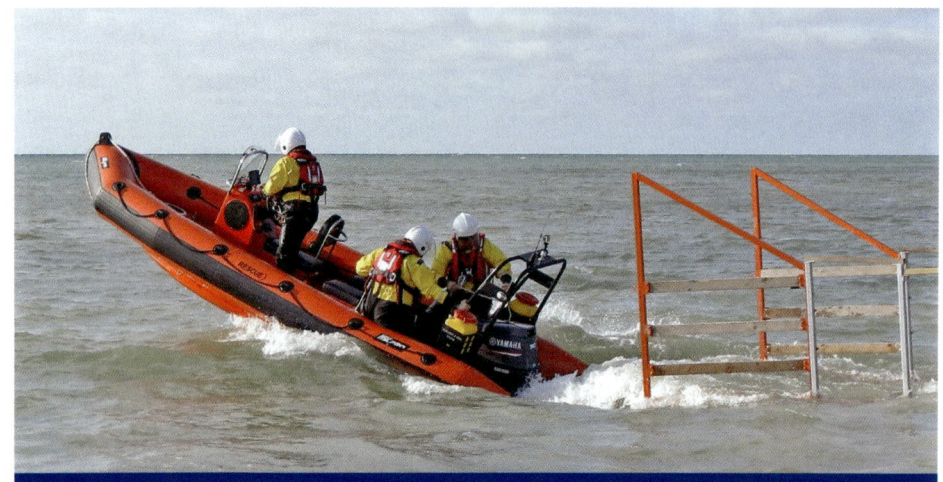

The current Pett Level lifeboat Margaret and John Pulfer being launched from the specially designed trailer. (Courtesy of Pett Level Independent Rescue Boat)

station, the new house was officially opened on 16 June. The building had an enlarged boat hall for the inshore lifeboats and launching vehicles, together with improved crew facilities and a lookout over the beach.

2015 A new Arancia IRB, powered by a Tohatsu 30hp outboard, was purchased as a second inshore rescue boat. The new boat was formally named John Pettifer AKA JP in June.

2016 A Zodiac Milpro Searider rigid inflatable was acquired, powered by a 90hp Yamaha outboard which provided an increased top speed to the previous lifeboat. A helm console was fitted, with seating for two crew. A naming ceremony took place in March 2017, when the High Sheriff of East Sussex, Michael Foster, named the boat Margaret and John Pulfer.

CURRENT ASSETS Zodiac Milpro Searider, named Margaret and John Pulfer, launched by bespoke 4x4 vehicle and trailer, on station 2016; Arancia IRB, named John Pettifer AKA JP, launched by trailer, on station 2015.

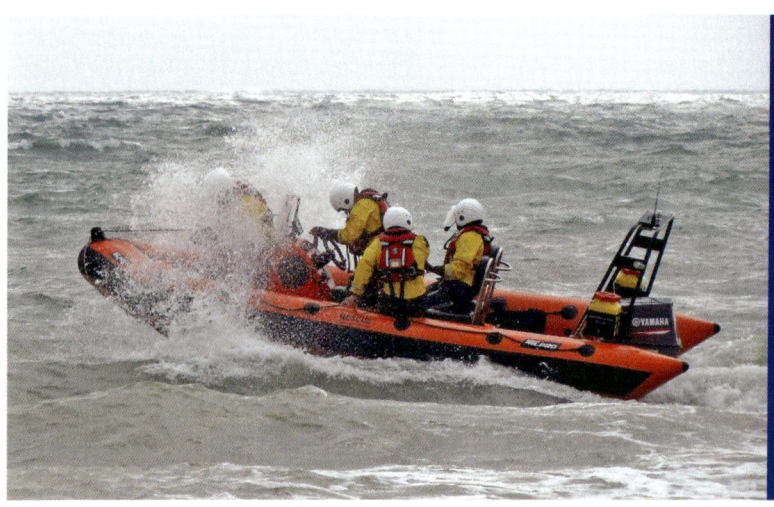

The Zodiac Milpro Searider rigid inflatable Margaret and John Pulfer at sea off Pett Level. (Courtesy of Pett Level Independent Rescue Boat)

PORTSEA

Hampshire

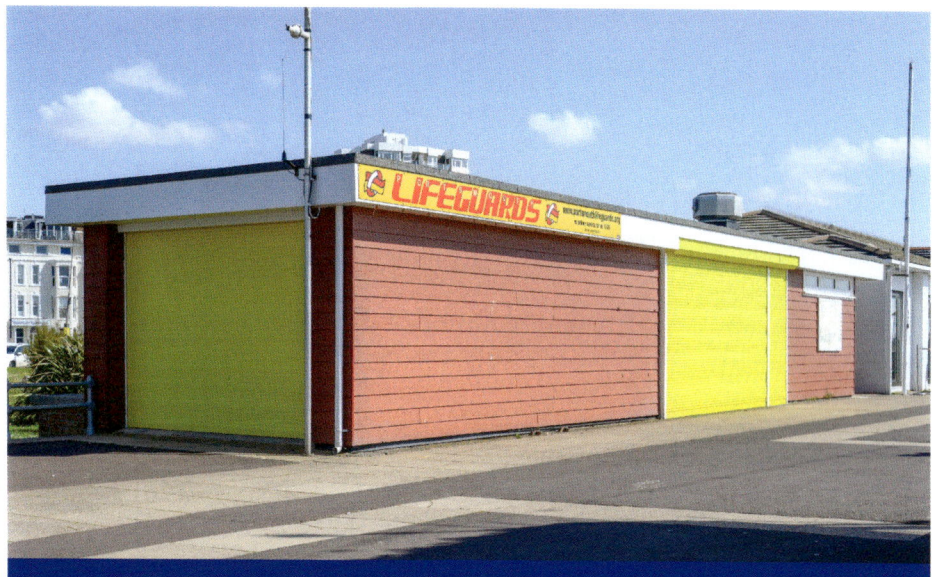

The current lifeguards' post at Southsea from where Portsea Rescue crews patrol during the season, with the lifeboat moored off the beach during the day when not being used for patrolling. (Maritime Photographic)

LOCATION Portsmouth, Hampshire
ORGANISATION Portsmouth and Southsea Voluntary Lifeguards (Portsea Rescue)
ESTABLISHED 1933
HISTORY Portsmouth and Southsea Voluntary Lifeguards is a beach lifeguard club based in Southsea, Portsmouth. Founded in 1933, the club is the oldest in the UK. It provides lifeguard cover for Southsea Seafront during weekends and bank holidays. The volunteers undertake shoreline, paddleboard, jet ski and boat patrols from May to October, and also provide safety cover for special events such as cross-Solent swims and pier to pier events.

Various rescue boats were operated prior to 1991, including a former RNLI inflatable Y boat, a Commando rigid inflatable and several dories. The boats are kept at Fort Cumberland,

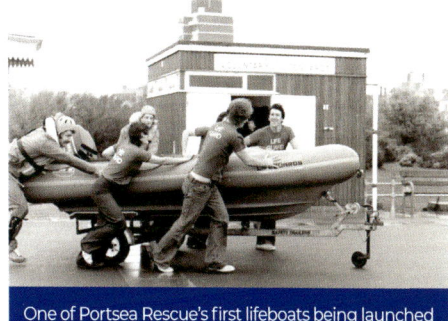

One of Portsea Rescue's first lifeboats being launched from the promenade beside the beach at Southsea.

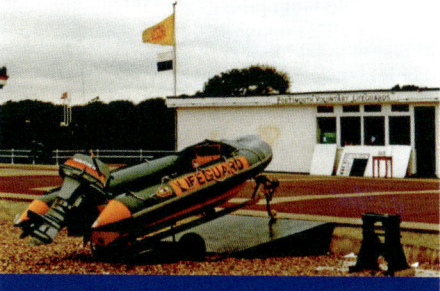

The Avon Searider on the beach outside the Voluntary Lifeguards' shore facility at Southsea.

Independent lifeboats of Britain

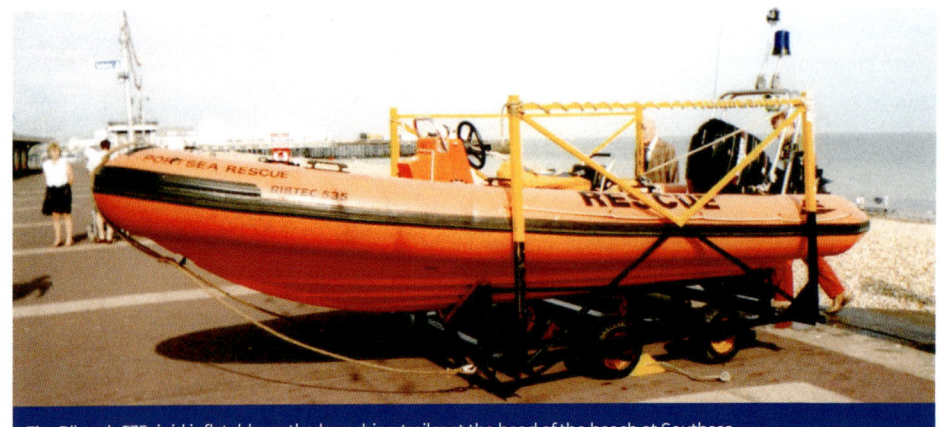

The Ribtech 535 rigid inflatable on the launching trailer at the head of the beach at Southsea.

east of Portsmouth, and taken to a slipway at The Camber Docks in Old Portsmouth to be launched. Once afloat, the boats are brought round to the headquarters, where they are put on a temporary mooring off Southsea when they are not on patrol. The boats are based here, and if required the crew swim out from the shore building and take the boat to sea. At the end of the day the mooring buoy is recovered and the boat brought ashore at The Camber.

PREVIOUS ASSETS
1991 A Ribtech 535 with a single 65hp Mercury engine, capable of 30 knots, was acquired. This boat was followed by an Avon Searider and a Zodiac Grand Raid Mk.3, which was a 5m tiller-steered boat powered by a 40hp Mariner two-stroke outboard. Around the same time the club also had a 4.8m Gemini with a 40hp long-shaft Mariner outboard, also with a tiller.
1997 The Club's first vehicle, a specialised yellow Land Rover, was purchased; prior to this, the boats were launched manually.
1998 Ribcraft 5.85, twin 60hp Yamaha engines, top speed 34 knots was acquired; sold to ICE-SAR in 2017 to continue lifesaving duties.
2003 A white Land Rover was acquired.
2007 Zodiac Grand Raid Inflatable, named Jobsite I – Portsea Rescue 2, acquired; beach-launched, it was withdrawn in 2017.
2008 Toyota Hilux vehicle was acquired.

CURRENT ASSETS Ribcraft 6.8m Professional, Portsea Rescue 1, twin 140hp four-stroke Suzuki engines, top speed 47 knots, on station 2017; two Mitsubishi Shogun 4x4 vehicles and trailer, one on station 2013 and the other in 2019, custom fitted with extra lights, radios and front winches; two Yamaha Waverunner Rescue Water Craft, launched by trailer.

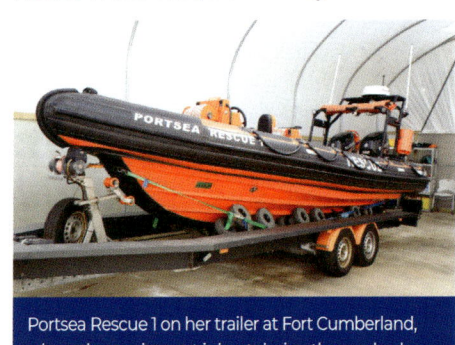

Portsea Rescue 1 on her trailer at Fort Cumberland, where the equipment is kept during the week when the assets are not in use. (Nicholas Leach)

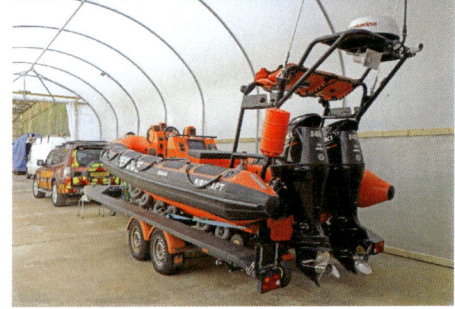

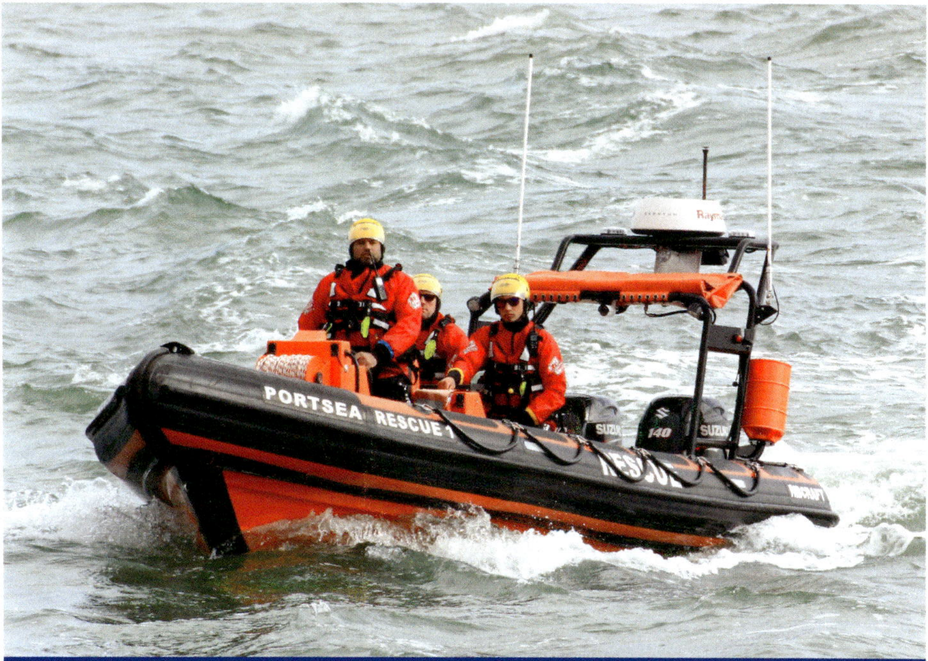

The 6.8m Ribcraft rigid inflatable Portsea Rescue 1 is powered by twin 140hp Suzuki outboards. (Andrew Cooke)

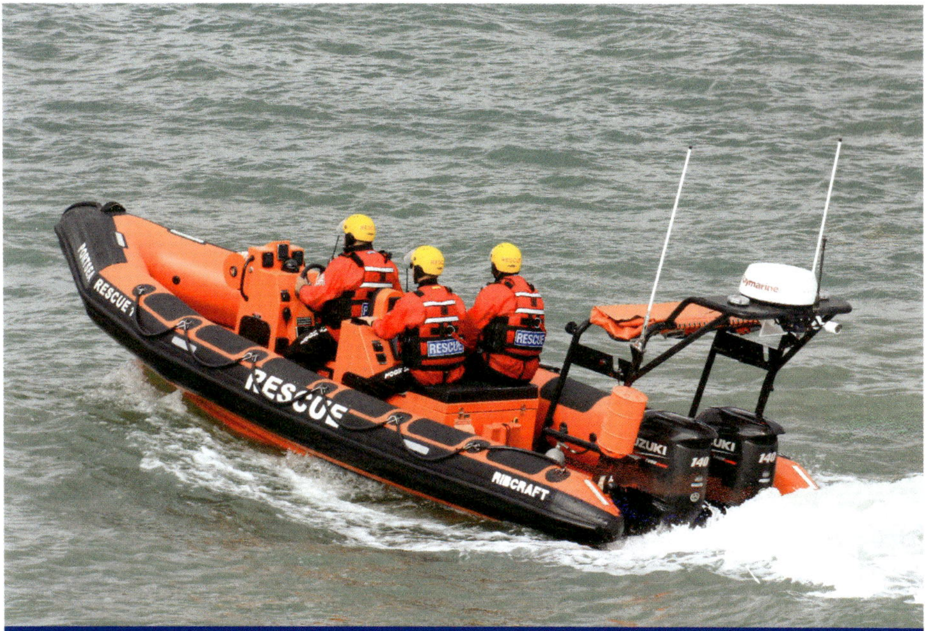

The 6.8m Ribcraft rigid inflatable Portsea Rescue 1 was funded with government support. (Andrew Cooke)

Independent lifeboats of Britain

GOSPORT
Hampshire

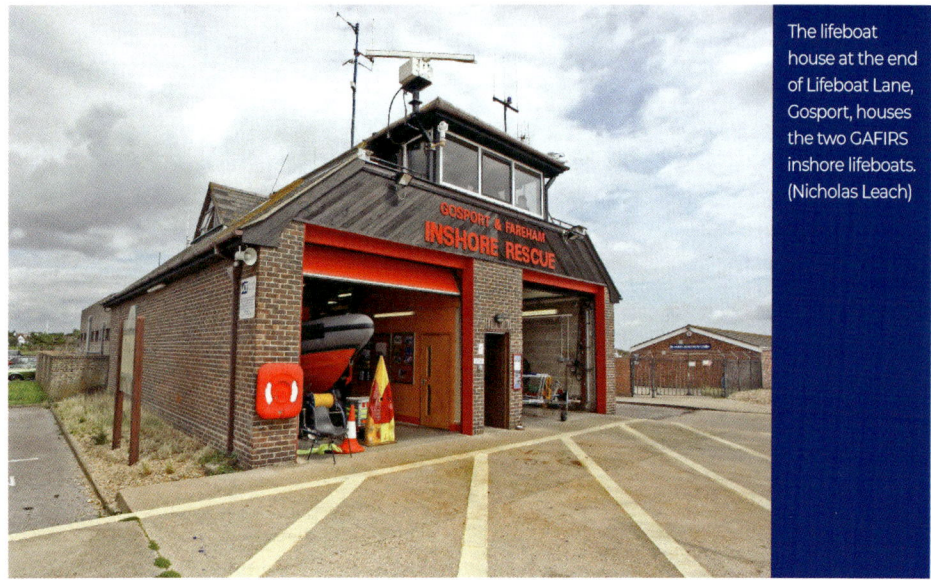

The lifeboat house at the end of Lifeboat Lane, Gosport, houses the two GAFIRS inshore lifeboats. (Nicholas Leach)

LOCATION Hampshire
ORGANISATION Gosport and Fareham Inshore Rescue Service (GAFIRS)
ESTABLISHED 1969
HISTORY In 1969 the inaugural meeting of the Gosport and Fareham Inshore Rescue Service (GAFIRS) agreed to set up an Independent Lifeboat Service to cover the Solent between Hill Head and the Forts, including Portsmouth Harbour. A local school teacher had witnessed a drowning in 1967 and worked to set up a service to help sailors. On average GAFIRS responds to about 100 emergency calls a year. The station is located to the south-west of Gosport, at the end of Lifeboat Lane. In 1970 Gosport Council agreed to the use of an old deckchair store as the GAFIRS HQ and the Royal Life Saving Society (Wessex Branch) part funded the purchase of a second-hand wooden rigid inflatable from Atlantic College, in Wales.
PREVIOUS ASSETS
1973 GAFIRS purchased two new rescue boats from Avon Ltd, a 5.4m and a 4m Searider, each powered by 30hp outboard motors.
1979 A new 6m Avon rigid inflatable, powered by twin 80hp engines, was acquired along with a new trailer, and an extension was built to the deckchair store.
1986 After raising £70,000 a new Lifeboat Station building was constructed, and was officially opened by Admiral of the Fleet, Sir John Fieldhouse; this has housed the operational lifeboats ever since, and is the operation's headquarters.
1993 A new 8.5m Avon Searider rigid inflatable, named David Brading, was acquired; powered by a 330hp Iveco turbo diesel engine, driving a Castoldi waterjet, it had a speed of 37 knots and served the station until September 2015.
2012 A new lifeboat was formally dedicated on 21 April at the lifeboat station. Named Jim and Mollie Newton in memory of a Shropshire couple whose legacy financed its purchase, the Halmatic Pacific 30 rigid inflatable was powered by twin 330hp Iveco 8061 six-cylinder inboard diesel engines, driving Castoldi 238

Independent lifeboats of Britain

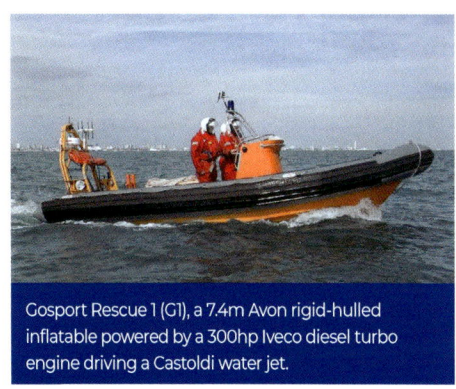

Gosport Rescue 1 (G1), a 7.4m Avon rigid-hulled inflatable powered by a 300hp Iveco diesel turbo engine driving a Castoldi water jet.

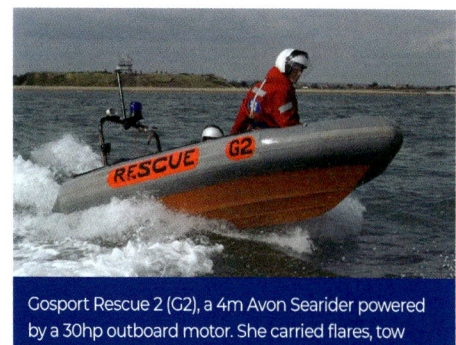

Gosport Rescue 2 (G2), a 4m Avon Searider powered by a 30hp outboard motor. She carried flares, tow lines, two VHF radios and first aid equipment.

waterjets, giving a speed of 45 knots. The electronic fit out included Raymarine HD radar and W90 chart plotter a sonar interface, VHF DF equipment and two Icom VHF radios.
2019 The 2nd ILB, Ian Fuller, was moved to a new location at Gosport Marina and operates from a Versadock berth. Premier Marinas provided the berth free of charge.
CURRENT ASSETS 9m Delta rigid inflatable Joan Dora Fuller, on station 2016, launched by Valtra tractor and carriage; 4.8m Ribcraft Professional Ian Fuller, on station 2016, launched by Versadock at Gosport Marina.

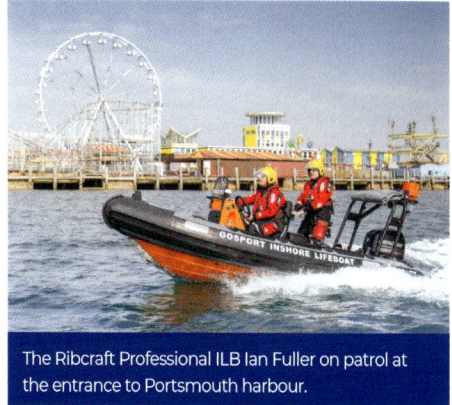

The Ribcraft Professional ILB Ian Fuller on patrol at the entrance to Portsmouth harbour.

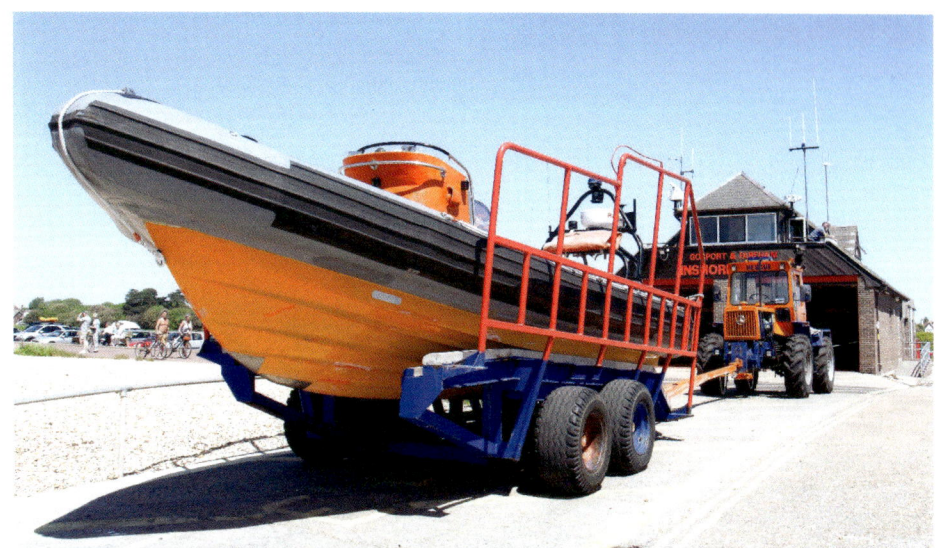

The 8.5m Avon Searider David Brading on her launch trailer outside the boathouse, May 2012. (Nicholas Leach)

Independent lifeboats of Britain

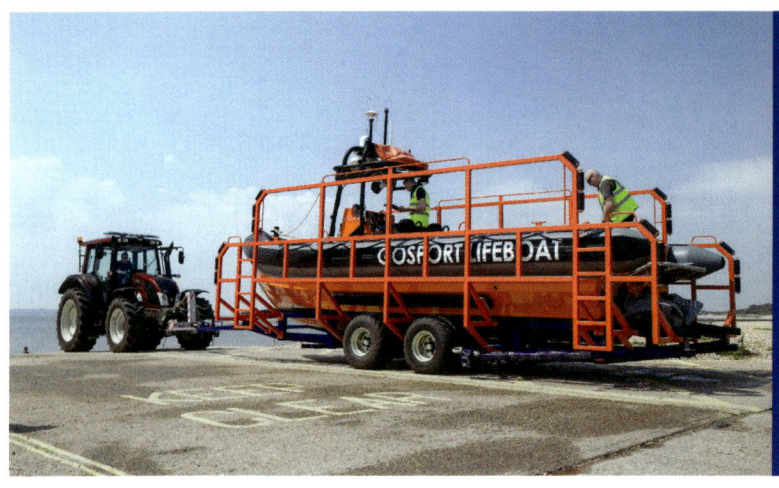

The 9m Delta rigid inflatable Joan Dora Fuller being launched (left and below). She is powered by two Yanmar 8LV 4.42-litre turbo diesel V8 engines, producing 320hp each, giving a top speed of approximately 43 knots.

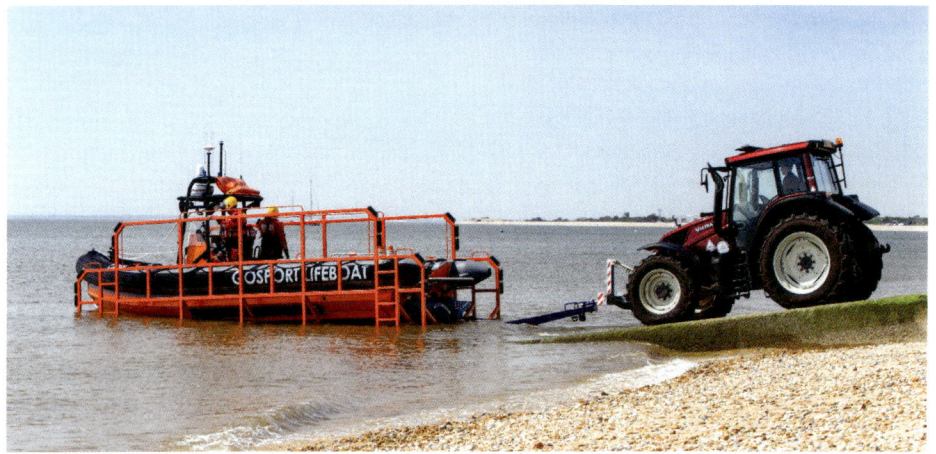

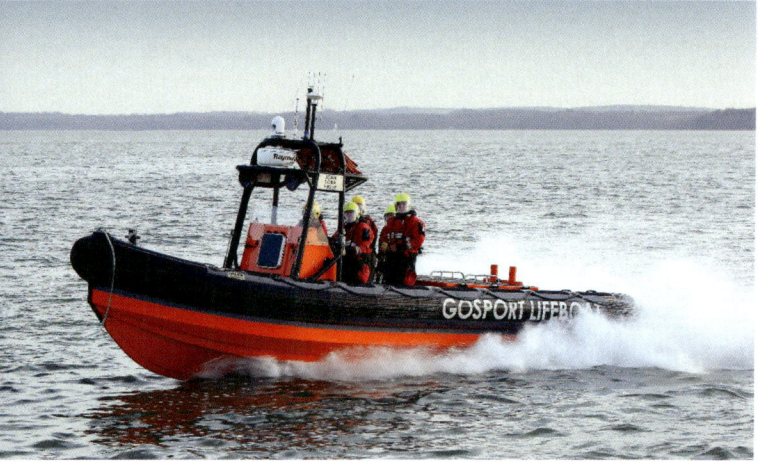

9m Delta rigid inflatable Joan Dora Fuller heading back to station following the annual get-together of Solent-based SAR assets in January 2020. (Nicholas Leach)

Independent lifeboats of Britain

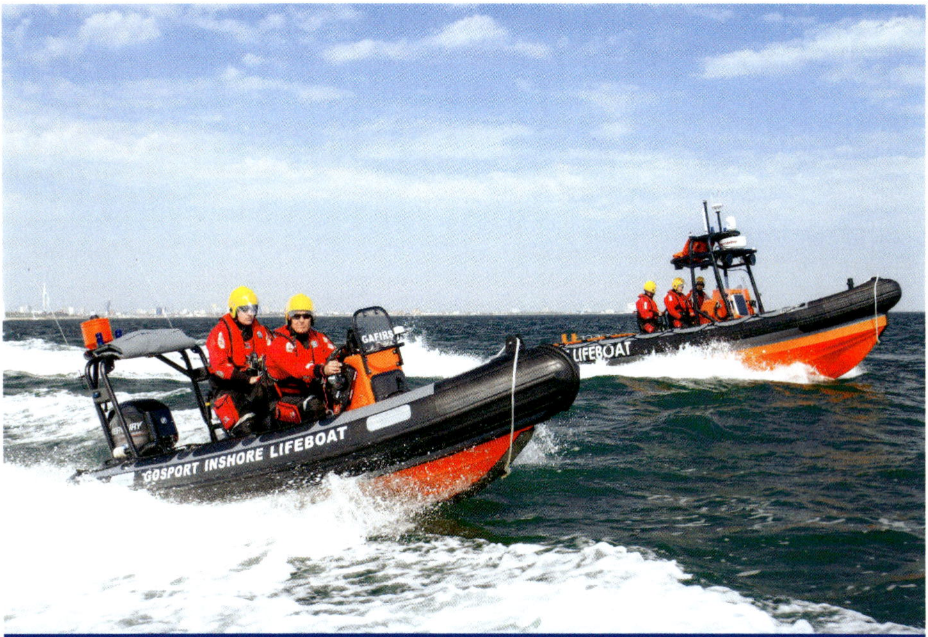

GAFIRS on patrol: 9m Delta rigid inflatable Joan Dora Fuller with the 4.8m Ribcraft Professional Ian Fuller.

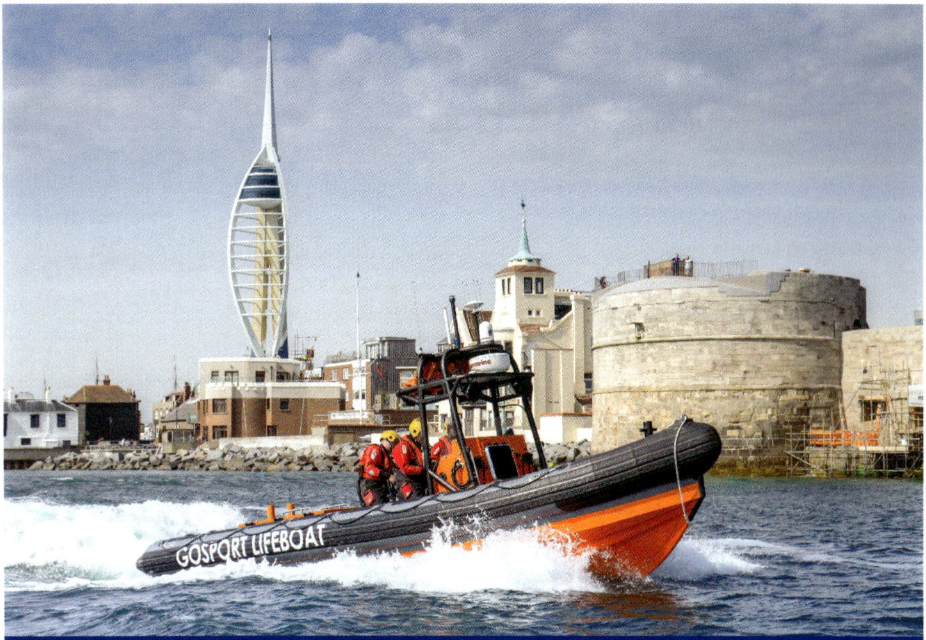

9m Delta rigid inflatable Joan Dora Fuller at the entrance to Portsmouth harbour, with Spinnaker Tower and the port's naval fortifications forming the backdrop.

Independent lifeboats of Britain

HAMBLE
Hampshire

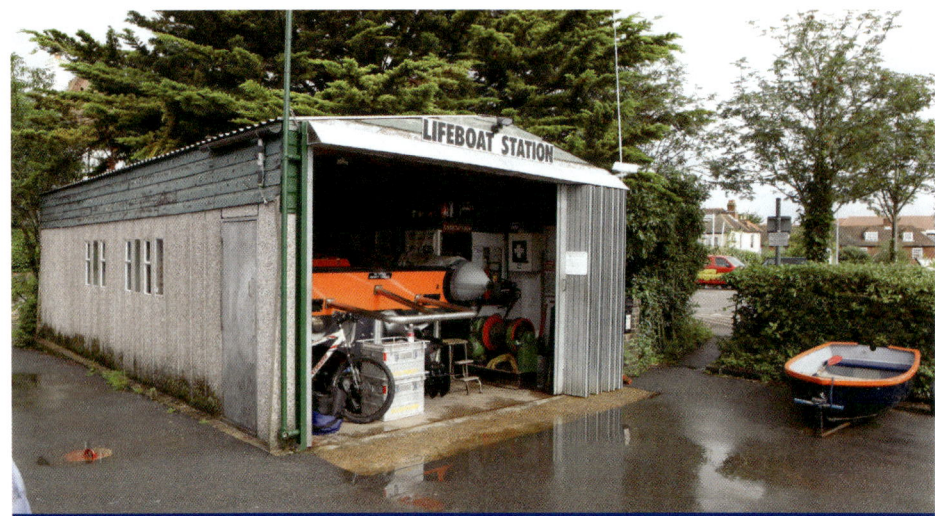

The boathouse on Hamble Foreshore, which housed the lifeboat from 1974. A new station building was erected on this site in 2017. (Nicholas Leach)

LOCATION Hampshire
ORGANISATION Hamble Lifeboat
ESTABLISHED 1968
HISTORY Hamble Lifeboat was formed in 1968 as the Southampton Water Inshore Rescue Service (Hamble Rescue) by local residents in response to the increasing number of casualties occurring in Southampton Water and the rivers Hamble, Itchen and Test, after there had been 19 deaths in one year. The RNLI, which at the time had lifeboats at Yarmouth and Bembridge, was approached but had no boat suitable for the area. A fast powerful boat, capable of operating in shallow water, was needed. Hamble lifeboat covers an area bounded by Lee-on-the-Solent, Cowes and the mouth of the Beaulieu River. It includes the central Solent, Southampton Water and the rivers Itchen, Hamble and Test.

PREVIOUS ASSETS
1968 The first rescue boat, St Andrew, was a small 17ft Dory with twin Mercury outboards, which went into service in 1969 and attended over 100 incidents in her first year.

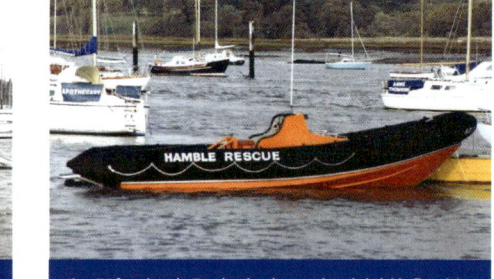

The 21ft Boston Whaler Outrage St Andrew II was the second lifeboat operated by Hamble Lifeboat.

The 30ft Atlantis Eagle single-engined rigid inflatable St Andrew III served from 1981 to 1988.

Independent lifeboats of Britain

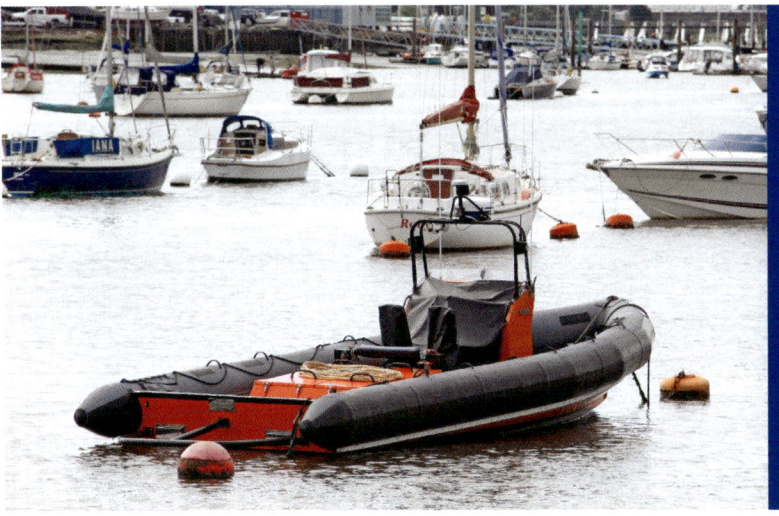

John and Violet Hurrell at moorings in the River Hamble, pictured in 2012. The service operates two lifeboats, usually in six month shifts, with one afloat in service and the other kept in the station for refit. (Nicholas Leach)

1972 The service moved from Petter's Slipway to its current base on Hamble foreshore.
1974 The first St Andrew was replaced by a 21ft Boston Whaler Outrage, named St Andrew II, powered by twin 50hp outboards.
1981 A 30ft Atlantis Eagle rigid inflatable, powered by a single 212hp diesel engine and Castoldi 06 waterjet, was acquired. Named St Andrew III, she had a top speed of 35 knots and could operate in very shallow waters.
1988 St Andrew III needed a major refit and so came out of service, leaving Hamble Rescue without a boat for nearly six months, so it was decided to purchase a reserve boat.

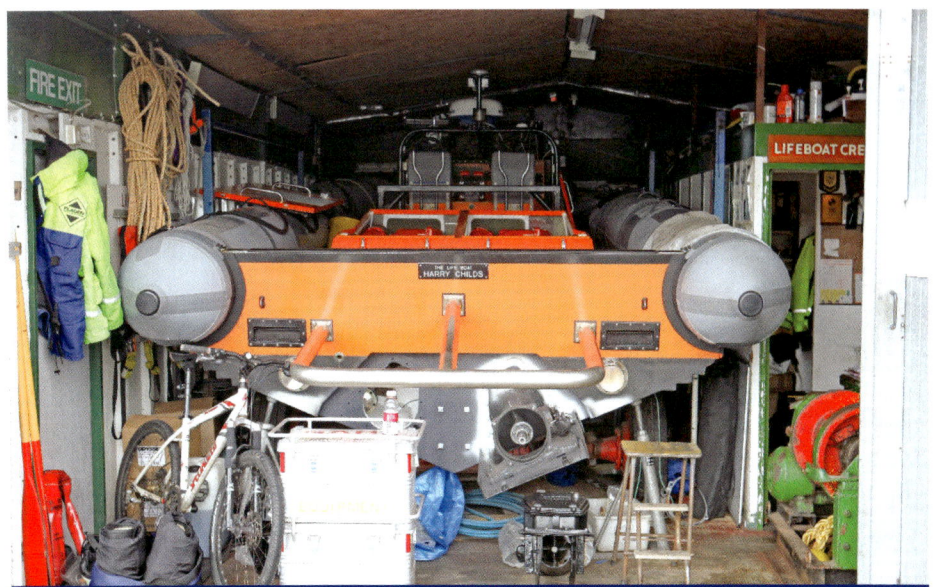

The lifeboat Harry Childs inside the boathouse; she is one of two Halmatic Pacific 32 rigid inflatables. The annual cost of running the two boats is in excess of £25,000 a year, which includes fuel and maintenance. (Nicholas Leach)

Independent lifeboats of Britain

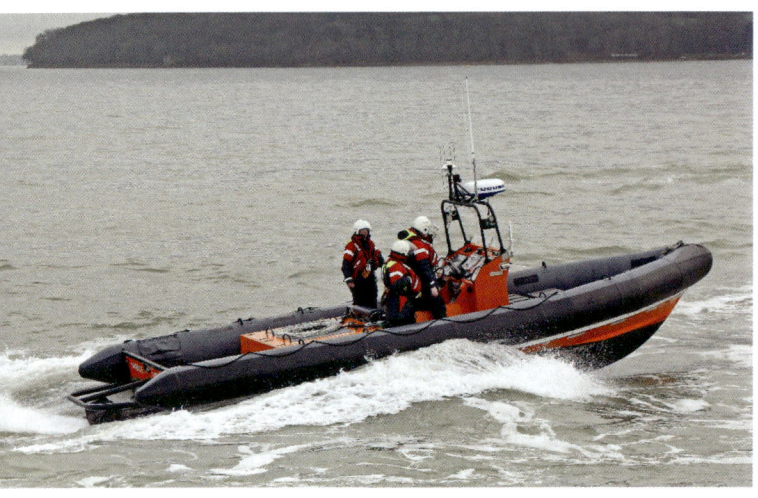

John and Violet Hurrell on exercise in the Solent in January 2018. (Nicholas Leach)

1989 After a year being fitted out by Chief Coxswain Colin Olden, the reserve boat St Mary went into service. A 7.4m Humber rigid inflatable powered by a single 250hp Iveco engine and Castoldi TD238 waterjet, she provided back up, but as she did not have the capabilities of the larger boat it was decided that two boats of equal size and capability were required.
1992 St Andrew IV, first of the current series of boats, went into service. A Pacific 30 rigid inflatable fitted with twin 250hp Iveco engines and twin TD238 waterjets, she was purchased as a bare hull and fitted out as funds permitted by the volunteer crew, with radar and GPS navigation systems.
1996 To work with St Andrew IV and after the sale of St Andrew III, a new boat, Harry Childs, was purchased. She was a Halmatic Pacific 32 with twin 330hp Iveco 8061 SRM 33 diesel engines and twin Castoldi TD238 water jets. She was purchased as a bare hull and fitted out on station, going into service in 1997.
2006 St Andrew IV was sold to become a Coast Guard boat in New Zealand and was

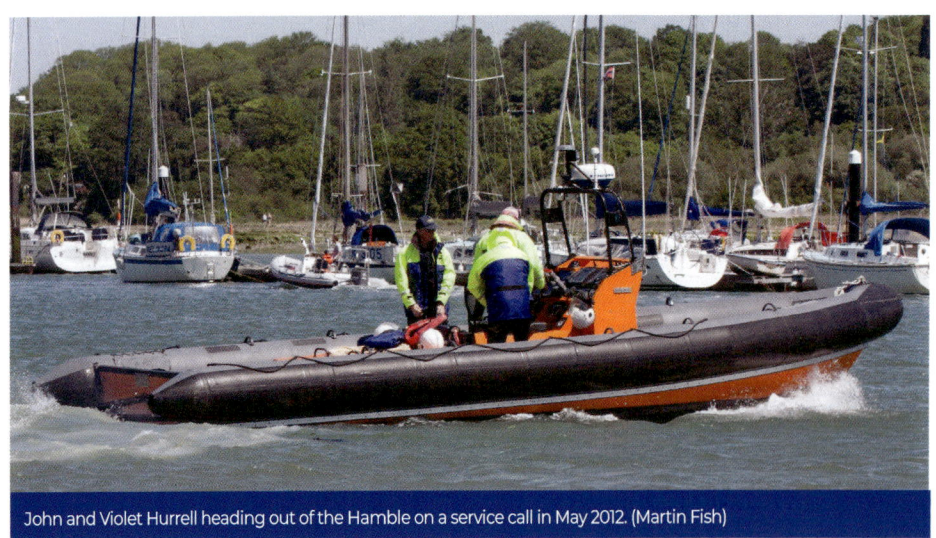

John and Violet Hurrell heading out of the Hamble on a service call in May 2012. (Martin Fish)

Independent lifeboats of Britain

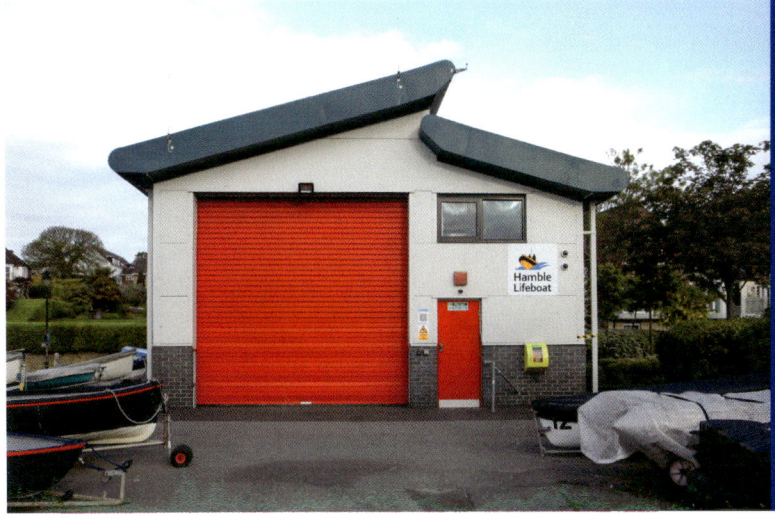

The shore building completed in 2017 provided much enhanced crew and storage facilities, and was built on the site of the previous building. (Martin Fish)

replaced by John and Violet Hurrell, another Halmatic Pacific 32 with twin 350hp Iveco diesel engines and Castoldi TD238 waterjets.
2015 John and Violet Hurrell was refitted with 400hp Iveco N60 M40 engines and Furuno NEXT integrated radar and navigation system.
2017 The small boathouse was replaced by a new building with enhanced facilities for crew training and space for maintaining the boats.
2019 An AirBerth boat lift was introduced to reduce maintenance downtime on the boats.

2021 The refit of Harry Childs was completed with new Castoldi TD238 jet drives, rebuilt Iveco 8061 SRM 33 engines, a new inflatable collar, and an updated Furuno radar and navigation system.

CURRENT ASSETS The service operates two lifeboats, with one afloat in service and the other kept in the station for refit. The current craft are both Halmatic Pacific 32 rigid inflatables: Harry Childs, on station 1997, and John and Violet Hurrell, on station 2006.

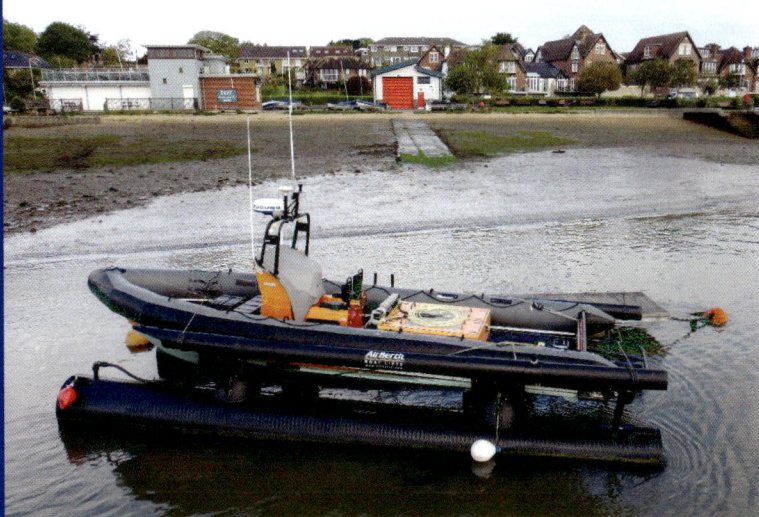

One of the Pacific rigid-inflatable lifeboats used by Hamble lifeboat in the AirBerth boat lift and pontoon used to lift the lifeboats out of the water; the boat lifts make undertaking maintenance and cleaning easier. (Martin Fish)

Independent lifeboats of Britain

SOLENT
Hampshire

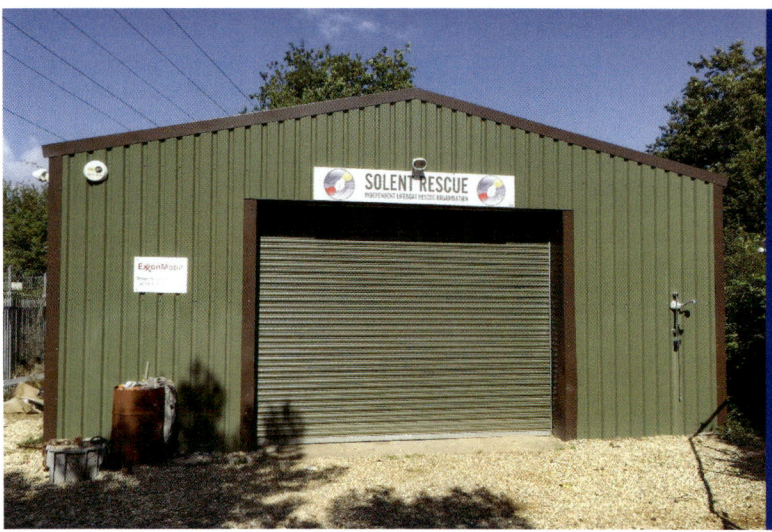

The shore facility used by Solent Rescue, located within Lepe Country Park, provides a base for the service's weekend patrols. (Nicholas Leach)

LOCATION Lepe Country Park
ORGANISATION Solent Rescue
ESTABLISHED 1971
HISTORY Solent Rescue was formed in 1971 by auxiliary coastguards as a beach rescue unit in response to a rising level of incidents in and around Lepe Country Park following increasing numbers of visitors. Gradually the unit transformed into an additional rescue asset for the Maritime and Coastguard Agency, providing an SAR service covering the Western Solent in the summer. The unit does not respond to pagers like the RNLI and independent lifeboats in the Solent, but instead is operational during busy times, operating at weekends and bank holidays from Easter to September, and for major events, as well as providing medical and safety cover for the country park.

One of the first lifeboats operated was a basic rigid-hulled inflatable with a tiller-controlled Mercury outboard engine. A Land Rover was used to launch the boat from a boat shed built at Lepe Country Park. The Service upgraded to a larger and more capable Avon Searider rigid inflatable, powered by twin Yamaha outboard engines, with a seated helm position. The next main lifeboat to come into service was a Delta

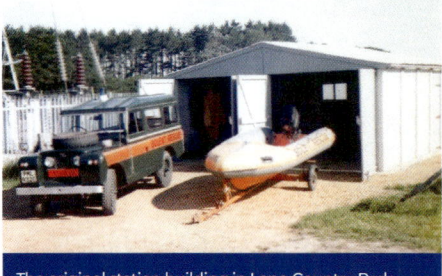

The original station building in Lepe Country Park with the Land Rover and one of the first rescue boats.

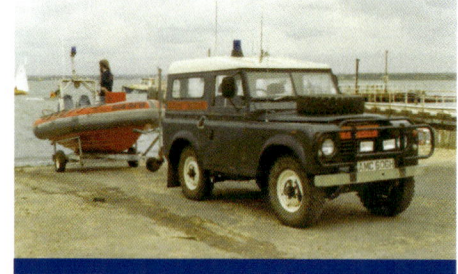

The twin-engined Avon Searider lifeboat being launched by the Land Rover at Calshot.

Independent lifeboats of Britain

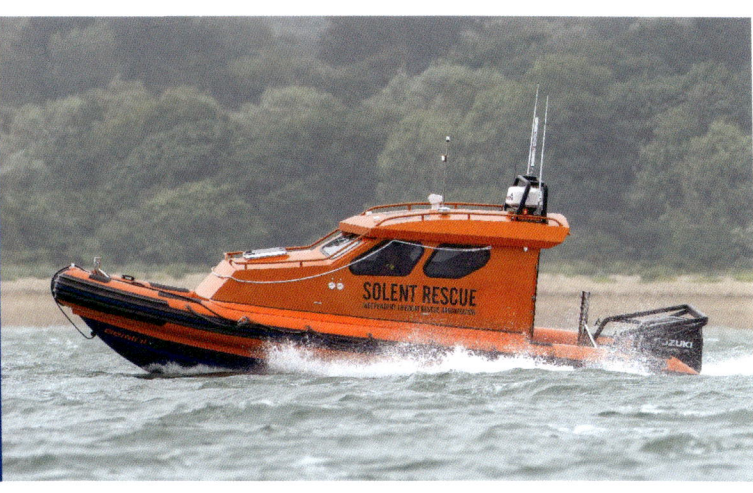

The 9m Gemini 880WA Rescue RIB, powered by Suzuki DF250 outboard engines, on exercise in June 2018. It was capable of speeds in excess of 45 knots. (Maritime Photographic)

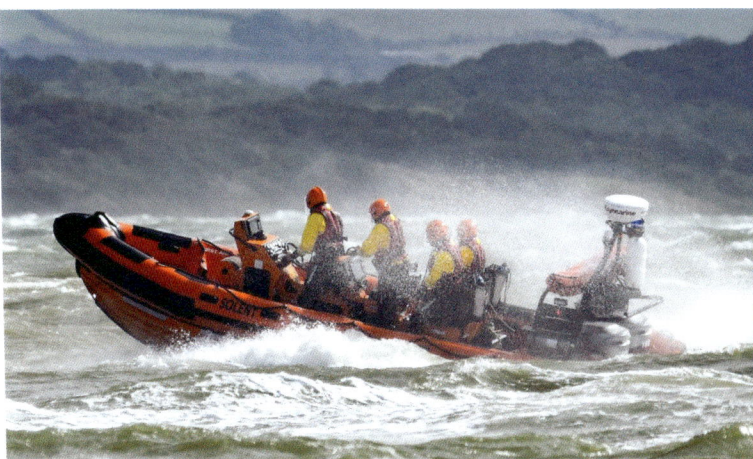

The Arctic 24 rigid inflatable Solent Rescue 1 on exercise off Lepe, from where she patrols the Western Solent. The boat has seating for four crew, is powered by twin Mariner 150hp outboards and has a top speed of 45 knots. (By courtesy of Solent Rescue)

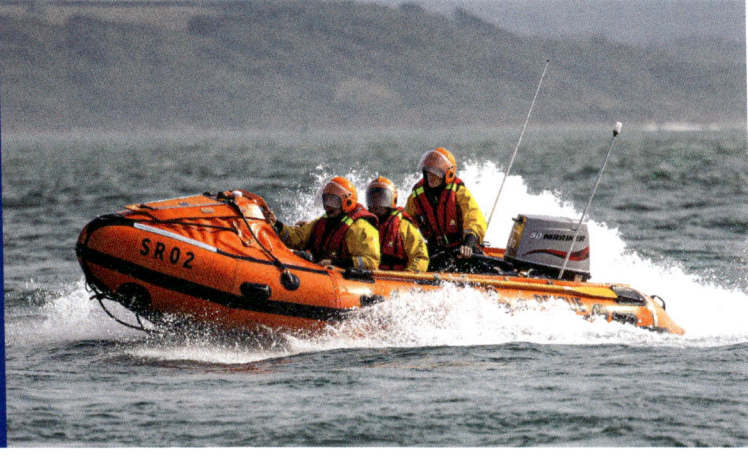

The D class inflatable Solent Rescue 2, formerly RNLI D class inflatable D-532, on exercise off Lepe. The service has operated a series of smaller ILBs, including single-engined Avon Seariders, launched from the beach by trailer at Lepe. (By courtesy of Solent Rescue)

rigid inflatable, which had twin Suzuki 55hp outboards, a seating console for the helm and two crew, and a simple roll bar.

Replacing the Delta RIB, was a Halmatic Pacific 22 rigid inflatable powered by an inboard diesel engine driving a single Castoldi waterjet. The Pacific was upgraded during its service life with a revised layout and new central console. A County tractor was used to launch it, stern first, from the beach at Lepe.

PREVIOUS ASSETS
2012 The main lifeboat was replaced with a 7.9m Delta 800SX Fire rigid inflatable, powered by twin Suzuki DF90 outboards giving a top speed of thirty-five knots. The Delta had been used as a fire boat by Kent Fire & Rescue Service, being commissioned in 1998. Before going into service with Solent Rescue, it underwent a refit and commissioning at Hythe Marina.
2013 The wooden boathouse at Lepe had been subject to break-ins and vandalism, so it was replaced by a new steel-frame building to house the lifeboats and launch vehicle.
2017 A 9m Gemini 880WA Rescue RIB, powered by Suzuki DF250 outboard engines, was obtained. The crew raised more than £100,000 in seven months to buy the new lifeboat, which was built to a unique design. The cabin had a watertight door, four Shoxs single jockey seats for the crew and bench seating forward. The new boat arrived from South Africa in May and was fitted out by Gemini UK in Lymington. As the Gemini boat was too large to be launched from Lepe beach, it was kept afloat in Hythe Marina, being moored off Lepe when on patrol at weekends. A smaller Gemini inflatable rescue boat with a Yamaha 25hp outboard was kept in the boathouse at Lepe, being launched and recovered by a Toyota Hilux 4x4 vehicle.
2019 The Gemini 880WA lifeboat was found to be unsuitable, so was sold and the lifeboats were based solely at Lepe. The former RNLI D class ILB D-532 (ex-Kingsand) was purchased, refitted and upgraded. In addition, as Sidmouth Lifeboat had acquired a new lifeboat, they donated their recently replaced Arctic 24 Pride of Sidmouth, which had been in use since 2004, to Solent Rescue in June.
2020 The timber-built lookout post was replaced with a larger timber-clad containerised building to provide a better crew area and improved views, with wraparound windows at the front.
2022 A new launching carriage for the Arctic 24 lifeboat was built to improve launch procedures. The Service purchased another former RNLI inflatable, ex-D-728, which was refitted before coming into service at Lepe.
CURRENT ASSETS Solent Rescue 1 (SR1), Arctic 24 named Pride of Sidmouth, previously with Sidmouth Lifeboat, built by VT Halmatic Ltd, launched by Massey Ferguson 8240 tractor and carriage, funded partially by a Morrisons Foundation Grant, on station 2019; Solent Rescue 2 (SR2), IB1 inflatable, formerly RNLI D class inshore lifeboat Braund (D-728), launched by tractor and trailer, on station 2022.

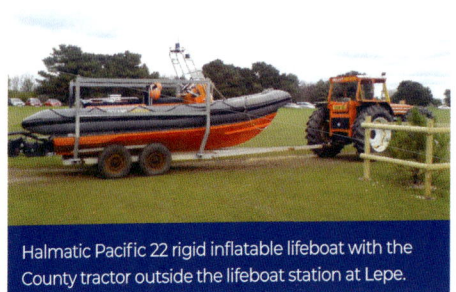

Halmatic Pacific 22 rigid inflatable lifeboat with the County tractor outside the lifeboat station at Lepe.

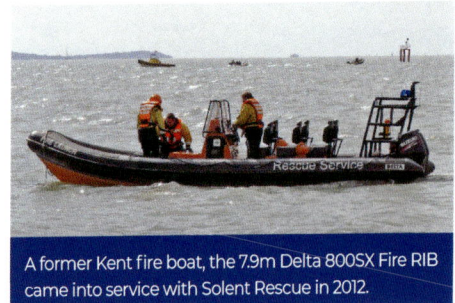

A former Kent fire boat, the 7.9m Delta 800SX Fire RIB came into service with Solent Rescue in 2012.

Independent lifeboats of Britain

SIDMOUTH
South Devon

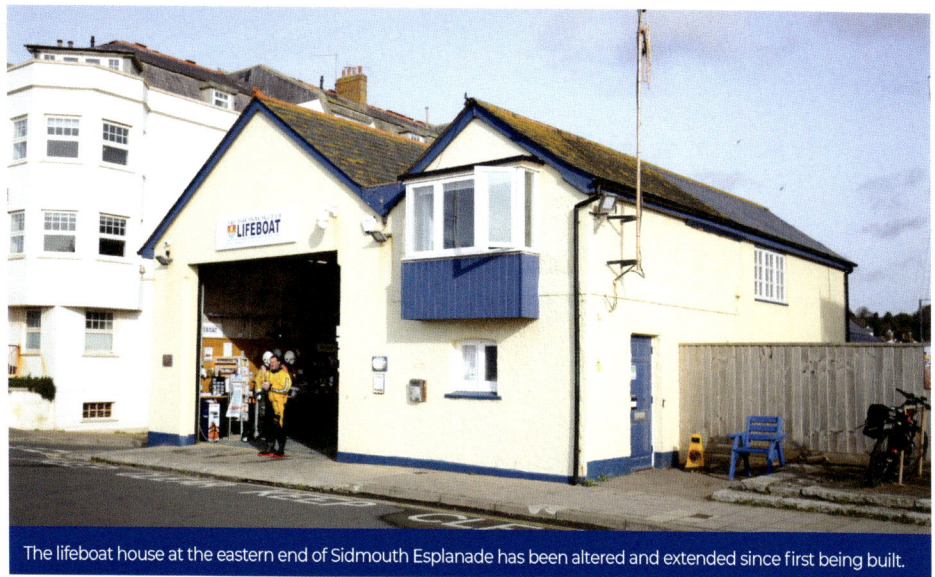

The lifeboat house at the eastern end of Sidmouth Esplanade has been altered and extended since first being built.

ORGANISATION Sidmouth Lifeboat
ESTABLISHED 1968
HISTORY Following the departure of the RNLI lifeboat from Sidmouth in 1912, lifeboat cover was provided by RNLI lifeboats at Exmouth and Lyme Regis, nine and twelve miles away respectively, with a motor lifeboat being placed at Exmouth in 1933, by which time Lyme Regis had also been closed.

However, in the mid-1960s leisure activities were increasing in Sidmouth, resulting in more people using the local beaches. In 1968 students from the local secondary school formed a surf life-saving organisation, forerunner of the Sidmouth Lifeboat organisation. Founder members included Keith Roberts and Alan Phillips, the latter going on to be involved for almost half a century.

Initially beach patrols were organised, covering Jacob's Ladder Beach during weekends in the summer. The first HQ was located at the Clock Tower above Jacob's Ladder Beach. In 1972 the level of cover was greatly improved following the purchase of a larger 16ft rigid inflatable with a 40hp outboard, which was used for daytime patrols and surf rescue, being able to cover Sidmouth and Jacob's Ladder Beaches.

In the late 1970s the level of cover was further improved to include evenings and eventually extended to 24-hour coverage. In 1982 Sidmouth Inshore Rescue Service became a declared rescue facility with the Coastguard.

PREVIOUS ASSETS
1985 The lifeboat Storm was purchased and dedicated at a ceremony presided over by the Rev Richard Sigrist. The lifeboat was named by crew member Robin Coop after his eleven-year-old daughter.
1991 A 5m Humber rigid inflatable was acquired, named Spirit of Sidmouth, powered by twin 40hp Mariner engines and equipped with GPS navigation, fixed-base radio and first aid.
1999 The Atlantic 21 Sidmouth Herald came on station, having been purchased from the RNLI (ex-B-577 Graham Hillier and Tony

Independent lifeboats of Britain

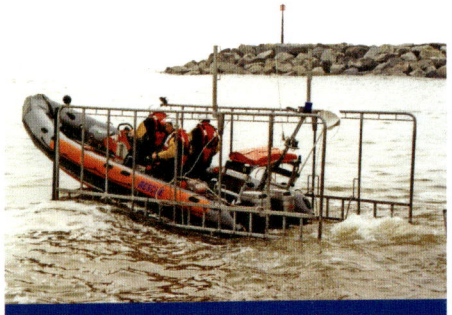

Atlantic 21 Sidmouth Herald (formerly the RNLI lifeboat B-577) being launched on exercise in 2001.

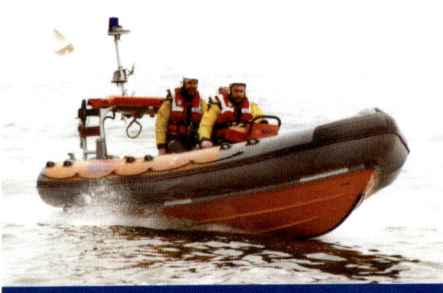

Atlantic 21 Sidmouth Herald on exercise. She served at Sidmouth from 1999 to 2004.

Cater). The lifeboat, which was stationed at Brighton from 1989 to 1997, was too large for the existing station and so a new building had to be built. A new drive-on drive-off launching system was also developed using a ballasted and marinised Renault tractor, complete with launching trailer, designed and constructed by crew member Barrie Whittock.

2004 The Arctic 24 rigid inflatable Pride of Sidmouth, built by VT Halmatic Ltd, was acquired in October, having been funded by donations from the local community and visitors. Powered by twin 115hp Mariner outboards, she had a range of ninety nautical miles and an endurance of two and a half hours at a top speed of forty-five knots. She was crewed by four, had a righting capability and carried a GPS chartplotter and night vision equipment. She was later upgraded with twin 135hp and then twin 150hp Mariner Optimax two-stroke outboards, all fitted with a PIRS (post immersion restart system).

2006 On 21 March Sidmouth Lifeboat took delivery of a new drive-on drive-off (do-do) launching and recovery system. The system comprises two units: a marinised tractor and a semi-submersible trailer unit. The tractor was a specially modified Renault agricultural

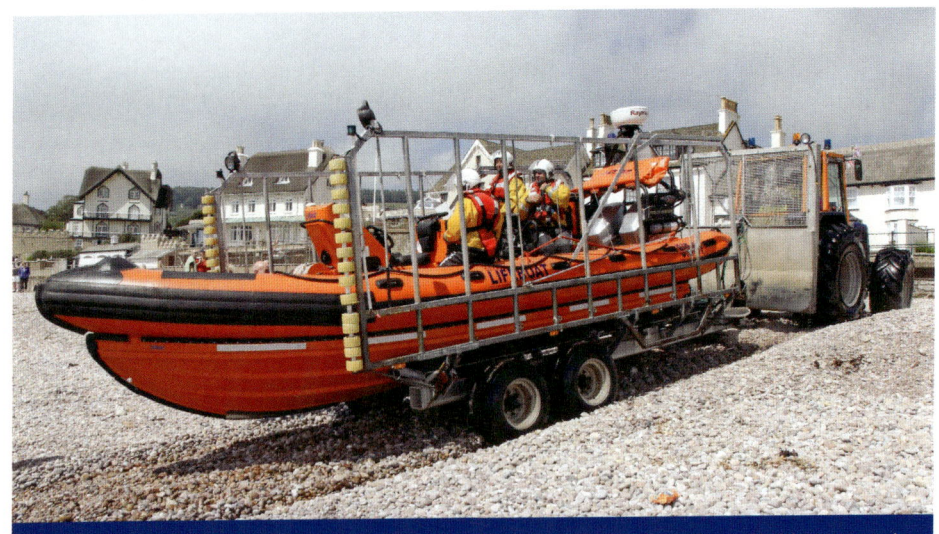

Pride of Sidmouth (on station 2004-19) being recovered on the shingle beach at the western end of the Promenade.

Independent lifeboats of Britain

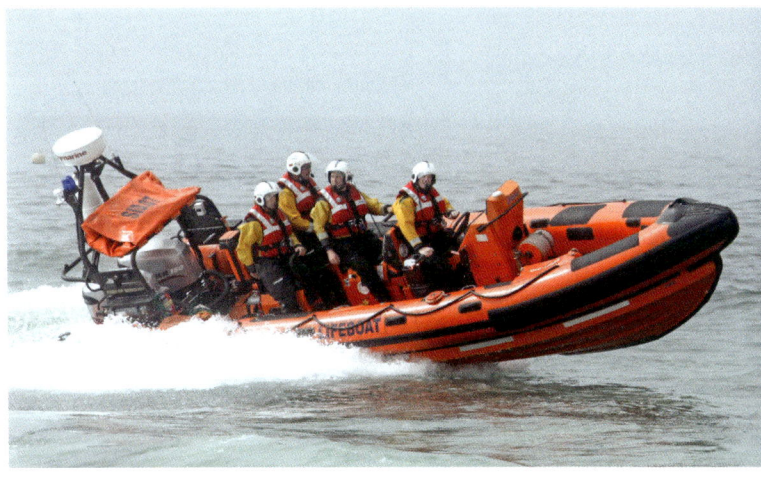

Pride of Sidmouth off the beach at Sidmouth during a routine Sunday patrol in July 2012. The station's area of coverage extends from Beer Head, east of Sidmouth, to Otterton Ledge in the west. (Nicholas Leach)

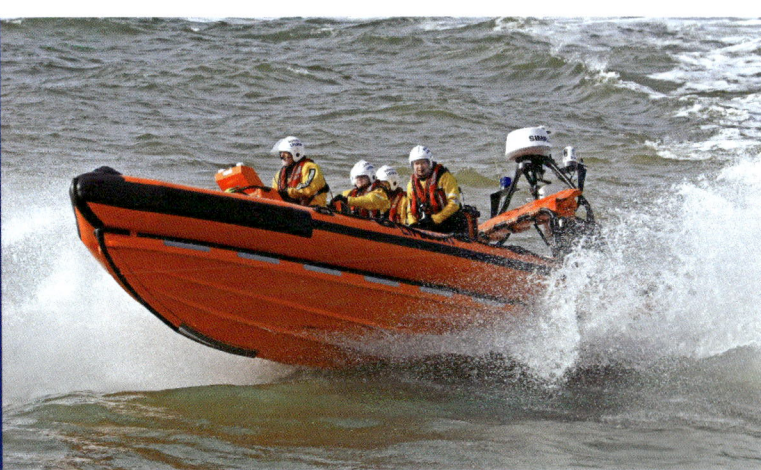

The Arctic 24 rigid inflatable Peter and Barbara Truesdale on exercise off Sidmouth, April 2022. (Nicholas Leach)

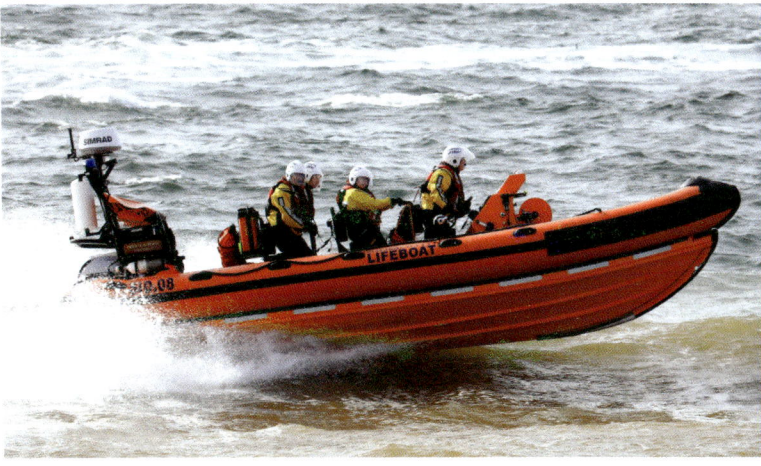

The Arctic 24 rigid inflatable Peter and Barbara Truesdale is an updated version of the previous boat Pride of Sidmouth, but is of a similar design and was built by BAE Systems at Portsmouth. (Nicholas Leach)

Independent lifeboats of Britain

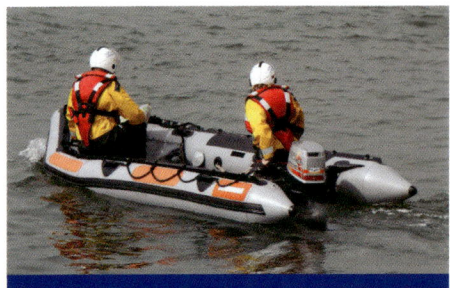
The single-engined Zodiac inflatable was used for crew training and inshore rescues until 2014.

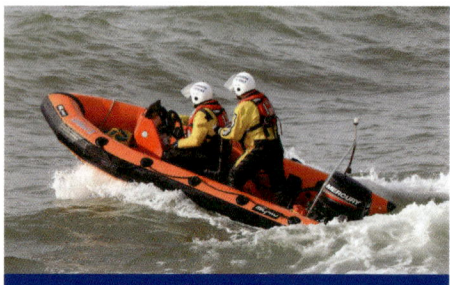
The Zodiac Milpro Searider Sidmouth 2 "Speedy Sid" on exercise off Sidmouth beach. (Nicholas Leach)

tractor that has been waterproofed and fitted with a fresh water washing facility. This modification was carried out by P. Bowler & Son. The trailer was built by Admiral trailers and features hydraulic lift capabilities, LED running lights and floodlights for night time operation.

2014 The second inshore lifeboat was replaced by a Zodiac Milpro Searider inflatable. Powered by a Mercury outboard, the ILB is light enough to be launched without the need for a tractor, and provides cover for the main lifeboat. The Zodiac replaced a previous Gemini RIB, which fulfilled a similar role.

2018 In May a Yamaha WaveRunner VX series personal watercraft was acquired. It could be launched and operated by just two crew. However, it was found that the craft did not meet Sidmouth's needs and it was sold to another rescue organisation.

CURRENT ASSETS Arctic 24 built by BAE Systems, named Peter and Barbara Truesdale, on station 2019; Valtra T140 launch tractor, named Mary Taylor, on station 2015; Zodiac Milpro Searider, named Sidmouth 2 "Speedy Sid", launched by trailer, on station 2014.

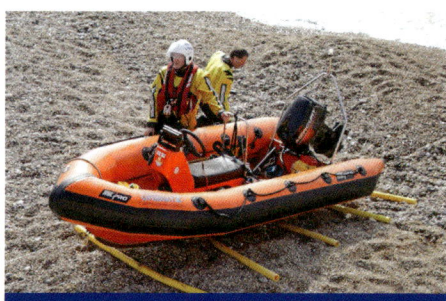
The small Zodiac Sidmouth 2 "Speedy Sid" being recovered on the beach using skids. (Nicholas Leach)

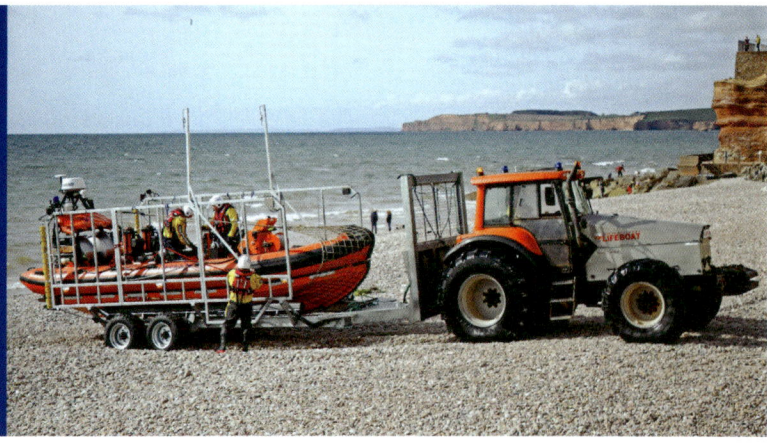
The Arctic 24 rigid inflatable Peter and Barbara Truesdale being recovered on the beach at the western end of Sidmouth sea front. (Nicholas Leach)

HOPE COVE
Devon

LOCATION South Devon
ORGANISATION Hope Cove Lifeboat
ESTABLISHED 2010
HISTORY The RNLI operated pulling and sailing lifeboats from Hope Cove from 1878 to 1930. From 1960 a rescue boat managed by the Maritime and Coastguard Agency (MCA), and operated by volunteers, was used to deal with the significant increase in the number of recreational craft in Bigbury Bay including yachts, dinghies, power boats, kayaks, windsurf and paddle boards. But in 2008 the boat was removed by the MCA following funding cutbacks which meant funding for the boat was no longer available.

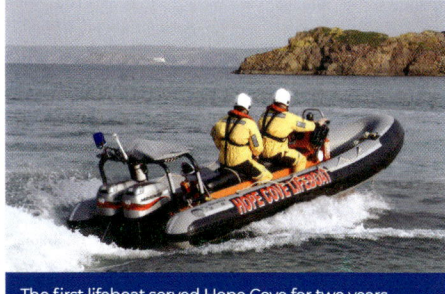

The first lifeboat served Hope Cove for two years.

Local concerns about the lack of a rescue boat came to a head in late summer and early autumn 2010, when negotiations took place between local people, MPs, representatives of the MCA and government ministers. It was agreed that there was a definite need for a rescue service based at Hope Cove and that a new boat was needed to cover the area.

A public meeting in October 2010 resulted in unanimous support for the formation of an independently-operated lifeboat service in Hope Cove. Following this meeting, directors and officers of the new company were elected. A proposal of how it would operate was sent to the MCA. On 1 December 2010 Hope Cove Lifeboat was registered as a limited company, and in January 2011 it was granted registered charity status.

Five launching authorities were appointed who, together with the senior coxswains, decide when the lifeboat is required. The boat's area of operation is from Soar Mill Cove

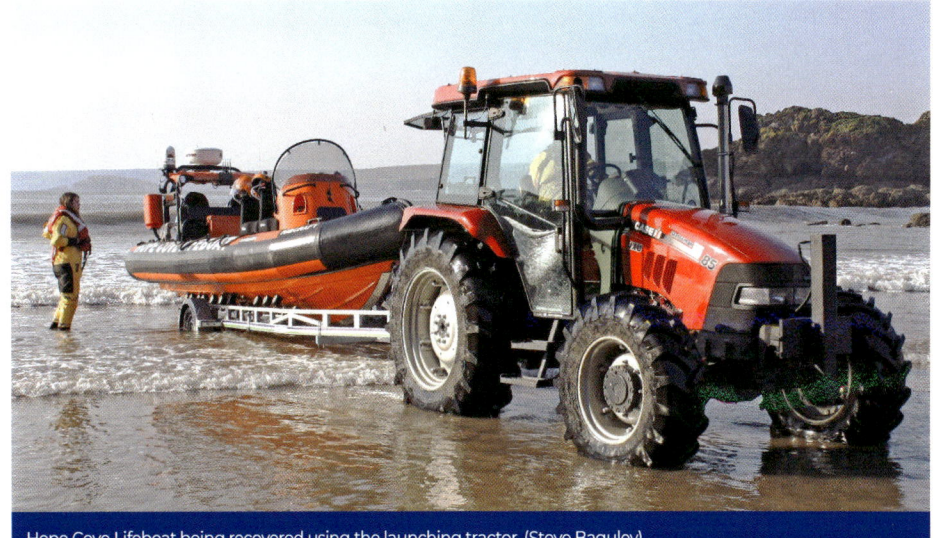

Hope Cove Lifeboat being recovered using the launching tractor. (Steve Baguley)

Independent lifeboats of Britain

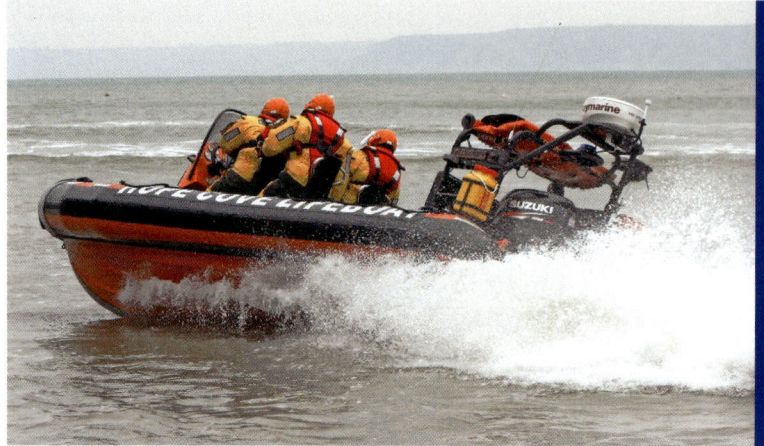

Hope Cove Lifeboat being put through her paces after being formally dedicated, March 2013. The boat was delivered to Hope Cove on 29 March 2013 and became operational after trials and crew training had been completed in May 2013. (Steve Baguley)

in the east to the River Erme in the west, extending two nautical miles offshore, with upper limits of wind speed. The lifeboat will also assist the Salcombe and Plymouth RNLI lifeboats as required beyond this area.

Following the creation of the Hope Cove Lifeboat charity, two years of fundraising resulted in sufficient finance to pay for a new lifeboat. This boat, a rigid inflatable built by Ribcraft of Yeovil, replaced an older boat which had been used by the service since May 2011. The new fully-equipped boat, specially designed for Hope Cove, is operated by four crew and able to carry up to eight casualties.

The new boat was dedicated and formally launched at a ceremony on Easter Sunday, 31 March 2013. The boat was blessed by the Bishop of Plymouth, the Right Rev John Ford, with the ceremony taking place outside the Hope and Anchor public house in Hope Cove.

CURRENT ASSETS 6.4m Ribcraft RIB, twin Suzuki DF90 four-stroke outboard engines, named Alexandra, on station 2013; Terex TA5 launching vehicle and carriage.

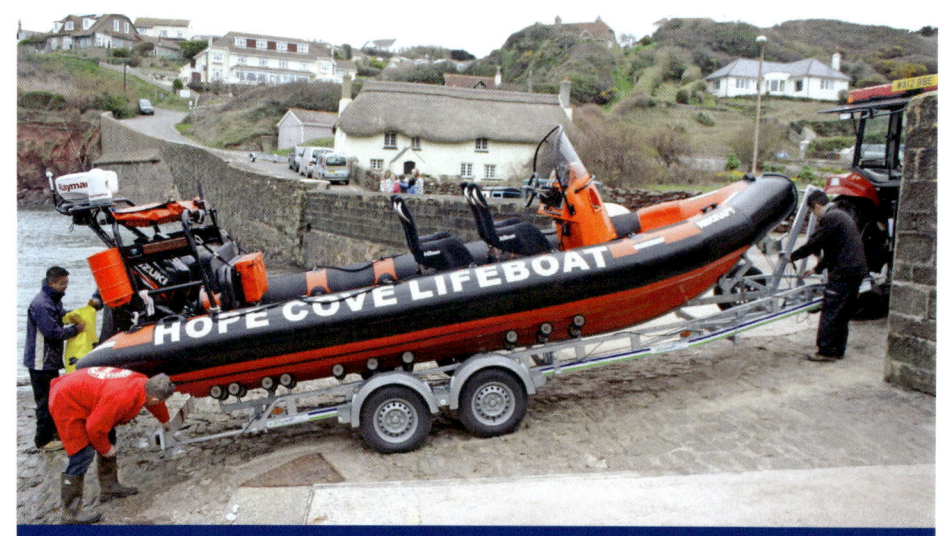

Hope Cove Lifeboat being recovered up the slipway, which was once used by the RNLI lifeboats. (Steve Baguley)

ISLE OF WIGHT AND CHANNEL ISLANDS

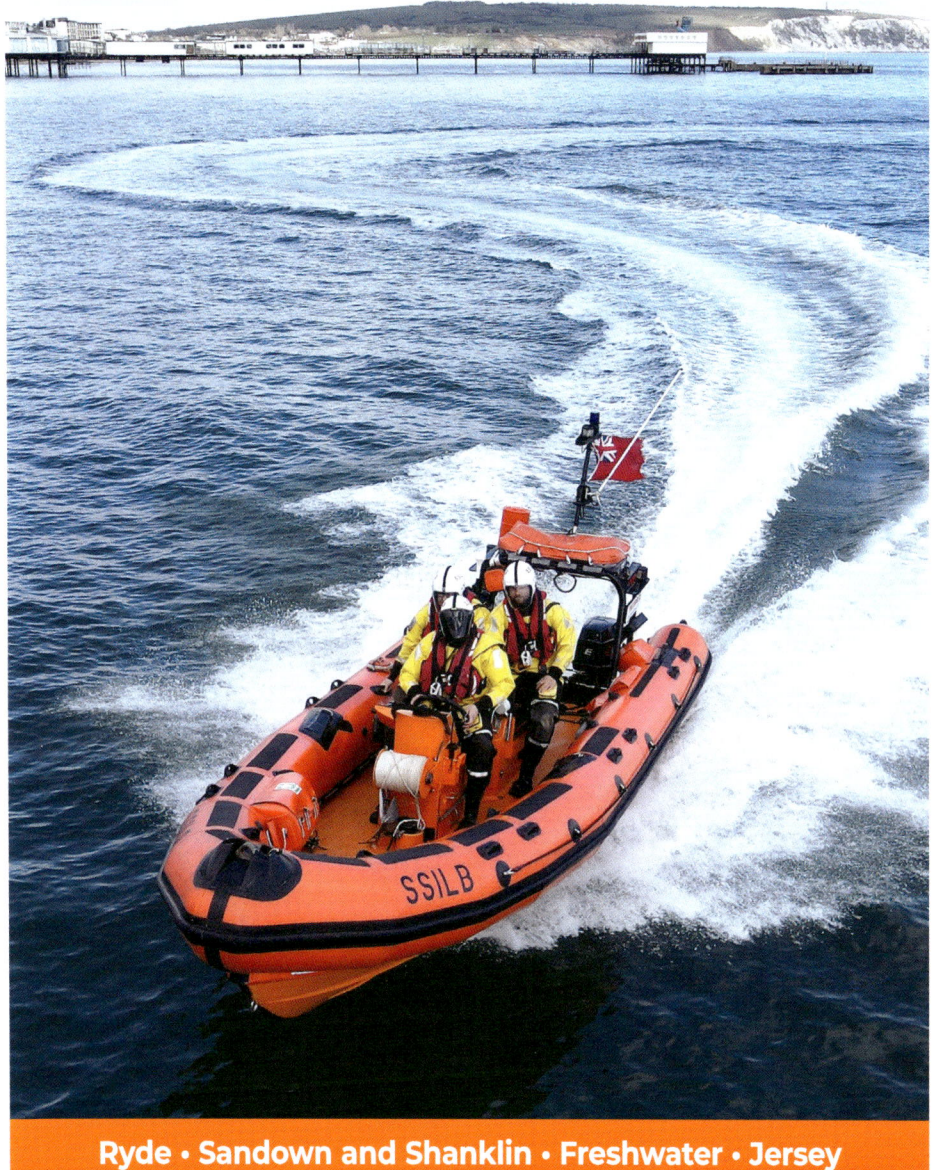

Ryde • Sandown and Shanklin • Freshwater • Jersey

RYDE
Isle of Wight

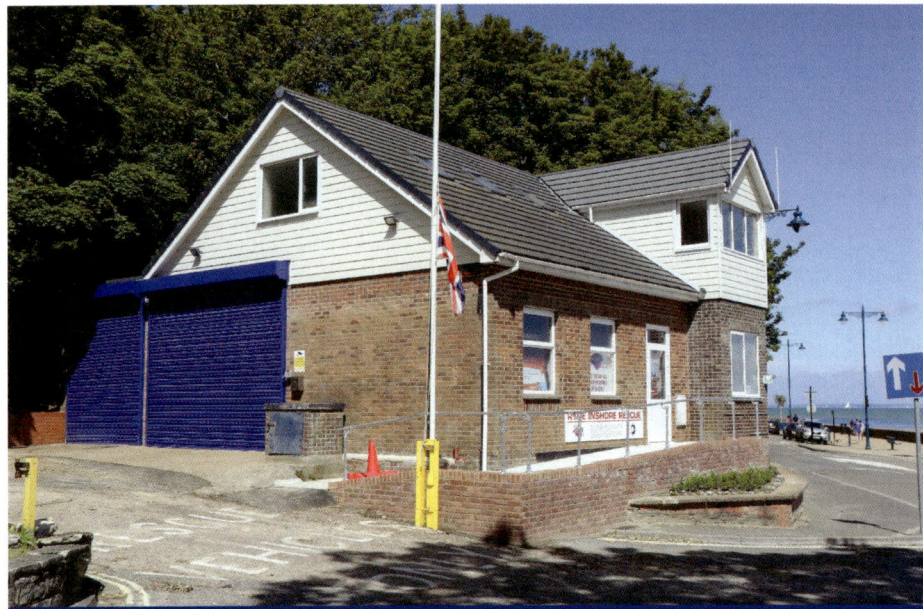

The lifeboat house situated on Appley Lane at the eastern end of Ryde Esplanade. This site has been used since 1978, with the building extended and improved since then. During the 1980s the organisation's primary role gradually changed from beach lifeguarding to becoming a full Inshore Rescue Lifeboat unit. This building was re-roofed and extended in 2013, providing enhanced crew facilities.

LOCATION Isle of Wight
ORGANISATION Ryde Inshore Rescue
ESTABLISHED 1969
HISTORY A sea rescue organisation at Ryde was established as a voluntary beach lifeguard club in 1956, being founded after two deaths by drowning at the end of Ryde Pier. The Ryde Sea Rescue Scheme, run largely by the Vectis Fishing Club which used 12ft dinghies powered by small Seagull outboards, operated from a base near the end of the pier, which had been the location of the RNLI's lifeboat station until it was closed in 1923.

The organisation's primary aim initially was to offer safety to swimmers and beach users, and under the title Ryde Life Guard Corps got underway in May 1956, assisted by the Shanklin Life Guard Corps, Sandown Lifeguard Corps, and the St John Ambulance Brigade. Further support came from the Borough of Ryde. The equipment consisted of a 9ft rowing boat loaned by the Borough, a reel and line, and a rocket line. Two beach huts, next to the Red Cross hut, were used for changing.

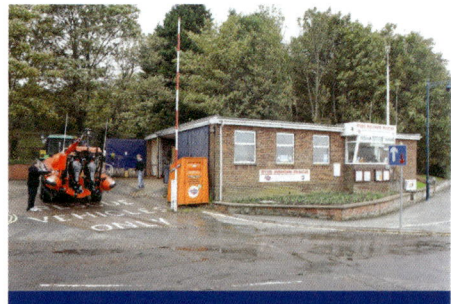

The lifeboat station on Appley Lane pictured in October 2012, before it was extended and modified.

Independent lifeboats of Britain

PREVIOUS ASSETS
1969 The first inshore lifeboat was acquired after vandals destroyed the rowing dinghy. The club raised money to fund a dory powered by a 40hp outboard.
1977 The unit changed its name to Ryde Voluntary Lifeguards following an edict from the Royal Life Saving Society. Although most of the work was by this time being done using a boat, rather than swimming, the main objective was ensuring the safety of swimmers on the beaches of Appley. The service was operating three boats: Miss Mobil, donated by the Mobil Oil Co and loaned from the RLSS; the main glass-reinforced plastic (GRP) lifeboat, named Carnival 71 as she was bought though collections at Ryde Carnival 1971; and the rigid inflatable.
1978 The station was vandalised and the boathouse was destroyed by fire. Through a major fundraising effort and help from the local council, a new building was erected at the Appley end of Ryde seafront and this is still in use as the organisation's headquarters, housing two lifeboats and crew facilities, and providing a look-out over the beach. A Q17 Dory powered by waterjets was bought, as a shallow draft boat was needed to cope with the sandbanks, where people were often cut off by the tide. The unit's second boat, named Carnival 71, was slightly damaged in the fire and so, with a donation from Medina Lions, was replaced by a 4m Avon Searider. To launch the boats over the soft sand, a Fordson Major tractor, ideal for the light GRP boats, was acquired.
1981 the main rescue boat was replaced by a slightly larger Taskforce Q18 Dory, which was fitted out by crew members Malcolm Lane and Colin Eggleton. The inboard diesel engine and waterjet arrangement was retained.
1995 An EA16 type inflatable inshore lifeboat was built specifically for the Service by Avon Inflatables in Llanelli to an RNLI standard

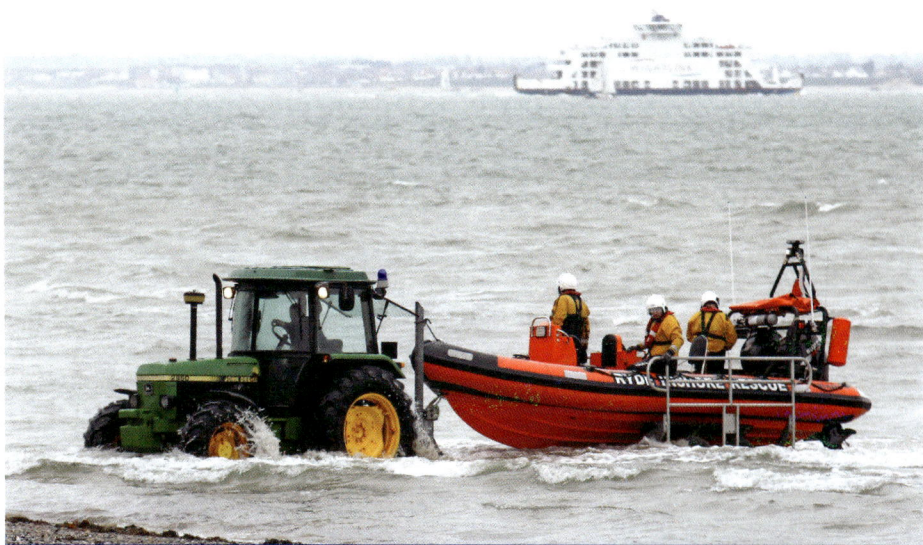

The 6.3m Ribcraft rigid inflatable Sir Norman Echlin Bt being launched in 2012. At low water it is necessary to tow the lifeboats out through nearly a mile of shallow water before they can be launched. The salt water environment is not kind to the standard agricultural tractor and they have to be replaced regularly, and at least seven different vehicles have been used. The most effective launch vehicle was purpose-built for the service by Bateman Engineering in 1995 and had the engine high up driving a hydraulic pump. (Nicholas Leach)

Independent lifeboats of Britain

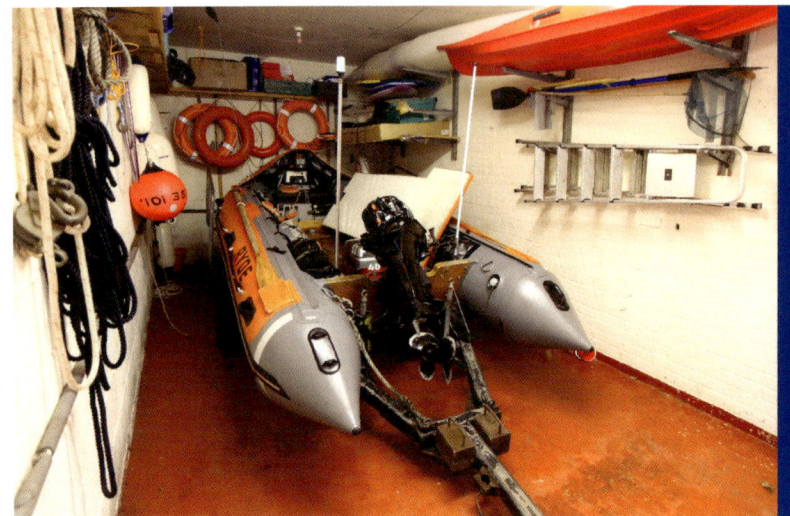

The single-engined EA16 type inflatable (on station 1995-2012) inside the boathouse. (Nicholas Leach)

design and went on station as the second ILB, primarily for shallow water rescues.

2008 A 6.3m Ribcraft twin-engined rigid inflatable, named Sir Norman Echlin Bt, was acquired. The boat was funded after the service, assisted by local businesses, organisations and individuals, raised £50,000 in a year.

2012 Ryde Rescue 2, an Avon EA16 inflatable, was replaced by a 4m Valiant rigid inflatable, powered by a single 25hp outboard, intended for shallow water rescues.

2014 Both boats were vandalised in July, and the sponsons badly damaged. In October a new Massey Ferguson launching tractor was acquired to replace the John Deere, and this was used for the second ILB.

CURRENT ASSETS Ribcraft 8.0 Inshore Lifeboat, named Ryde Rescue 1, launched by John Deere 6820 tractor and trailer, on station 2019; Ribcraft 4.8m Professional, named Ryde Rescue 2, launched by John Deere 2850 tractor and trailer, on station 2021.

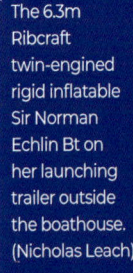

The 6.3m Ribcraft twin-engined rigid inflatable Sir Norman Echlin Bt on her launching trailer outside the boathouse. (Nicholas Leach)

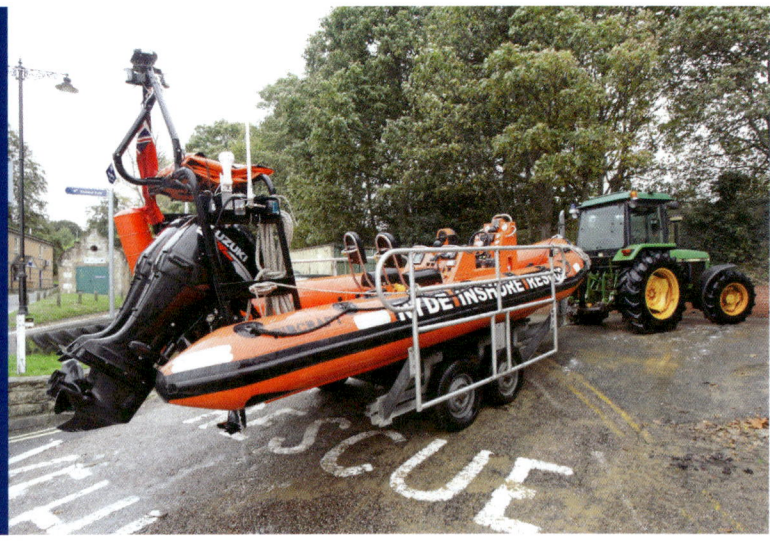

Independent lifeboats of Britain

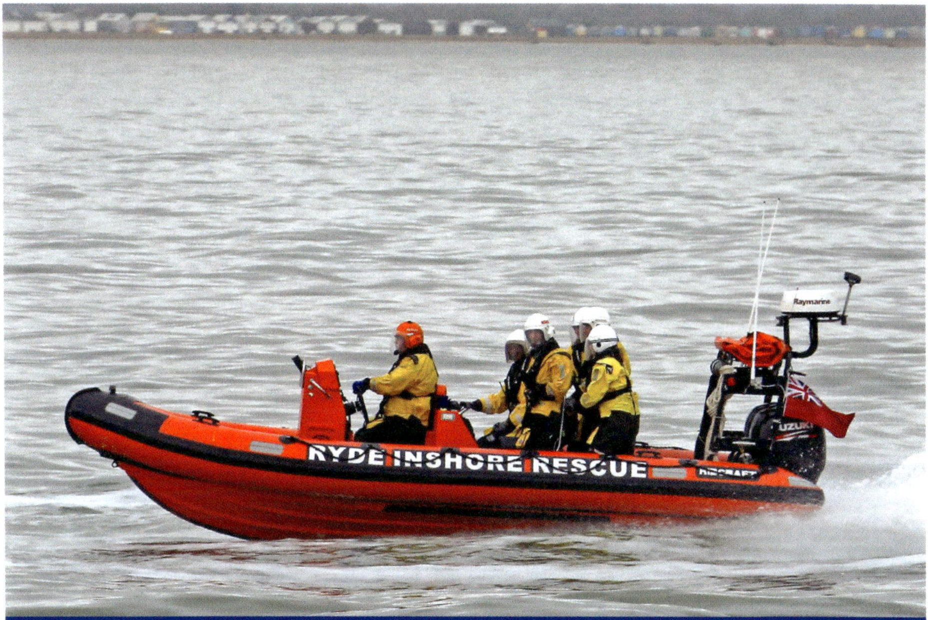

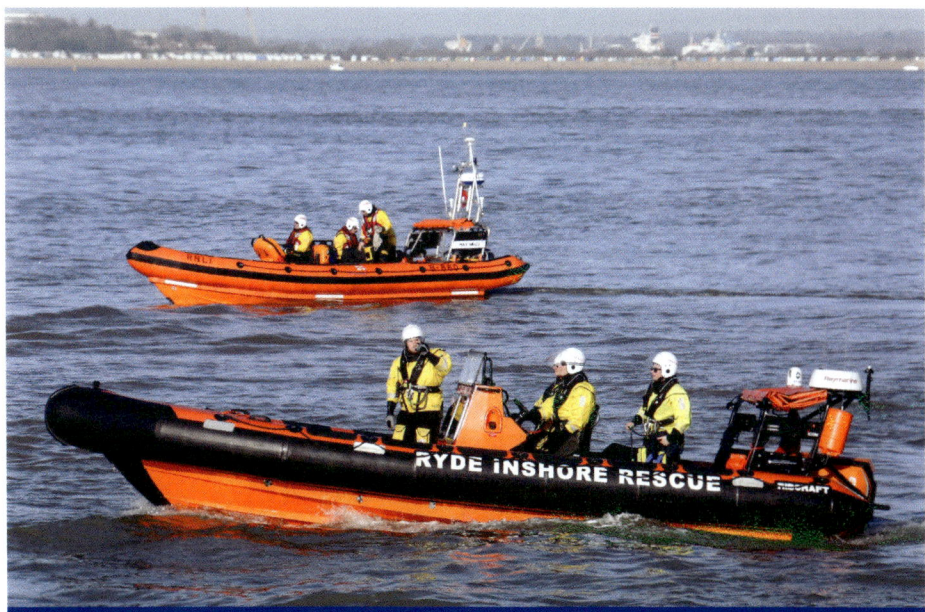

The 6.3m Ribcraft twin-engined rigid inflatable Sir Norman Echlin Bt was on station from 2008 to 2019. She is pictured on exercise in the Solent in January 2018. (Nicholas Leach)

The 7.8m Ribcraft rigid inflatable Ryde Rescue 1 is powered by two 150hp Evinrude Etec outboards giving her a speed of 40 knots, has four Ullman Shock Absorbing Seats, and carries a thermal imaging camera. She is pictured off Cowes, with the RNLI Atlantic 85 lifeboat from Calshot, Max Walls (B-860). (Nicholas Leach)

Independent lifeboats of Britain

SANDOWN AND SHANKLIN — Isle of Wight

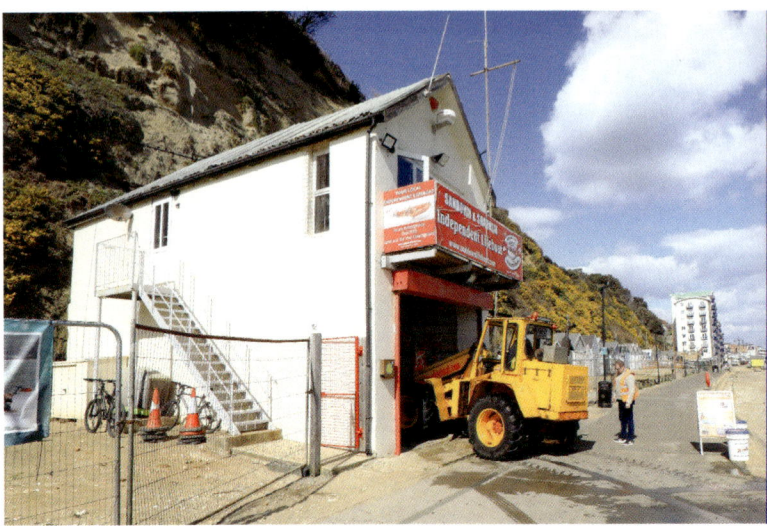

The boathouse on the Western Esplanade, which has been home to Sandown & Shanklin Independent Lifeboat since the 1970s.

LOCATION Sandown, Isle of Wight
ORGANISATION Sandown & Shanklin Independent Lifeboat
ESTABLISHED 1972
HISTORY The first lifeboat to cover Shanklin Bay was built in 1884, but unlike almost all other lifeboats of that era was not supplied or funded by the RNLI. A lifeboat for Shanklin was deemed necessary after the naval training ship HMS Eurydice was wrecked on 25 March 1878 after being caught in a sudden squall and over 300 men lost their lives. Following this, an appeal was made locally to fund a lifeboat and in 1884 the pulling lifeboat Dove was introduced at Shanklin, funded by the Sunday school children of the Island. Dove served at Shanklin until 1916, when it was washed away in a storm.

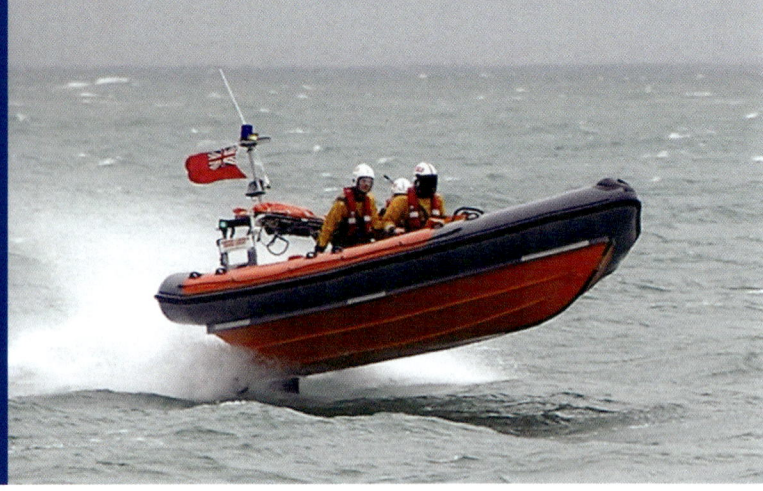

The first Atlantic 21 used at Sandown, ex-RNLI B-553, served the independent rescuers from 1999 to 2011. (By courtesy of SSILB)

Independent lifeboats of Britain

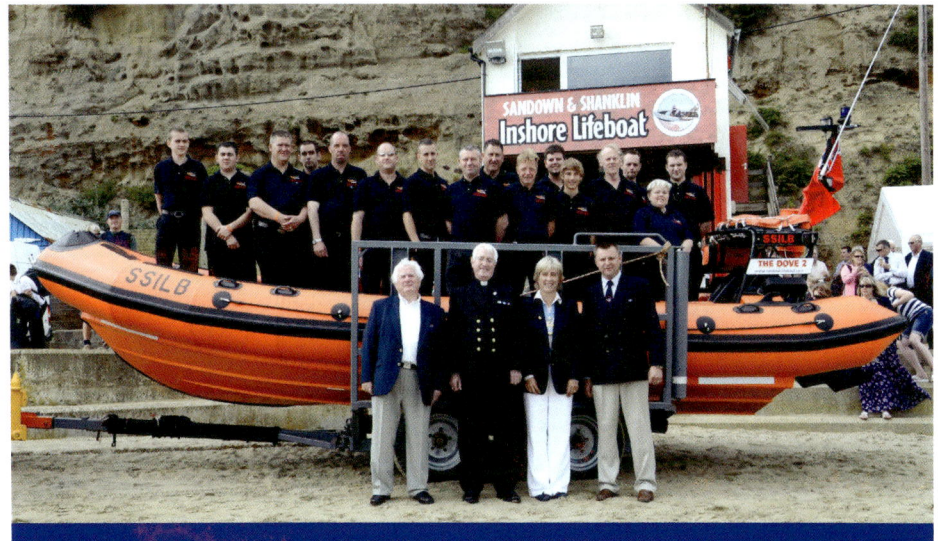

Crew and station officials on the launch day for Atlantic 21 The Dove II, 3 September 2011. (By courtesy of SSILB)

Sandown & Shanklin Independent Lifeboat began operations in the 1970s. Various small inshore lifeboats were used during the 1970s, with the first larger ILB entering service in 1988. The current boathouse was built in 1988 on Sandown's Western Esplanade. However, after a cliff fall the council decided that the station needed to be moved away from the cliff and a new station was planned. This will provide extra space for a larger lifeboat, a sales outlet and training area for the crew. Planning permission was received, and the work is

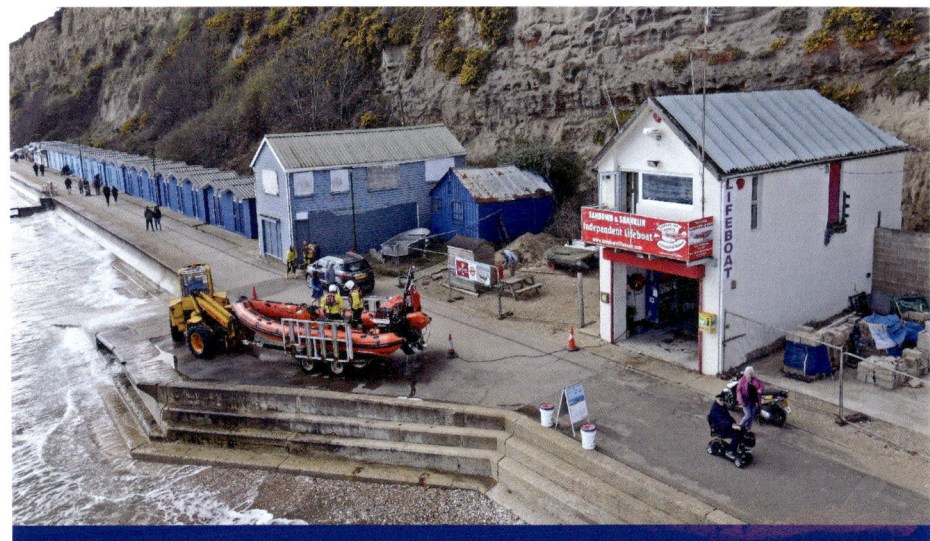

Atlantic 21 The Dove II and launching tractor outside the boathouse on the Western Promenade, beneath the cliffs. The service covers the sea between Bembridge Ledge and St Catherine's Point, to six miles offshore, totalling about seventy square miles. (Nicholas Leach)

Independent lifeboats of Britain

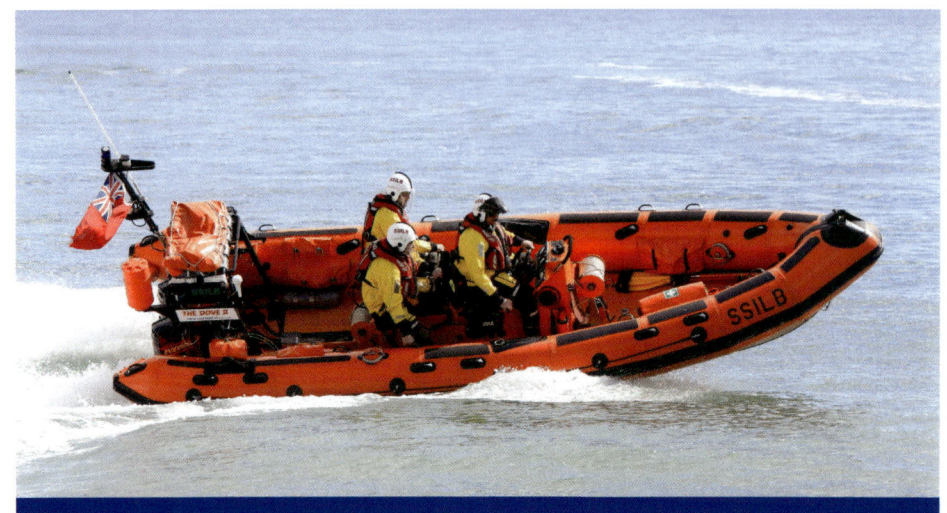

Atlantic 21 The Dove II being put through her paces off Sandown Pier. (By courtesy of SSILB)

estimated to cost about £180,000, but raising the necessary funds is challenging.

PREVIOUS ASSETS
1988 A 6m Halmatic type ILB was in service.
1991 A twin engined Avon Searider rigid inflatable was acquired which had a central helm console and seating for the crew.
1999 In September an ex-RNLI Atlantic 21 rigid inflatable, B-553, was purchased for about £10,000. This boat, which was built in 1981 and served at the Newbiggin station for seventeen years, gave good service at Sandown before being replaced. She subsequently went to

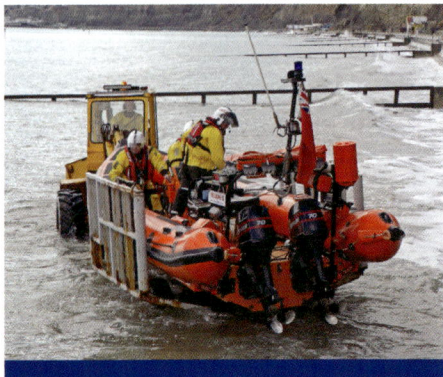

Atlantic 21 The Dove II being launched on exercise at high tide. (Nicholas Leach)

serve with Lagan SAR in Belfast.
2010 Another ex-RNLI Atlantic 21, B-590, was purchased for about £12,000. This boat, which was fitted out at the RNLI's Inshore Lifeboat Centre at Cowes and used as a relief lifeboat by the RNLI, was refitted and rebuilt by crew members during 2010 and 2011, and entered service on 3 September 2011. She was powered by twin 70hp Evinrude outboard engines, giving a speed of over 30 knots, and was named Dove II. Equipment includes a satellite navigation, GPS chart plotter and radio, and 148 litres of fuel gives an endurance of three hours at full speed. The boat also has a righting air-bag.
2015 The Service acquired a second hand Atlantic 75 from the RNLI, B-768, and the fitting out is an ongoing process. This boat is unable to be accommodated in the current lifeboat station and cannot be commissioned until extension work on the building is complete. When commissioned, the Atlantic 75 will become the main boat and the existing boat, The Dove II, will provide backup.
CURRENT ASSETS Atlantic 21 The Dove II (ex-RNLI B-590 Wolverson X-Ray, built 1992), launched by Matbro teleporter and carriage, refitted and on station 2011.

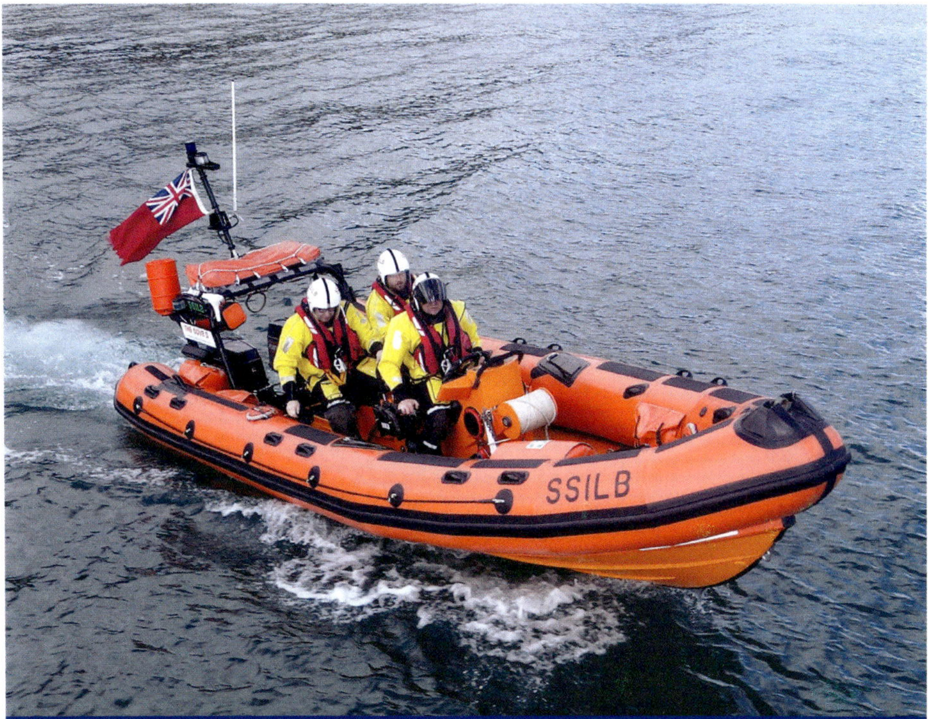

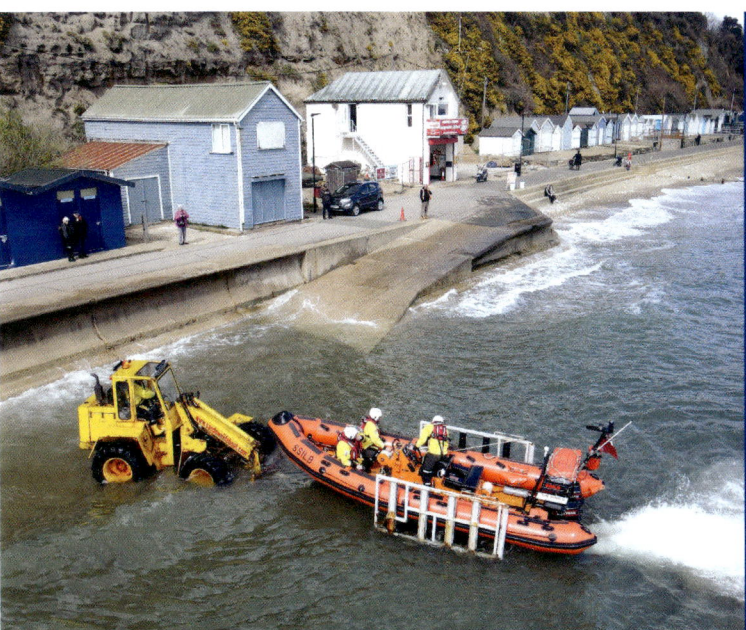

Atlantic 21 The Dove II was built by the RNLI in 1992 but has been extensively refitted since then. (Nicholas Leach)

Atlantic 21 The Dove II being recovered onto her carrriage, outside the boathouse. The slipway runs alongside the promenade. (Nicholas Leach)

Independent lifeboats of Britain

FRESHWATER
Isle of Wight

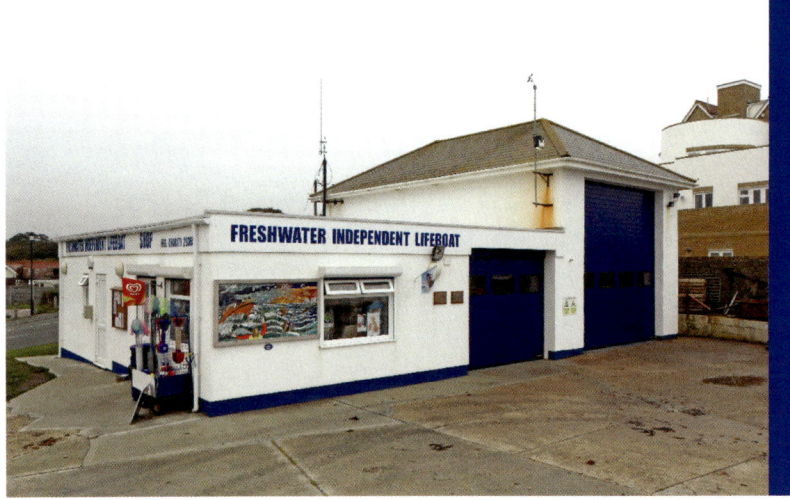

The boathouse at Freshwater Bay pictured in 2012. The building started life as a basic garage for the 16ft inflatable and has been progressively extended. (Nicholas Leach)

LOCATION Freshwater Bay, Isle of Wight
ORGANISATION Freshwater Independent Lifeboat
ESTABLISHED 1972
HISTORY Freshwater Independent Lifeboat was founded in 1972 in response to an increase in waterborne activities which showed the need for an inshore patrol to cover the south-west of the island. The Council obtained a second-hand single-engined 16ft inflatable, and the crew raised the money for another boat as the Coastguard were concerned about a single-engined craft working alone. So Freshwater Lifeguards, with two 16ft RFD PB16 type inflatables, became Freshwater Bay Inshore Rescue, and began patrolling an area from The Needles to St Catherine's Point.
PREVIOUS ASSETS
1981 A larger and faster boat was required, so a 6m Avon Searider twin-engined rigid inflatable was purchased. An extension to the boathouse was built by the crew and other volunteers to accommodate the new boat, with a gift shop also added to help raise funds.
1992 A 7.4m Avon Sea Rider rigid inflatable was purchased. The crew added a small cabin to accommodate the navigator and electronic equipment. This boat, named Spirit of West Wight, by Countess Mountbatten of Burma, served for ten years during which time the area covered was extended to mid-Channel.
2000 With the enlarged area of coverage, improved protection was deemed necessary for the crew when the boat was on service in cold nights in mid-Channel, and so an 8.8m Barbarian class rigid inflatable with a cabin was purchased. Built by Island Plastics and named Spirit of the West Wight II, she was powered by twin 225hp Yamaha outboards and launched from a purpose-built trolley.
2005 A new 16ft EA16 inflatable, named Berry B and built by Avon Inflatables, was placed on station. It was powered by a 40hp Yamaha outboard and launched by trolley.
2014 A new 9.6m rigid inflatable, named Spirit of the West Wight III, was built by Ribcraft and placed on station in May following an official naming ceremony. Equipped with radar and thermal-imaging camera, it has seating for four crew and is powered by twin inboard

Independent lifeboats of Britain

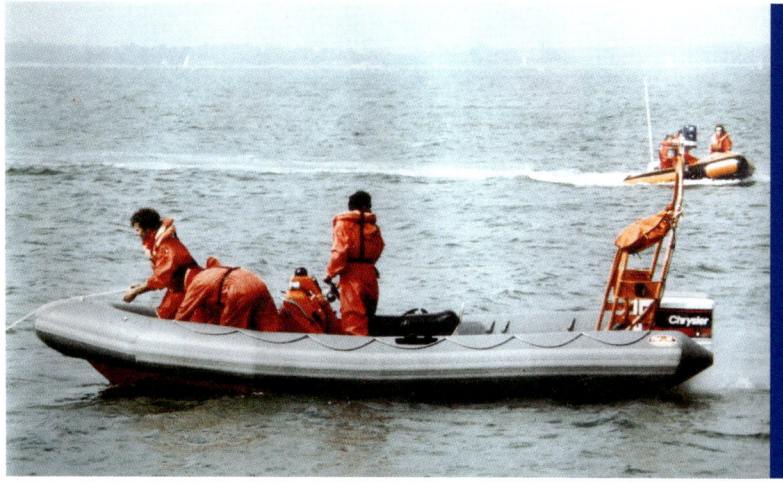

The Avon Searider rigid inflatable was placed on station in 1981. The RFD PB16 type inflatable is background right. (By courtesy of Freshwater Independent Lifeboat)

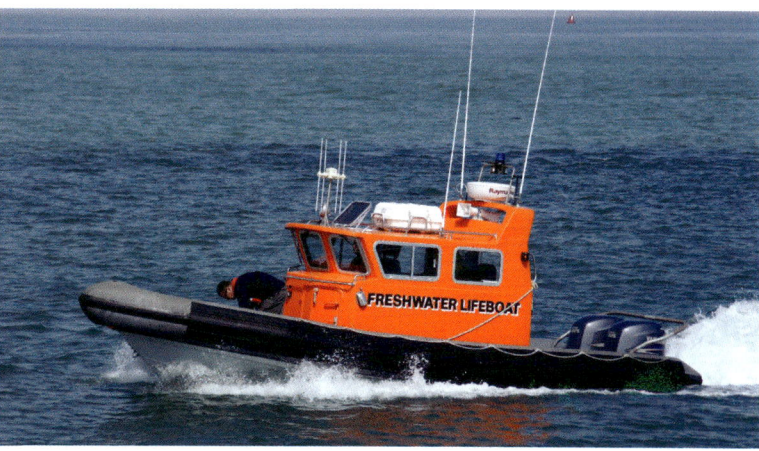

The 2000-built Barbarian RIB Spirit of the West Wight II at sea in Freshwater Bay in May 2012. (Andrew Cooke)

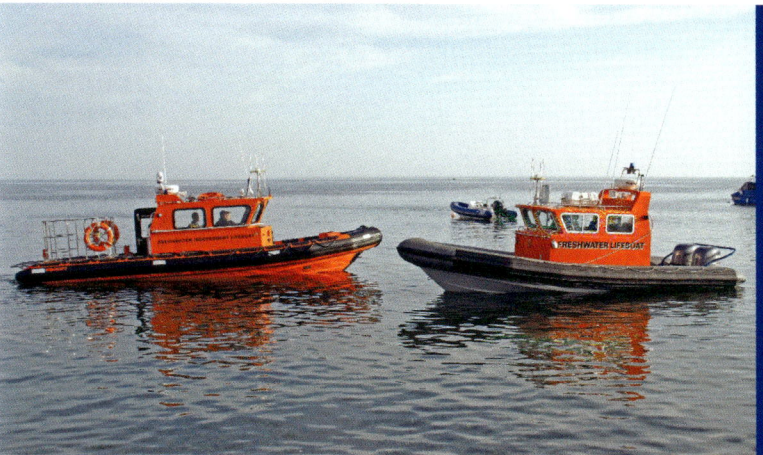

Spirit of West Wight III (left) replaced Spirit of West Wight II (right), in Freshwater Bay, July 2013. (Andrew Cooke)

Independent lifeboats of Britain

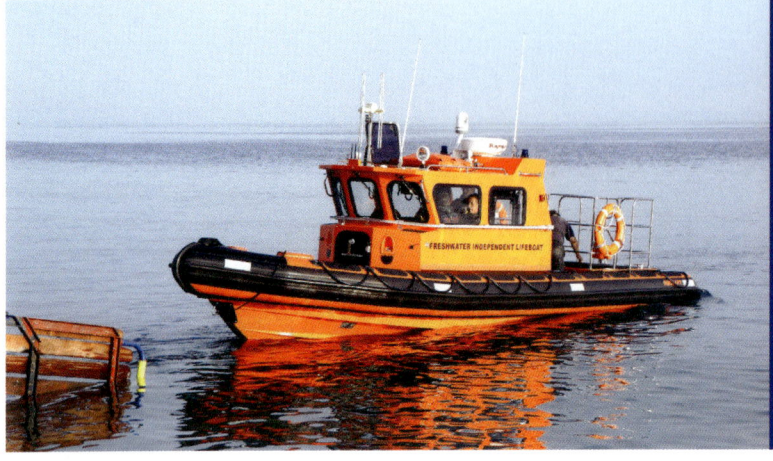

The 2014-built Spirit of the West Wight III being recovered into the launching cradle. (Andrew Cooke)

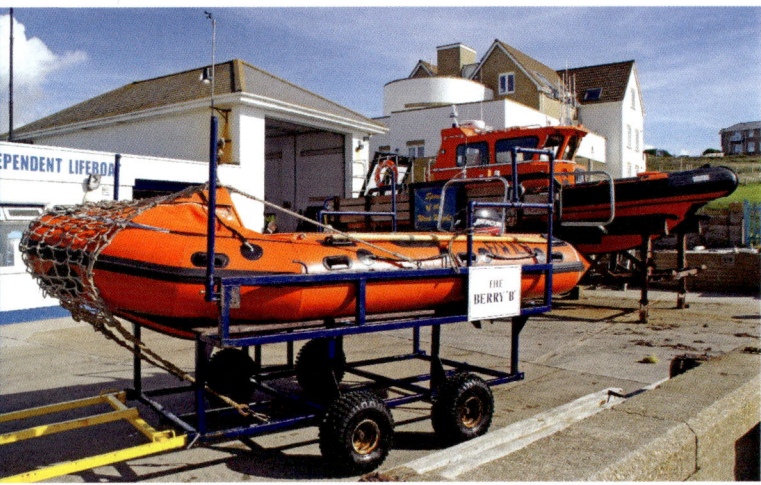

EA16 inflatable Berry B and Spirit of the West Wight III outside the boathouse, October 2013. Berry B was on station from 2005 to 2016, and was then given to the Sea Scouts, who sold her on to Drogheda River Rescue in Ireland. (Andrew Cooke)

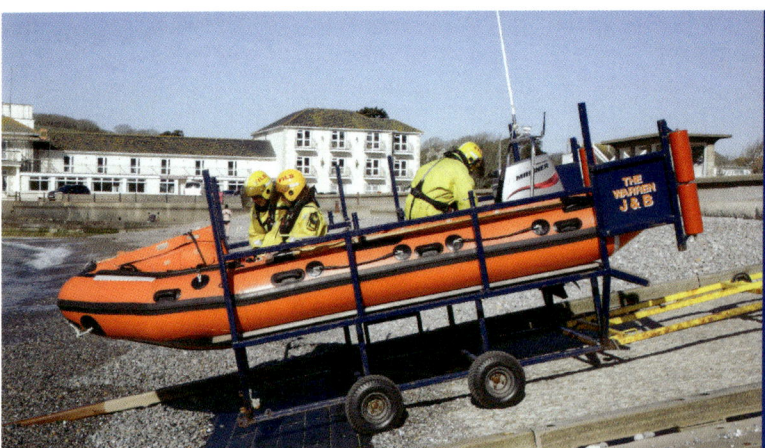

IB1 inflatable inshore lifeboat Warren J&B being launched on exercise, April 2022. The ILB was purpose-built for the service by the RNLI in 2016. (Nicholas Leach)

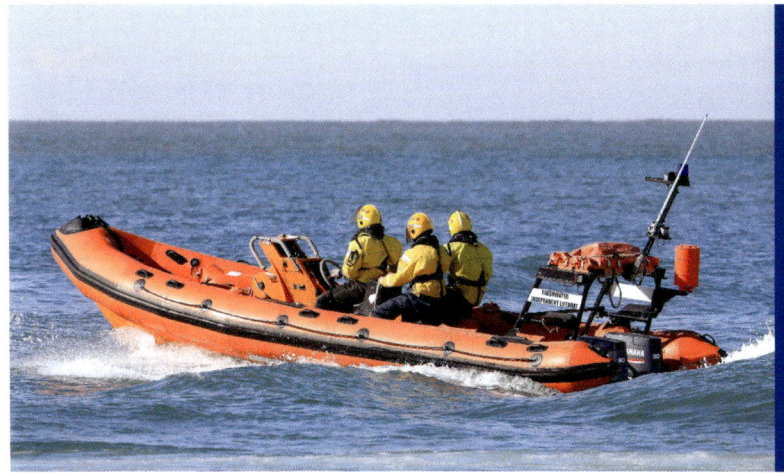

The former RNLI Atlantic 75 (ex-B-784) on exercise in Freshwater Bay, April 2022. The Atlantic was built by the RNLI at Cowes in 2002 and was acquired for service at Freshwater in 2021. (Nicholas Leach)

Yanmar 315 V8 engines, delivering a total of 630hp and giving a cruising speed of 34 knots.

2016 An IB1 inflatable was purchased new from the RNLI, and named Warren J&B; it has an electronics console and upgraded 50hp Yamaha electric start outboard.

2020 9m Ribcraft cabin rigid inflatable, named Spirit of the West Wight III, on station since 2014, was taken off operational duty; it was sold in 2022.

2021 A former RNLI Atlantic 75 ILB was acquired; powered by twin 90hp Yamaha outboard engines, it is launched down the slipway from a drive-off carriage. Problems with the slipway resulted in the service launching a major fundraising drive to finance rectification works and make the launch and recovery procedure safer.

CURRENT ASSETS RNLI-built D class inflatable IB1, named Warren J&B, launched by slipway, on station 2016; ex-RNLI Atlantic 75 rigid inflatable B-784 (ex-Lymington), acquired from RNLI in August 2021; two Yamaha fast rescue craft, named Rescue Craft 1 and Rescue Craft 2, launched by trailer, both on station 2017, used as safety craft.

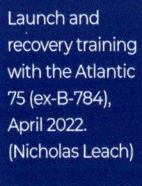

Launch and recovery training with the Atlantic 75 (ex-B-784), April 2022. (Nicholas Leach)

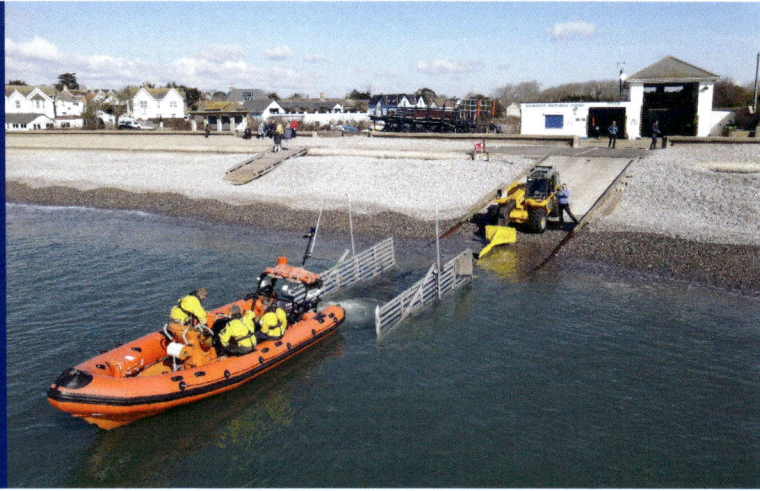

Independent lifeboats of Britain

JERSEY FIRE & RESCUE
Channel Islands

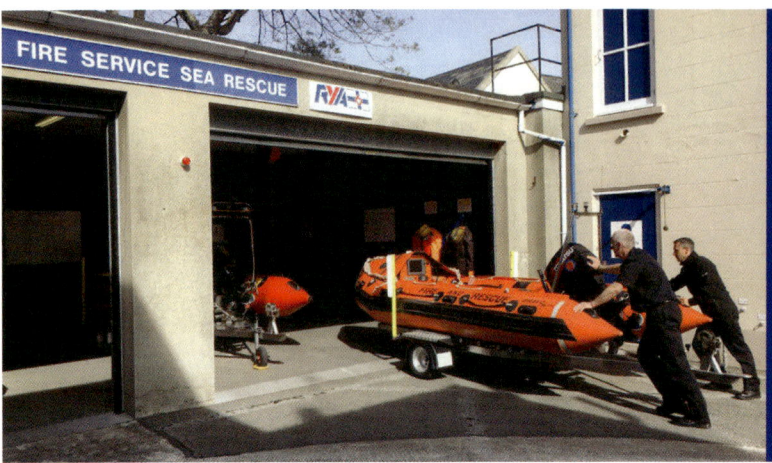

The two inshore rescue boats operated by Jersey Fire and Rescue Service are housed in a dedicated garage behind Jersey's main fire station in St Helier.

LOCATION St Helier, Jersey
ORGANISATION States of Jersey Fire & Rescue Service
ESTABLISHED 1960
HISTORY The inshore rescue service in Jersey, operated by the island's Fire and Rescue Service, can trace its foundation back to the late 1950s. At 4.25am on 3 September 1958 St Helier's RNLI lifeboat Elizabeth Rippon launched on service to three men stranded on Grande d'Azette rock, three-quarters of a mile south-east of her station. Police officers had attempted a rescue using a lifeline, but it was too short, and the police and harbour master could not find a suitable boat. The lifeboat crew succeeded in rescuing the men using the boarding boat, which the lifeboat towed to the scene. Although a rescue was effected, the incident demonstrated the need for a small rescue craft and the States Police approached the Defence Committee with a view to purchasing a suitable boat to be available from the shore.

The St John Ambulance Service in Guernsey was operating a small inflatable craft in conjunction with the RNLI St Peter Port lifeboat at the time so, after consultation with St John Ambulance, and verifying that there was a need for such a craft, the Defence Committee agreed to purchase one. It was decided that Jersey's Fire Service, not the Police, would operate the craft. The original inshore rescue boat, purchased in 1960, was a Zodiac inflatable which, in its first year, undertook thirty-five inshore rescues.

PREVIOUS ASSETS
1960 A Zodiac inflatable powered by a 40hp Evinrude outboard entered service in May.
1961 In October a Cheetah catamaran was provided as an additional rescue craft. This boat has the advantages of the Zodiac but with added stability and reliability. However, the catamaran proved to be underpowered and did not match the capabilities of the inflatable rescue craft.
1966 The Zodiac was replaced by an RFD (Reginald Foster Dagnall) PB16 type inflatable, powered by a 40hp Evinrude outboard.
1968 A second RFD PB16 boat was bought in February to replace the catamaran.
1971 The RFDs' Evinrude outboards were replaced by 50hp Mercury outboards. These were manually started but later changed to electric starting, which proved more reliable.
1982 A new RFD PB16 inflatable, named Grève

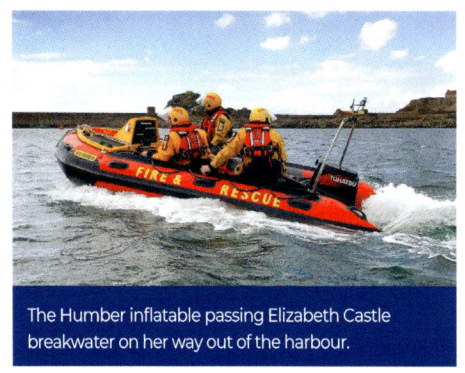

The Humber inflatable passing Elizabeth Castle breakwater on her way out of the harbour.

de Lecq, was acquired.

1993 After various types of craft were considered, an Avon EA16 inflatable, built to the same specifications as those used by the RNLI and fitted with a 40hp Mariner outboard, was purchased in June.

1994 In June another Avon EA16, to the same specifications, was acquired. The boats' call signs had been RL1 and RL2 (Rescue Launch), but these were later changed to IRB 1 and IRB 2 (Inshore Rescue Boat).

1996 The Avon EA16 remained in service, but was fitted with a 50hp Tohatsu outboard.

2000 The first orange Avon EA16 inflatable, named Fire Alpha, arrived.

2001 The second orange Avon EA16 inflatable, named Fire Bravo, arrived.

2014 Jersey Fire and Rescue commissioned DPM Trading, a Jersey-based manufacturer specialising in custom fabrications, and Humber RIBs (a UK-based manufacturer) to build a new rescue boat. The hull was based on Humber's standard 16i Workboat. A heavy-duty transom enabled a 50hp engine to be installed, and an A frame was fitted.

2019 While the DPM Humber performed well at incidents with fair sea conditions, her manoeuvrability and responsiveness were found to suffer in heavier seas so JF&RS purchased a new IB1 inflatable from the RNLI to replace the DPM Humber. The vessel was fitted with a 50hp Mariner immersion-proofed engine as well as a 'pod' containing a complete RNLI electronics package.

2020 A second immersion-proofed 50hp Mariner was bought and replaced the Tohatsu on Fire Bravo, the older EA 16 inflatable.

CURRENT ASSETS IB1 purchased in 2019 from RNLI (D-831 in RNLI build schedule), fitted with 50hp Mariner immersion proof engine and RNLI pod including SIMS package; call sign 'Fire Alpha'; Avon EA16 inflatable, purchased in 2001, call Sign 'Fire Bravo', with 50hp Mariner immersion proof engine purchased in 2020; main towing vehicle is a Land Rover purchased in 2019; second towing vehicle is Toyota Land Cruiser purchased in 2020, call sign 'Fire Tango'; both ILBs are launched via trailer using the vehicles. The States of Jersey Fire and Rescue Service also provides a specialist Rope Rescue Team. All firefighters in the JF&RS are trained to crew the Inshore rescue boats.

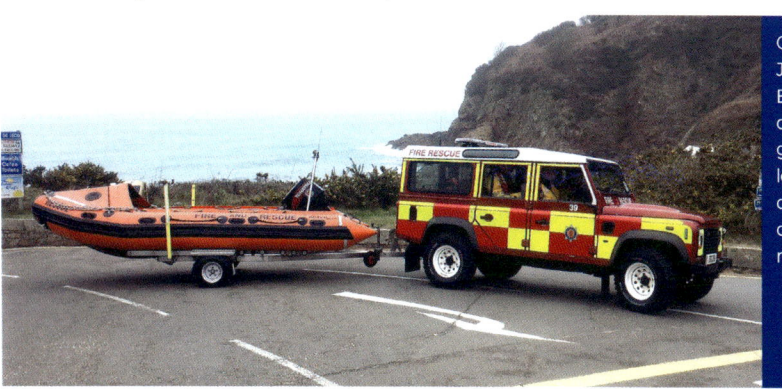

One of the JF&RS' Avon EA16 inflatables on its road-going trailer, leaving Grève de Lecq, a bay on Jersey's north coast.

Independent lifeboats of Britain

JERSEY

Channel Islands

LOCATION Jersey, Channel Islands
ORGANISATION Jersey Lifeboat Association
ESTABLISHED 2018
HISTORY The Jersey Lifeboat Association was established in 2018 by a number of former RNLI volunteers. Its formation was approved by the Royal Court of Jersey on 2 February 2018, after which efforts were made to acquire a lifeboat, with the former RNLI 47ft Tyne class lifeboat Max Aitken III, built at Cowes in 1987 for Bembridge, being bought and renamed Sir Max Aitken III.

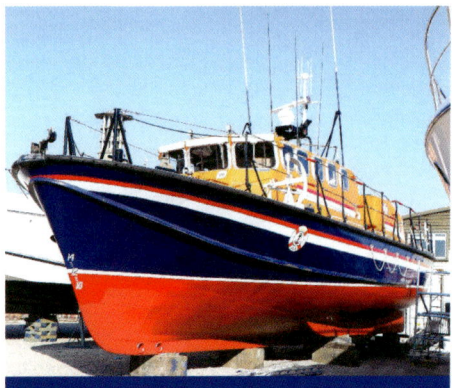

Sir Max Aitken III out of the water at St Helier prior to entering service for the Jersey Lifeboat Association.

The boat had been sold out of RNLI service in May 2014 to Rea Associates Ltd for resale and was stored at Gosport. She was sold in July 2015 and shipped by road to Goodchild Marine, Burgh Castle, in Norfolk for a refit, remaining out of the water there for three years. The JLA had her surveyed so that she could be used as an independent lifeboat at St Helier and on 11 June 2018, carrying no name or number, she sailed from Burgh Castle. She arrived in Jersey two days later, and lifted out for painting and refurbishment.

The lifeboat was declared operational in April 2019 after an assessment process overseen by the Island's Harbourmaster. Moorings for the lifeboat were found in St Helier, near the harbour entrance. A shore

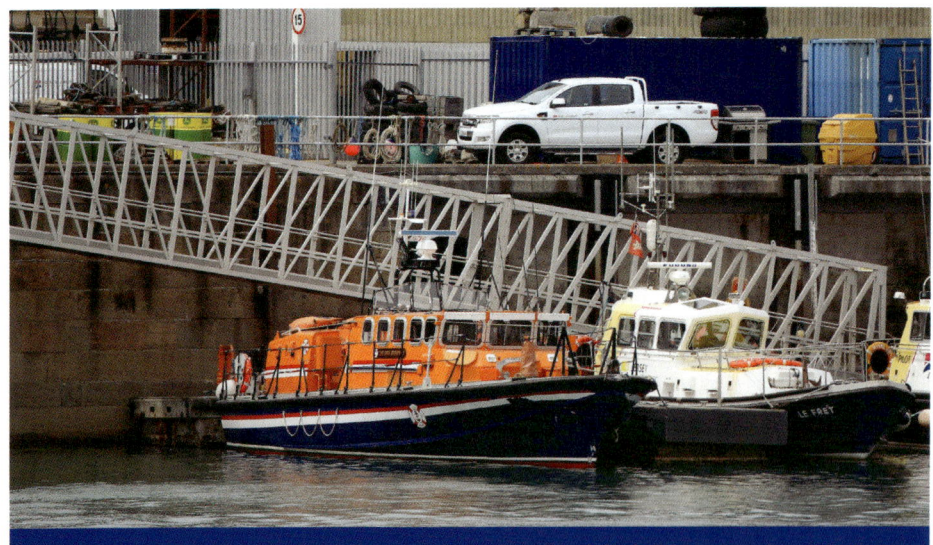

47ft Tyne Sir Max Aitken III moored in St Helier harbour, in JLA livery. An existing building was made available by the Ports of Jersey at the Albert Pier in St Helier to provide a support facility and accommodation for crew clothing and equipment, close to the lifeboat's pontoon. (Nicholas Leach)

Independent lifeboats of Britain

facility was established in an existing building made available by the Ports of Jersey, on the harbourside at Albert Pier in St Helier to provide a support facility and accommodation for crew clothing and equipment.

The JLA expanded its capabilities in 2021 with the addition of a fats rigid inflatable boat. The service purchased a Gemini Waverider 880 CR lifeboat constructed at the Gemini factory in South Africa and fitted out by Berthon Boat Company in Lymington. The 8.8m boat, which is named Albert Pinel, has a top speed of forty-five knots and features some advanced technology, including a FLIR thermal camera and an advanced water ballast system to ensure stability in rough seas. A floating Versadock pontoon was installed close to the all-weather boat on a temporary basis to keep the boat out of the water.

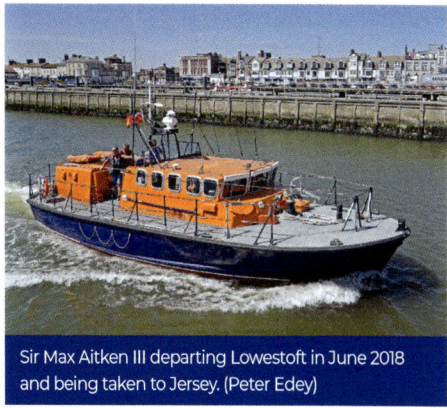

Sir Max Aitken III departing Lowestoft in June 2018 and being taken to Jersey. (Peter Edey)

2021 The JLA expanded its capabilities with the purchase of a Gemini Waverider 880 CR lifeboat constructed at the Gemini factory in South Africa and fitted out by Berthon Boat Company in Lymington. The 8.8m boat has a top speed of 45 knots and has advanced

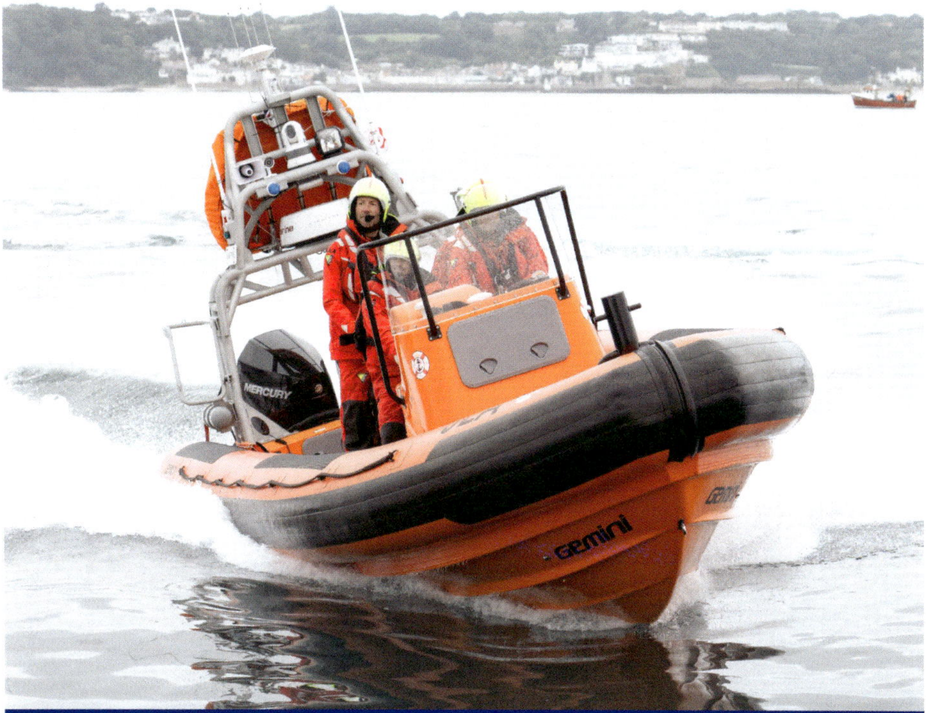

The Gemini rigid inflatable Albert Pinel arriving at Jersey on 3 July 2021. (By courtesy of Andy Habin)

Independent lifeboats of Britain

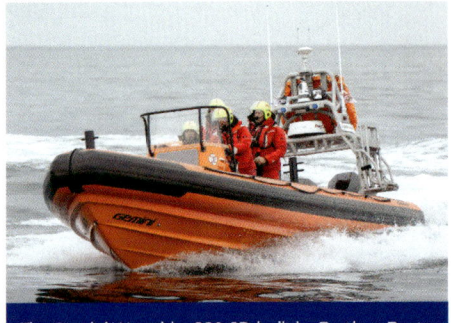

The Gemini Waverider 880 CR, built by Berthon Boat Co, Albert Pinel at Jersey. (By courtesy of Andy Habin)

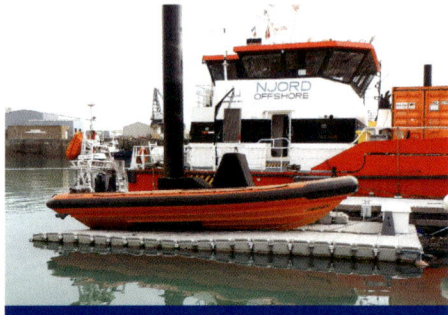

The Gemini Waverider 880 CR Albert Pinel in her berth at St Peter Port. (Ian Moignard)

technology including an FLIR thermal camera and an advanced water ballast system. The boat is kept clear of the water on a platform, being hauled out of the water by an electric winch, designed and installed by VersaDock.

2022 The 47ft Tyne was damaged on service, and was temporarily withdrawn, being sent to Berthon Boat Co at Lymington for repairs. She returned to the station in July following the completion of the repairs.

CURRENT ASSETS 47ft Tyne (ex-RNLI 47-018), named Sir Max Aitken III, built in 1987 by Fairey Marine, Cowes, moored afloat, operational April 2019; Gemini Waverider 880 CR, fitted out by Berthon Boat Co, Lymington, named Albert Pinel, on station 31 August 2021.

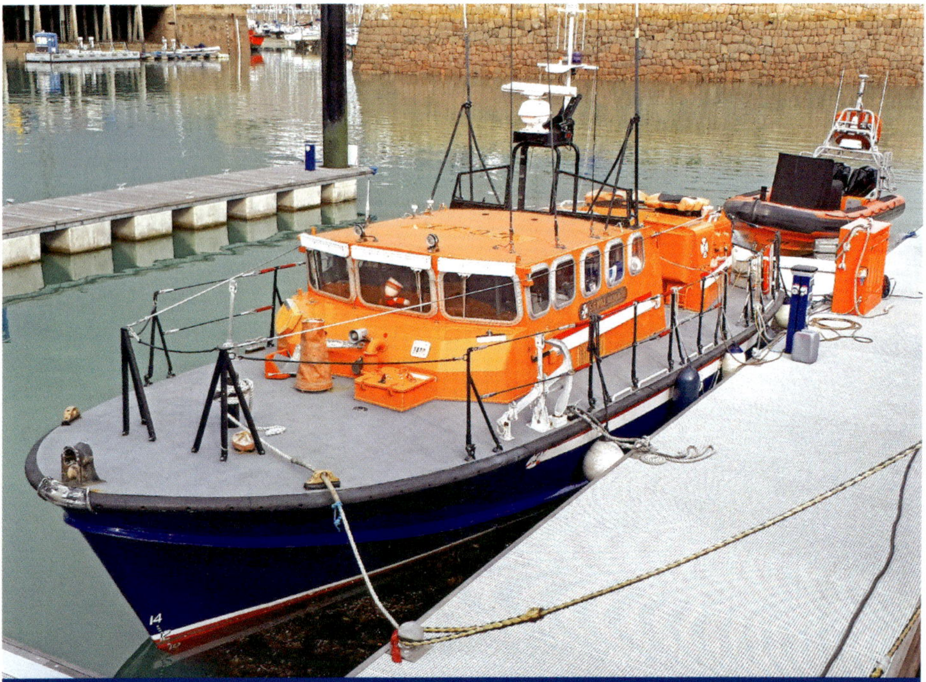

The 47ft Tyne class lifeboat Sir Max Aitken III (ex-RNLI 47-018, stationed at Bembridge) and the rigid inflatable Albert Pinel at the berth at St Helier harbour in October 2022. (Ian Moignard)

BRISTOL CHANNEL AND SOUTH WALES

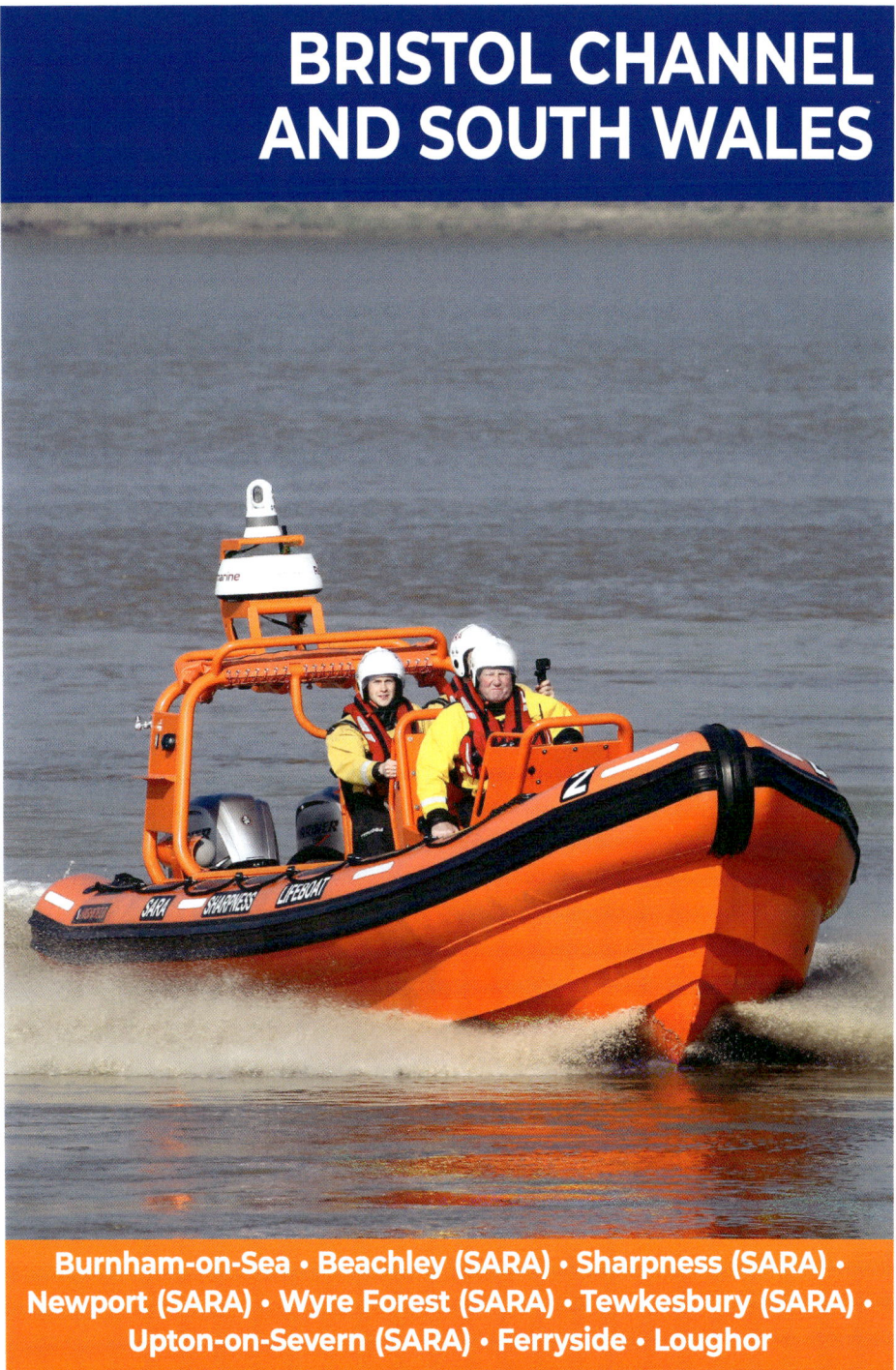

Burnham-on-Sea • Beachley (SARA) • Sharpness (SARA) • Newport (SARA) • Wyre Forest (SARA) • Tewkesbury (SARA) • Upton-on-Severn (SARA) • Ferryside • Loughor

BURNHAM-ON-SEA
Somerset

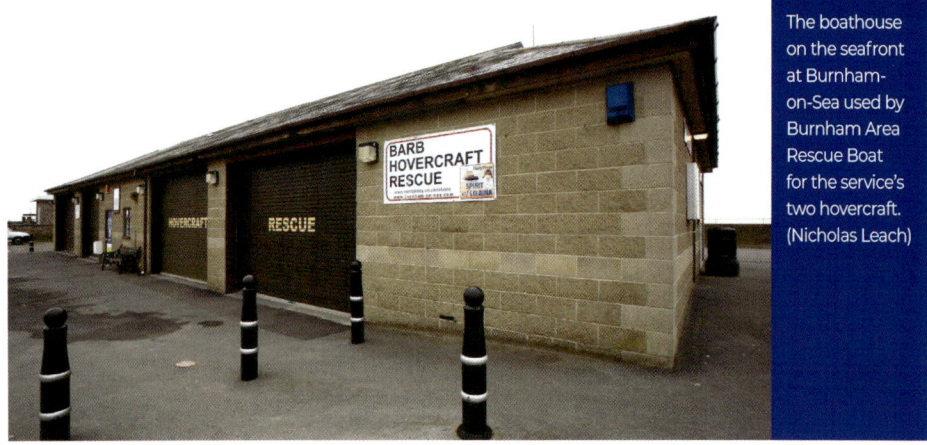

The boathouse on the seafront at Burnham-on-Sea used by Burnham Area Rescue Boat for the service's two hovercraft. (Nicholas Leach)

LOCATION Burnham-on-Sea
ORGANISATION BARB Search & Rescue (Burnham Area Rescue Boat)
ESTABLISHED 1992
HISTORY Burnham-on-Sea is situated on the southern shore of the Bristol Channel. RNLI pulling lifeboats served the town from 1836 until 1930, when a motor lifeboat at neighbouring Weston-super-Mare was deemed sufficient to cover the area. However, in 1992 plans to provide an inshore rescue boat for the town were made with the formation of Burnham Area Rescue Boat (BARB). The service bought a Ribcraft rigid inflatable, powered by twin Yamaha outboards. Initially the boat was kept at a facility inland.

In June 1994 a new boathouse was built in the space of three days by Anneka Rice and a team of builders from the BBC TV programme Challenge Anneka. The building on the promenade, on a site made available by the local council, provided a permanent home for BARB as well as facilities for HMCG rescue team.

In addition to the Ribcraft, an EA16 D class ILB built by Avon inflatables and powered by a Yamaha outboard was used, being launched and recovered using a Massey Ferguson tractor down the slipway onto the beach.

PREVIOUS ASSETS
2002 In June a five-year-old holidaymaker, Lelaina Hall, was drowned on the mudflats at Berrow, north of the town. An appeal was launched in conjunction with the Association of Search and Rescue Hovercraft and with the backing of the Western Daily Press. This raised £115,000 to buy a rescue hovercraft, which could operate on mud and in shallow water.
2003 The hovercraft Spirit of Lelaina arrived on 22 March. The six-seat BBV-6 craft was designed by Bill Baker Vehicles and built by Ivanoff Hovercraft AB in Sweden. It was 5.25m long, initially powered by a 110hp engine, and had a cruising speed of 20 knots over water. In November 2010 it was re-engined with a new 135hp engine donated by MG Motor.
2003 The charity approached the RNLI to take over the ILB service, and on 23 December 2003 an Atlantic 75 and D class ILB entered service, operating from a site a short distance from the launch slipway. BARB refocused its service on hovercraft operations.
2006 To supplement the BBV-6 hovercraft, BARB introduced Light of Elizabeth in August. The four-seat BBV-4 craft was used for crew training and to reach sites on the River Parrett

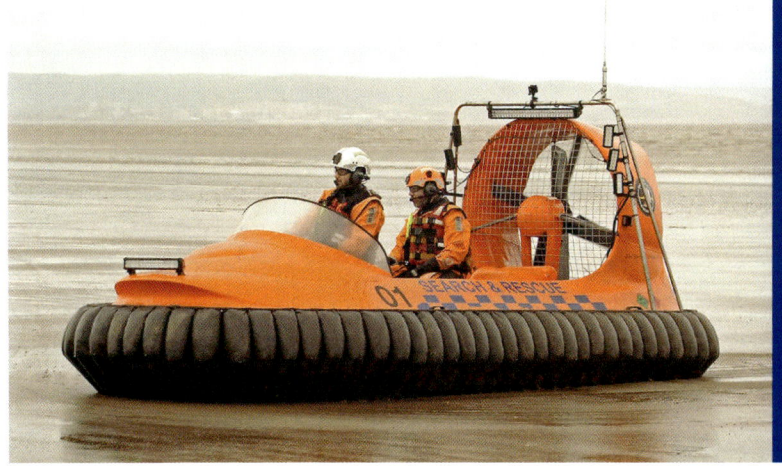

BARB01, one of the two BBV-5 type rescue hovercraft used to cover the extensive sandbanks at Burnham-on-Sea.

where the larger hovercraft could not operate.
2011 BARB introduced an inland water and flood rescue capability. One of the first rescue boats was a Zodiac inflatable, named Premila Ilsley, powered by a Mariner outboard. A new Rigilex Newmatic inshore rescue boat was acquired for rescues on lakes and rivers, and was named Seren in a ceremony in August.
2013 A new larger 5.2m Italian-designed hovercraft replaced Light of Elizabeth. It was funded by donations from local individuals and groups. Built by HTI, it had a 988cc four-stroke engine giving a top speed of 60mph.
2015 The inflatable was upgraded with a more powerful engine and new steering console. The Rigiflex boat was used during flooding on the

Somerset levels, crewed by BARB volunteers.
2017 BARB purchased two 3.8m Arancia inflatables, powered by 30hp Mariner outboard engines, for use by BARB Swift Water Team, and to support local wildlife charities with wildlife rescues on inland waters.
CURRENT ASSETS Two 5.25m x 2.5m BBV-5 type rescue hovercraft, named Spirit of Lelaina II and Light of Elizabeth II. A 13.5hp lift engine and 35hp thrust engine power the hovercraft, and a frame over the rear thrust fan carries lighting and VHF radio aerial. They are launched using road-going trailers, and two Isuzu Denver 4x4 vehicles are used to move the hovercraft across the sands. A Mercedes Vito crew cab van is used for a flood rescue service.

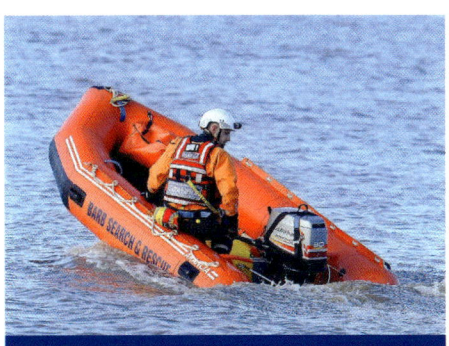

One of two Arancia IRBs operated by BARB as part of Surf Life Saving GB flood response capability

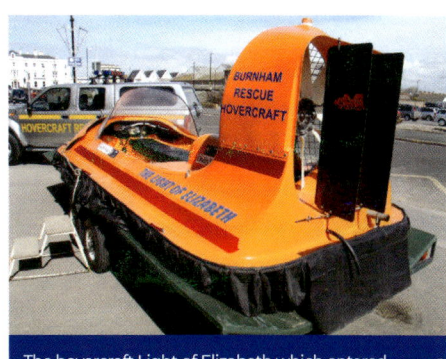

The hovercraft Light of Elizabeth which entered service in 2006. (By courtesy of BARB)

Independent lifeboats of Britain

SARA (Beachley) Somerset

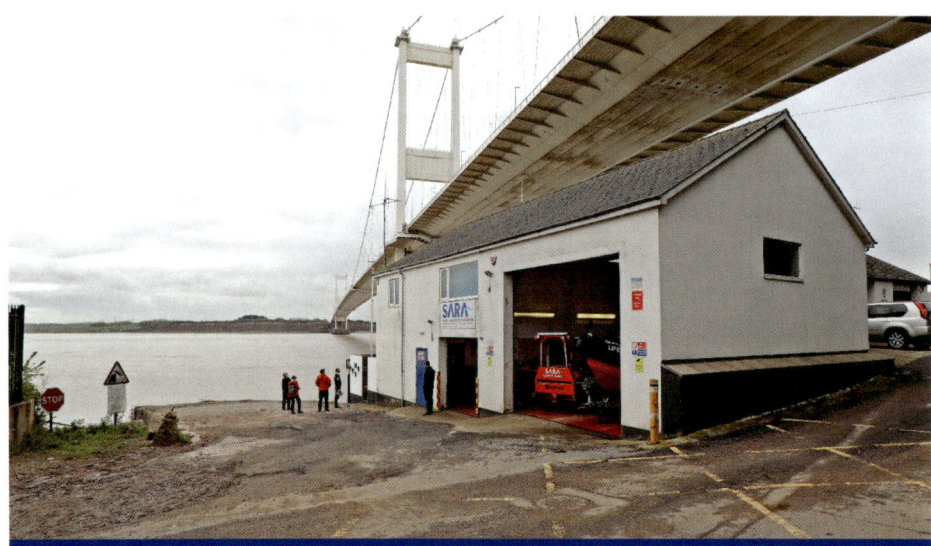

The boathouse at Beachley stands beneath the M48 motorway bridge. The ILBs are launched down the old ferry slipway.

LOCATION The Severn Estuary, including the tidal lengths of the rivers Wye and Usk
ORGANISATION Severn Area Rescue Association
ESTABLISHED 1973
HISTORY The Severn Area Rescue Association (SARA) is an inshore rescue boat and land search organisation covering the Severn Estuary and upper reaches of the river Severn, including the rivers Wye and Usk. It is multi-disciplinary organisation which operates three lifeboat stations with five lifeboats, as well as providing a range of inland search and rescue services, including both flood and cliff rescue,

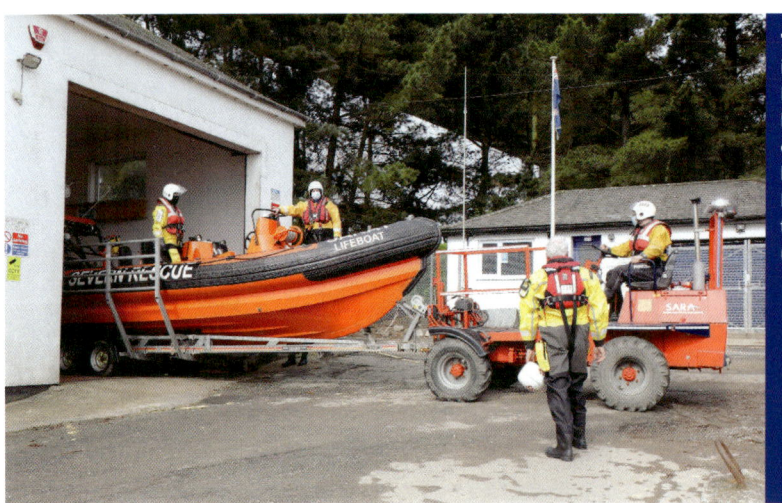

7m Delta rigid inflatable Jim Hewitt (SARA 1) being brought out of the boathouse at Beachley for a training exercise. (Nicholas Leach)

Independent lifeboats of Britain

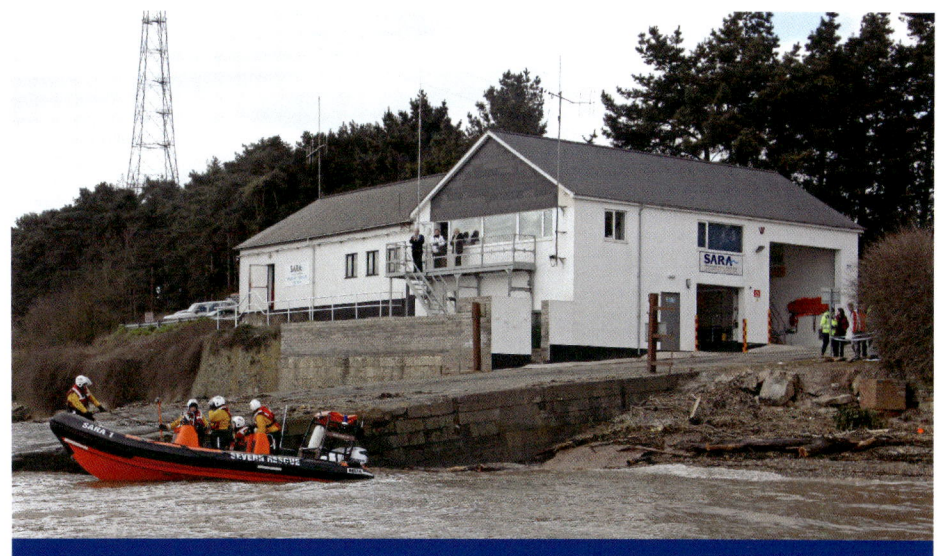

The rigid inflatable Joe Harris (SARA 1) alongside Beachley slipway, with the lifeboat station behind.

and all-terrain missing person searches. SARA is the largest independent lifeboat service in the UK, and, with 12 operational boats of varying sizes and approximately 220 personnel, all of whom are volunteers, as a sea rescue organisation is second only to the RNLI.

SARA was founded in 1973, with headquarters at Tutshill, close to the current Beachley station. In 1976 it became a registered charity and in 1977 purchased its first boat. In 1985 SARA became an official Mountain Rescue

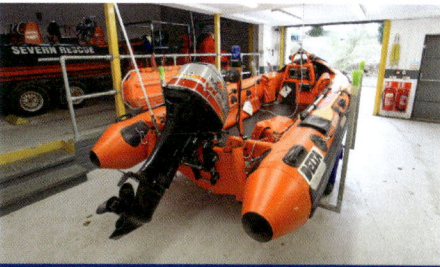

The rigid inflatable Swift and Bold (SARA 3) inside the boathouse at Beachley. (Nicholas Leach)

The Delta rigid inflatable Jim Hewitt (SARA 1) being launched into the River Severn at Beachley beneath the M48 motorway bridge. (Nicholas Leach)

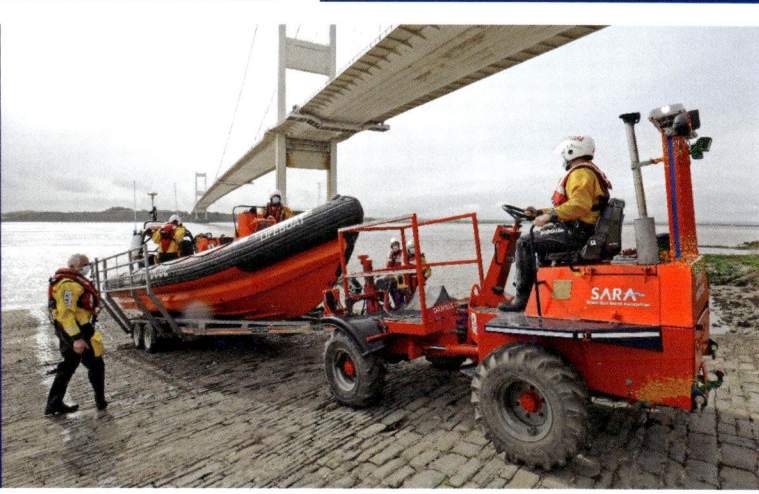

Independent lifeboats of Britain

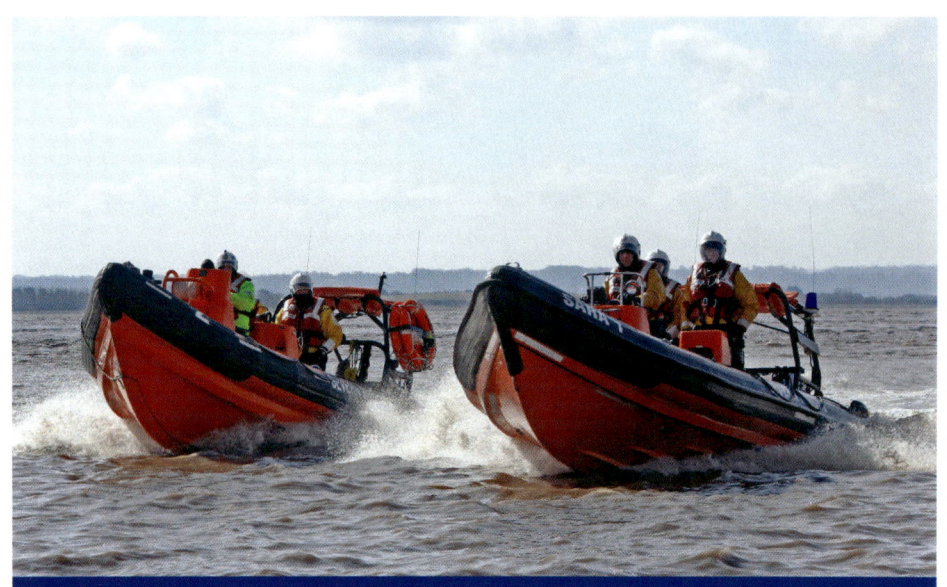

The rigid inflatables Joe Harris (SARA 1) and Dave Moore (SARA 2) together off Beachley in 2013. (Nicholas Leach)

Team, undertaking the role of cliff rescue for the Wye Valley. The organisation has operated from its primary station at Beachley since its founding, where a purpose-built boathouse beneath the M48 motorway bridge has been in use for much of that time.

SARA operates three lifeboat stations, at Sharpness in Gloucestershire, Beachley, near Chepstow in Monmouthshire, and Newport, and three inland flood rescue stations, at Tewkesbury, Wyre Forest, at Kidderminster, and Upton-upon-Severn. The operational

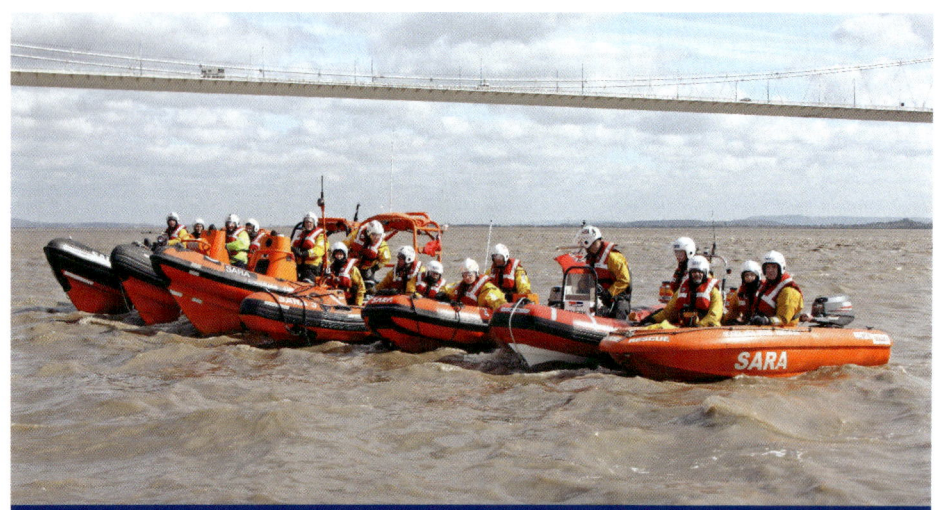

A line-up of seven of SARA's rescue craft in the river Severn off Beachley. From front to back: SARA 5, Beachley flood boat; SARA 16, Tewkesbury flood boat; SARA 4 from Sharpness; SARA 3 from Beachley; SARA 6 from Sharpness; SARA 2 from Sharpness; and SARA 1 from Beachley. (Nicholas Leach)

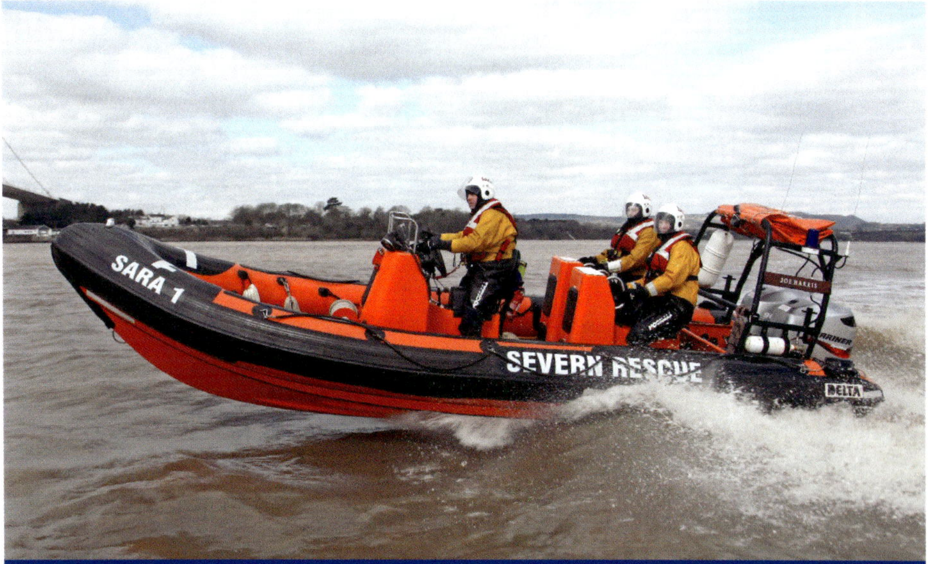

The 7m Delta rigid inflatable Joe Harris (SARA 1) on exercise off Beachley. (Nicholas Leach)

area for these stations includes large parts of the upper Severn estuary, as well as the rivers Severn, Wye, Avon and Usk. SARA is the designated rescue service for these areas. During flooding and other similar events, SARA personnel and equipment has often operated away from its core area to provide assistance when requested. SARA has six flood rescue teams dedicated to National Resilience.

BEACHLEY The first SARA lifeboat station was established at Beachley in 1973, and was located on a site beneath the Severn Crossing motorway bridge, on the eastern side of the estuary. In 1998 SARA acquired a 7m Delta X-Craft rigid inflatable, powered by twin 90hp outboards, named Joe Harris (SARA 1) and funded by local donations, for service at Beachley. An additional building was added to the original station in 2010, with a new boathall for the station's two lifeboats, as well as incorporating better crew facilities, an operations room and a training room. In 2015 SARA acquired the current SARA 1 through the first annual grant from the Department for Transport Rescue Boat Grant. The £200,000 boat was formally named at a ceremony on 17

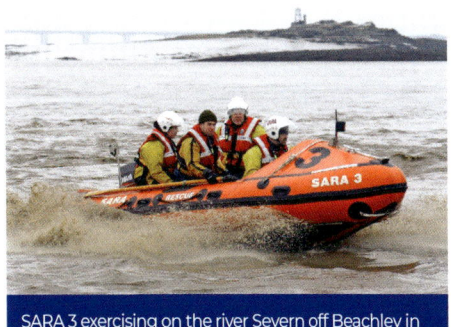

SARA 3 exercising on the river Severn off Beachley in March 2006. (Nicholas Leach)

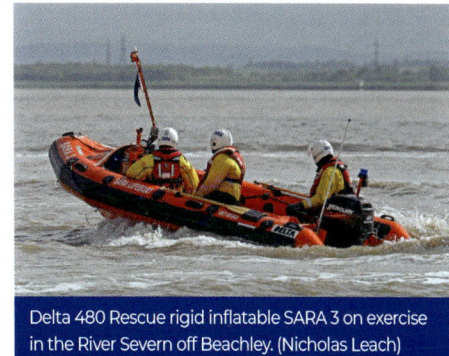

Delta 480 Rescue rigid inflatable SARA 3 on exercise in the River Severn off Beachley. (Nicholas Leach)

Independent lifeboats of Britain

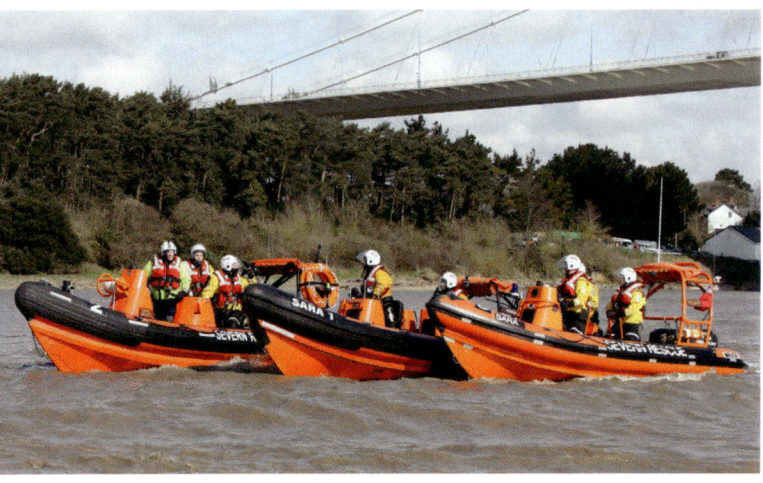

SARA lifeboats Dave Moore (then SARA 2, current SARA 6), Joe Harris (then SARA 1) and Marion Shaw (then SARA 6) together on the Severn, off Beachley in 2013. (Nicholas Leach)

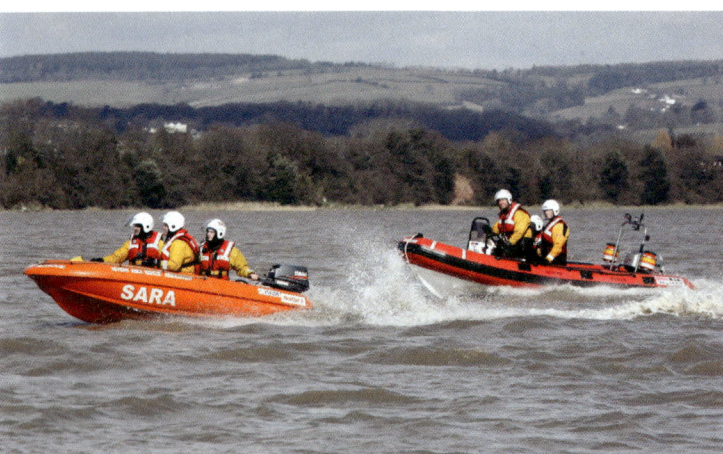

SARA flood response craft: the red Valiant RIB is based at Tewkesbury for inland and flood work (the SARA Station is housed in Gloucestershire Fire and Rescue flood response station); the plastic boat is one of four Rigiflex 360/400 craft, one stationed at each station specifically for flood work.

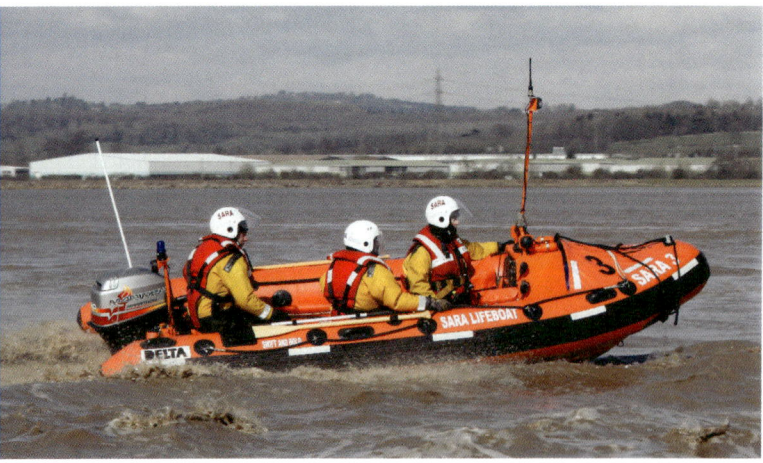

The small rigid inflatable Swift and Bold (SARA 3) on exercise in the river Severn.

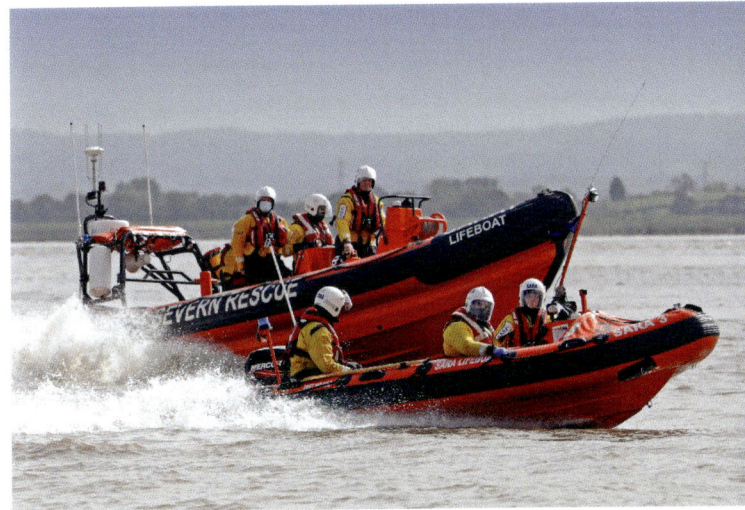

The Delta lifeboat Jim Hewitt (SARA 1) and Swift and Bold (SARA 3) in the River Severn together off Beachley, May 2021. SARA lifeboats are tasked to incidents in the dangerous waters of the Severn, which has one of the highest tidal ranges of anywhere in the world. (Nicholas Leach)

October 2015, being christened Jim Hewitt after the primary founder of SARA more than 40 years previously. The 8m Delta rigid inflatable is powered by twin 150hp outboard engines, giving a top speed of over 40 knots. The lifeboats are launched by a bespoke launch tractor, converted by volunteers in the SARA team.

CURRENT ASSETS Delta 800X rigid inflatable, named Jim Hewitt (SARA 1), launched by Benford launch vehicle and carriage, on station 2015; 5m Delta 480 Rescue rigid inflatable with single 40hp Mariner outboard, named Swift and Bold (SARA 3), funded by local donations and named for the motto of the Rifles Regiment which is based at Beachley Barracks, launched by trailer, on station 2011; Rigiflex 360, built by Rigiflex Boats, UK, named Rescue 5, launched by trailer.

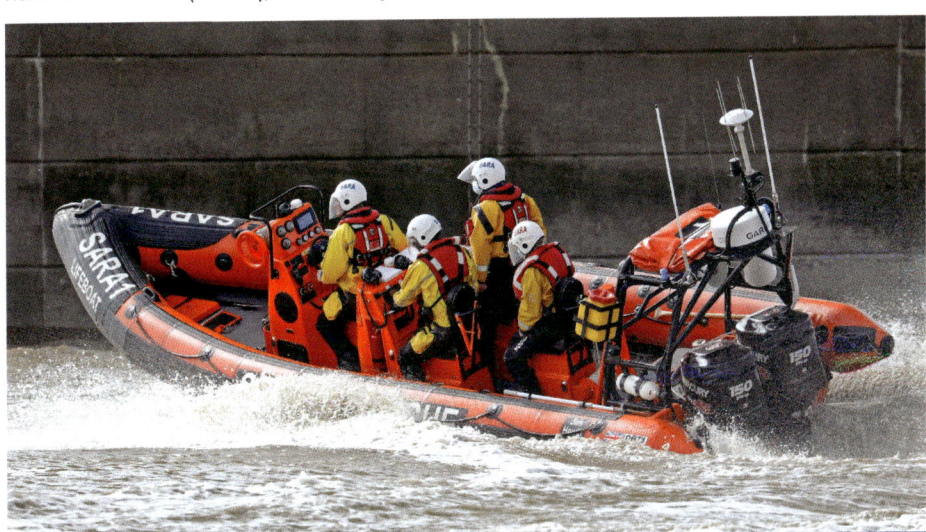

The Delta lifeboat Jim Hewitt (SARA 1) on exercise off Beachley. Funded by a grant from the Department of Transport, she was built by Delta Power Group of Cheshire to SARA's own design. (Nicholas Leach)

Independent lifeboats of Britain

SARA (Sharpness)

River Severn

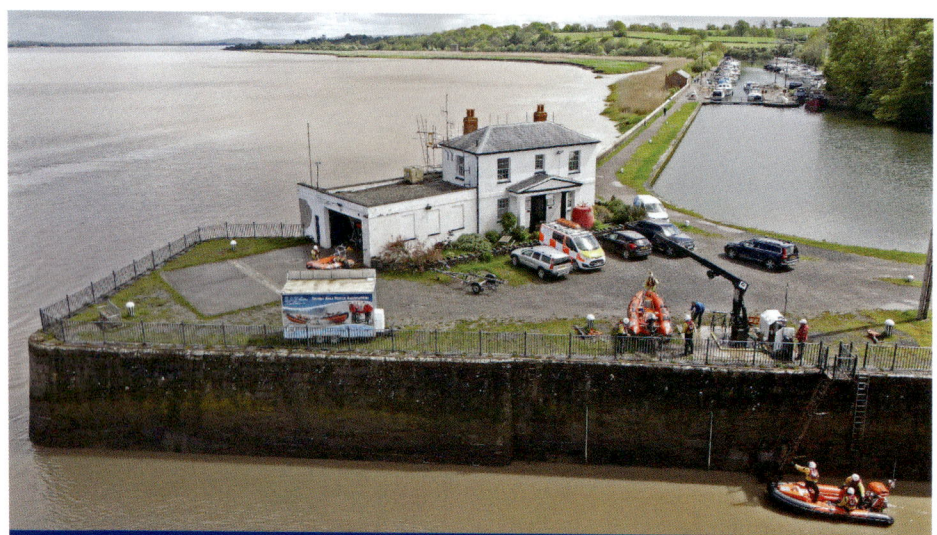

The Old Dock House at Sharpness is home to the SARA operation on the south bank of the river. (Nicholas Leach)

LOCATION The Severn Estuary, including the tidal lengths of the rivers Wye and Usk
ORGANISATION Severn Area Rescue Association
ESTABLISHED 1984
HISTORY A lifeboat station at Sharpness was established in 1984 in response to two incidents in which four people died: a family of three and a young man lost their lives within the space of a short time, prompting the opening of the station as the Beachley lifeboat could not get to the area as fast as was needed. The new station started working from portacabins and subsequently used the Old Dock House as a shore facility. A dedicated boathouse was added to this building, on the river side, with space for two boats and launch vehicles. An old crane on the quayside was used to launch the boats into the river; this was replaced in 2013 by a purpose-built davit, which was safer and more powerful.
PREVIOUS ASSETS
2008 A larger craft was needed at Sharpness, which could cope better with the speed and strength of the tides in the Severn, as well as deal with an increasing number of larger leisure boats that were using the river. A new boathouse and slipway were built at Sharpness Point, with a launch directly into the river, to accommodate the larger craft. SARA 6 was initially moved into this building, and stayed there until 2012, when the new and

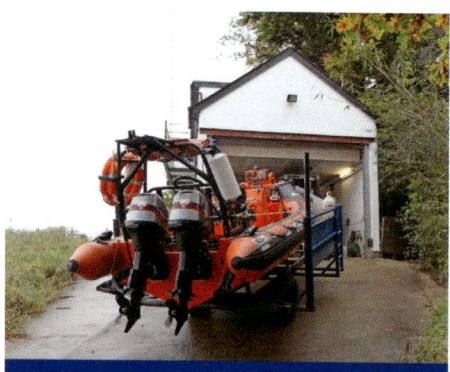

The 7m Delta rigid inflatable Dave Moore (SARA 2) on her trolley outside the boathouse at Sharpness Point.

Independent lifeboats of Britain

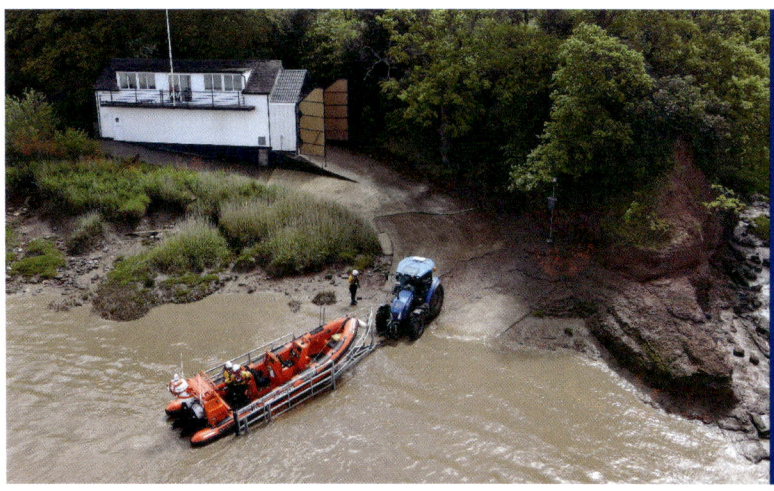

The boathouse at Sharpness Point built in 2008 with a launchway directly into the Severn. It was extended in 2019 to accommodate the new SARA2 lifeboat, which is being recovered. (Nicholas Leach)

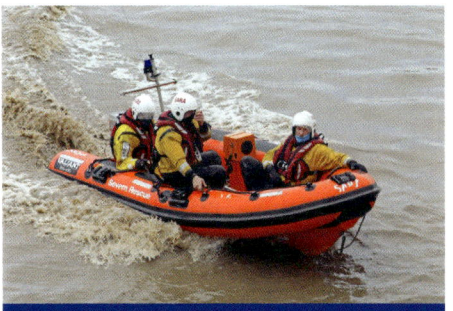

SARA 15 off Sharpness; she and the smaller Zodiac SARA 12 move between Sharpness and Gloucester.

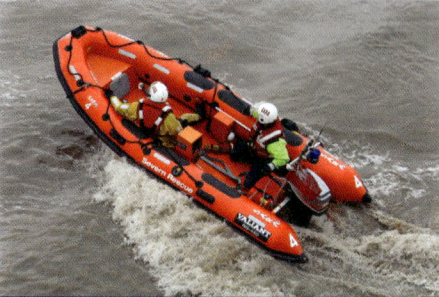

Alan Bibby (SARA 4) exercising on the River Severn near the Sharpness station.

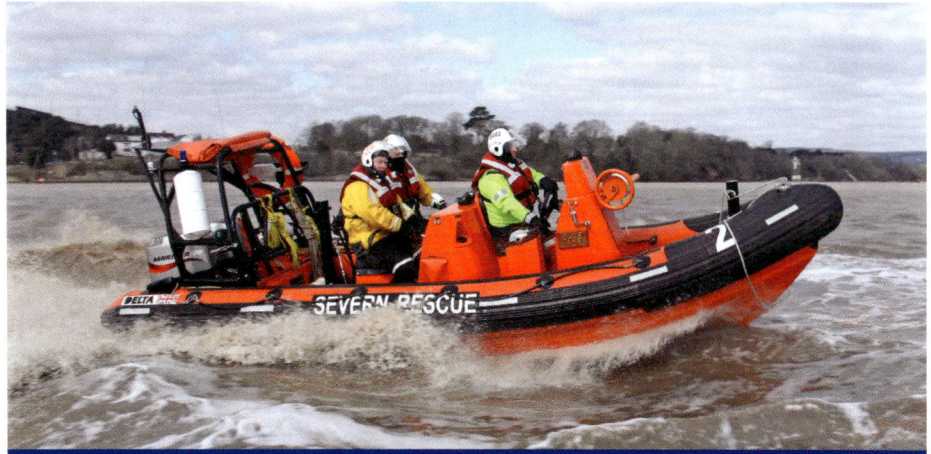

The 7m Delta rigid inflatable Dave Moore (SARA 2), which served at Sharpness until 2019, in the River Severn. In 2019 she was rebadged SARA 6, and became the service's training/reserve lifeboat.

Independent lifeboats of Britain

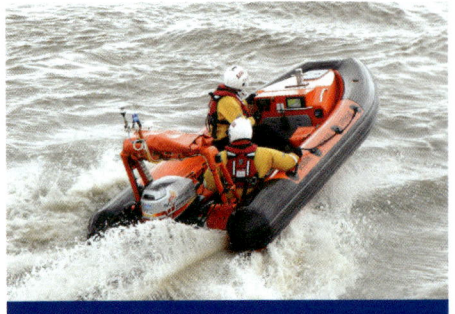

SARA 4 on exercise off Sharpness in May 2021. (Nicholas Leach)

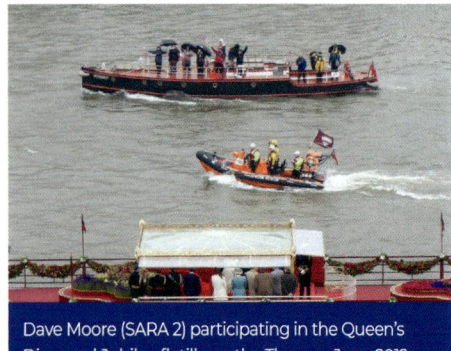

Dave Moore (SARA 2) participating in the Queen's Diamond Jubilee flotilla on the Thames, June 2012.

larger rigid inflatable was purchased.
2010 SARA celebrated the 25th anniversary of the opening of the Sharpness station and a special open day was held on 15 August. The event included lifeboat station tours and demonstrations, a sponsored swim by the crew, a barbecue and cake stall, and dinghy sailing. Work on the second boathouse at Sharpness was completed to coincide with the anniversary. The stations average about 120 services a year, helping a wide range of casualties, including yachts, jet skis and motor vessels which get damaged going aground, and people getting cut off by the tide.
2012 The new lifeboat was officially blessed and named Dave Moore, after a former coxswain who died in 2003 and left a legacy to the charity. The £137,000 Delta 6.5X craft also took part in the Queen's Diamond Jubilee flotilla on the river Thames on 3 June.
2014 In November Gloucestershire Fire and Rescue Service donated a hovercraft to SARA for use at Sharpness.
2019 A new aluminium-hulled lifeboat was built for SARA by Highfield Boats, the UK representative of Hendy Marine, with help

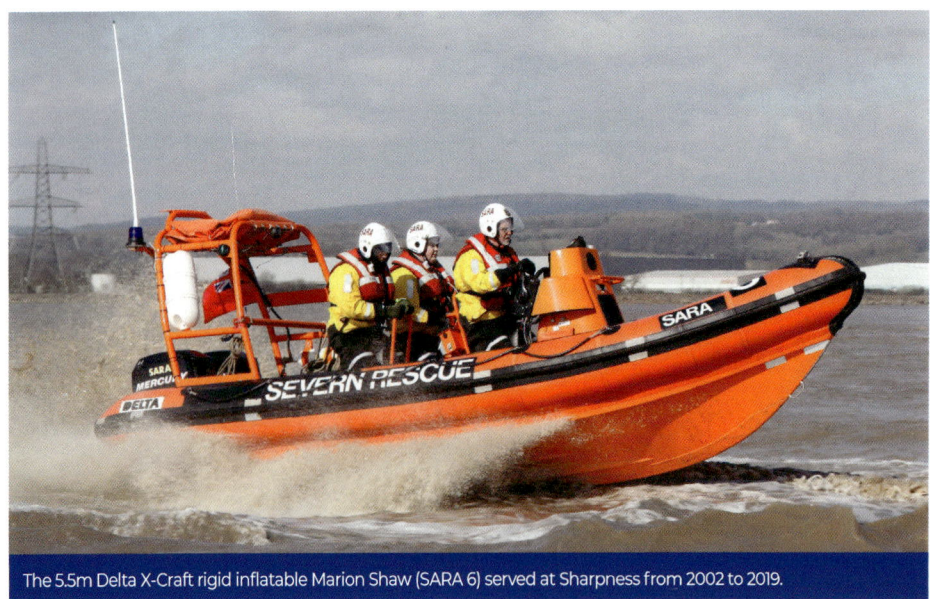

The 5.5m Delta X-Craft rigid inflatable Marion Shaw (SARA 6) served at Sharpness from 2002 to 2019.

Independent lifeboats of Britain

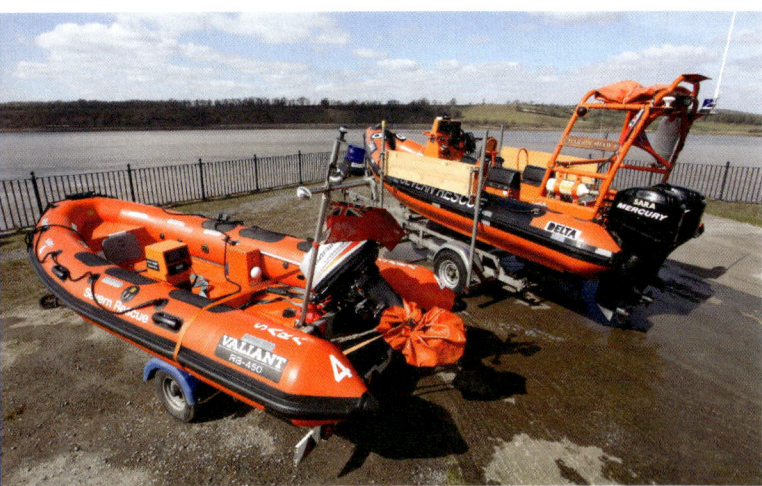

Marion Shaw (SARA 6) and Alan Bibby (SARA 4) on their respective trailers outside the boathouse at Sharpness, which is part of the Old Dock House. SARA 6 was taken out of service in 2019.

from Vortec Systems, a bespoke design company, and the RNLI. Due to the vagaries of the Severn, with its steep short wave patterns, rapid tidal flows, and massive standing waves, the hull needed to be strong and seaworthy. The hull had a very high sheer bow and double skin thick stem and keel area, with reverse chines to give extra lift and a softer ride. Ullman Biskaya hydraulic seats were fitted for crew. Power came from twin 115hp counter rotating Mariner XLS four-stroke outboards, fitted with a Barrus PIRS system.

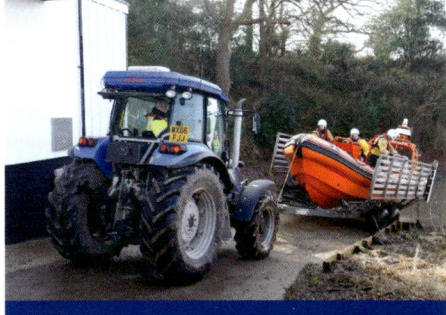

The 2018-built Pride of Sharpness being recovered at Sharpness after her naming ceremony, February 2019.

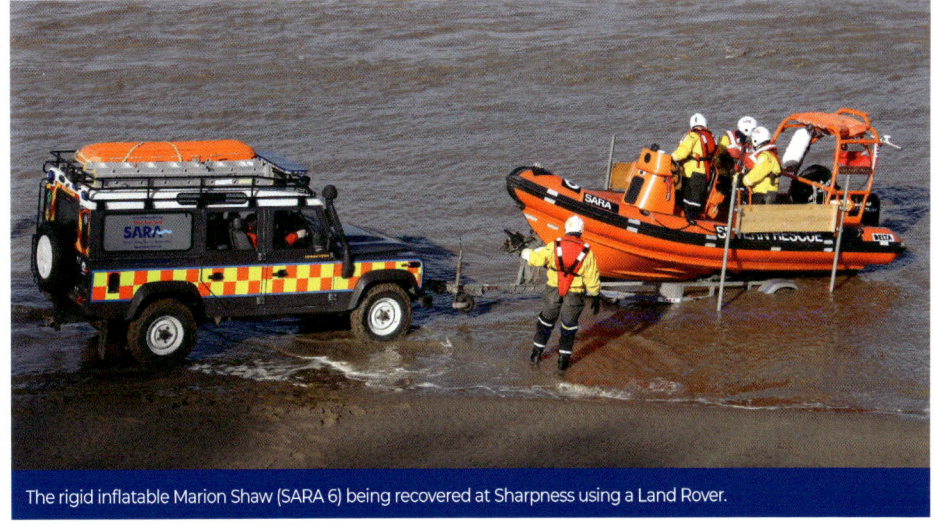

The rigid inflatable Marion Shaw (SARA 6) being recovered at Sharpness using a Land Rover.

Independent lifeboats of Britain

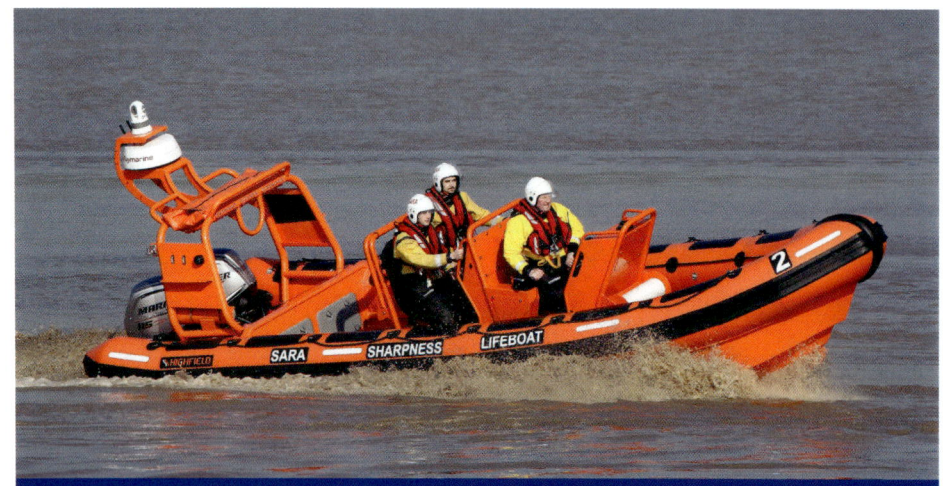

The 2018-built Pride of Sharpness at sea after her naming and dedication ceremony at Sharpness on 23 February 2019. The lifeboat, specially designed for SARA, has a crew of three, with a fourth removable Biskaya seat. Funding for the lifeboat came from the Department of Transport grant fund, and funds for the infrastructure were donated by the Masons, Rotary Clubs and other business supporters. (Nicholas Leach)

CURRENT ASSETS Highfield Ocean Master 460 rigid inflatable, named Pride of Sharpness (SARA 2), launch by New Holland T5.105 tractor and carriage, on station 2019; 7m Delta X-Craft rigid inflatable, twin 90hp outboards, named Dave Moore, built 2012, legacy of Dave Moore (former Coxswain), together with local donations and fund-raising events, on station 7.2012, launched by tractor and trolley; Highfield rigid inflatable, named Norman & Amy Watkins (SARA 4), launch by trailer/davit, on station 2015; Rescue Association SARA 12; Highfield Flood Boat (grey); Hi Tech International HTI-425 hovercraft (ex-Gloucestershire Fire & Rescue Service – 2008), launch by trailer, on station 2014.

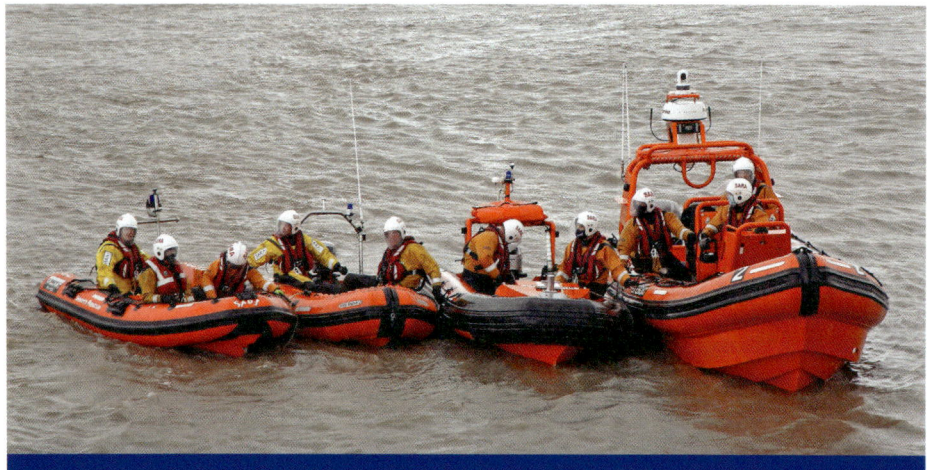

The SARA lifeboats based at Sharpness, from left to right, SARA 15, SARA 12, SARA 4 and SARA 2, line up in the River Severn off their base during a routine training exercise, May 2021. (Nicholas Leach)

Independent lifeboats of Britain

SARA stations — Somerset

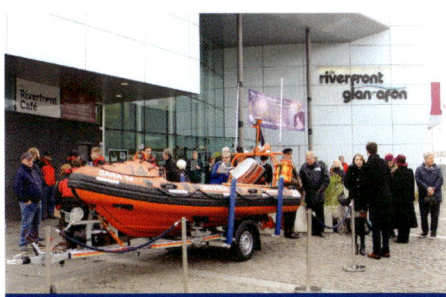

SARA 14 Maureen Easton at her dedication ceremony on 22 October 2016. (Supplied by SARA)

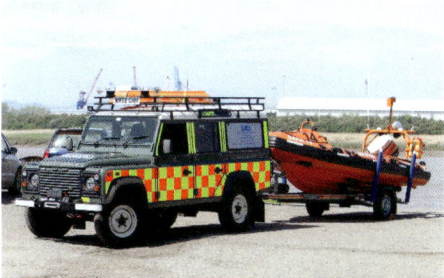

Newport's Mobile 20 Land Rover and SARA 14 at the Uskmouth launch site. (Supplied by SARA)

Newport

LOCATION Newport, South Wales
ESTABLISHED 2015 as a base, became a full SARA lifeboat station in 2019
HISTORY The SARA Newport Lifeboat Station is based in the Malpas Fire and Rescue station, on the north side of Newport city. The station is home to the Gwent lifeboat Maureen Easton (SARA 14) and a rigid flood boat SARA Rescue 20, a Rigiflex 400 fitted with navigation lights. One of the Swift Water Rescue Teams that specialise in technical water and flood rescue is also based at Newport. The station has a Land Rover, Mobile 20, which is used to deploy the team and the boats. The lifeboat is usually launched at Uskmouth. In October 2014 a Rescue Equipment Hub was established within the Newport city area for lifeboat, swift water or flood emergencies and incidents on the Rivers Usk, Ebbw and Afon Llwyd.

The Team has been located in the Malpas Fire and Rescue station since 2014, and they maintain a strong working relationship with South Wales Fire & Rescue Service, which provided room to expand the SARA rescue capability. SARA 14 was launched in October 2016, funded through a substantial bequest from the estate of the late Ms Maureen Easton, who lived in the West Midlands and holidayed in the Newport area. The donation also enabled a new vehicle (Mobile 20) to be purchased, and provided funds to cover general running costs.

SARA (inland rescue)

OVERVIEW Inland search and rescue crew are trained to Swiftwater and Flood Rescue Technician (SRT) and Swiftwater and Flood Rescue Boat Operator (SFRBO) standards, and regularly support local communities in areas which are frequently at risk of flooding.

WYRE FOREST In June 2005 a new station was opened at Upper Arley in the Wyre Forest. SARA Wyre Forest operates in the largest geographical area of the four stations, covering Shropshire, Worcestershire and parts of Herefordshire and the West Midlands county. SARA Wyre Forest operates three rescue boats, a 4x4 vehicle and a road ambulance, as well as housing the organisation's Incident Command Unit. Its assets consist of: SARA 9, Pioneer Double-walled Polyethylene craft, on station 2009; SARA 10, Eurocraft Inflatable; Whaly 435R Professional, SARA 26, named Stuart Frost, on station 2016; Pioneer Multi SARA 8 (on long-term loan from Hereford and Worcester Fire & Rescue Service), on station 2019; FC470 Inflatable (on long-term loan from Hereford

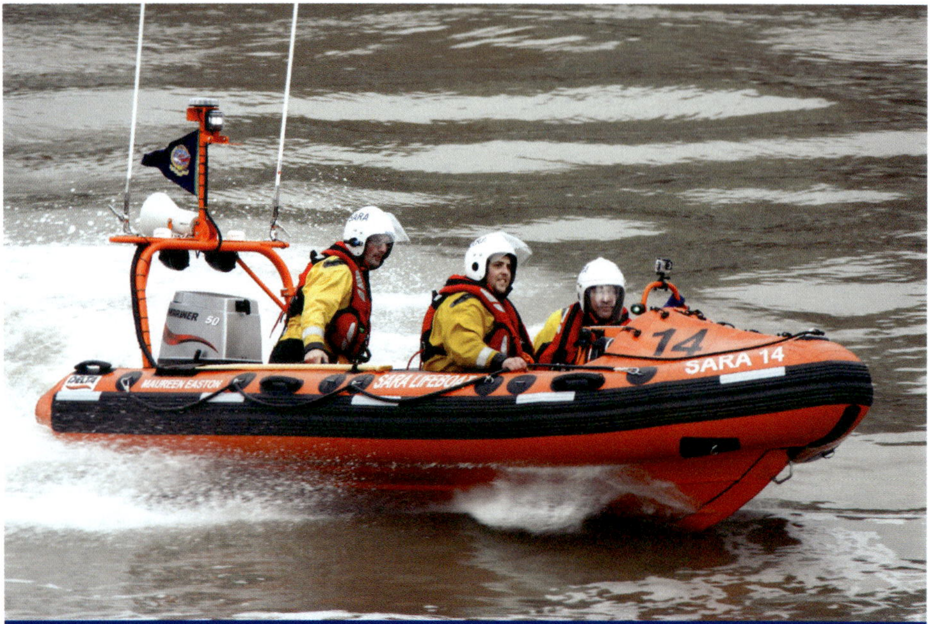

Maureen Easton (SARA 14) has been in service at Newport since 2016. (Martin Fish)

and Worcester Fire & Rescue Service), on station 2019; all launched by trailer.

UPTON-UPON-SEVERN A new station at Upton was opened on 1 January 2020, as an acquisition of the former WEIR Team. The station is home to the office complex, kit room for PPE, SRT equipment, three rescue sleds and four rescue boats: Rescue 21, a 3.4m Zodiac 0340; Rescue 22, a modified 3.6m Rescue Runner; Rescue 23, a 4m rugged Poly Fusion; Rescue 24, a 5.3m console Pioneer Multi; and Mobile 14, a modified Land Rover Defender 110.

TEWKESBURY The SARA station at Tewkesbury was established in 2007. The volunteer search and rescue team is based at the town's Fire and Rescue Station, embedded with Gloucestershire Fire Service, but funded solely by public donations. The station has the following assets: Zodiac Milpro Grand Raid Inflatable SARA 16; Rigiflex 360; Rigiflex 400; all launched by trailer; two Land Rovers for launching the boats and a twin-cab van.

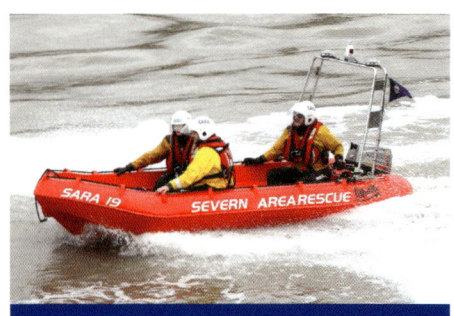

SARA 19 is based at Newport, which became a full SARA lifeboat station in 2019. (Martin Fish)

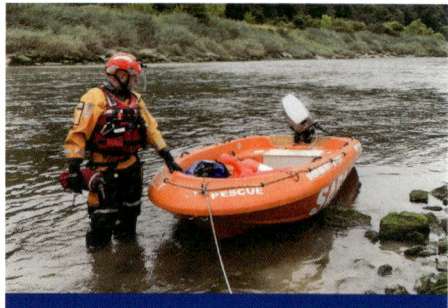

Rescue 5 at Tintern on the Wye at low water. (By courtesy of SARA)

Independent lifeboats of Britain

LOUGHOR
Glamorgan

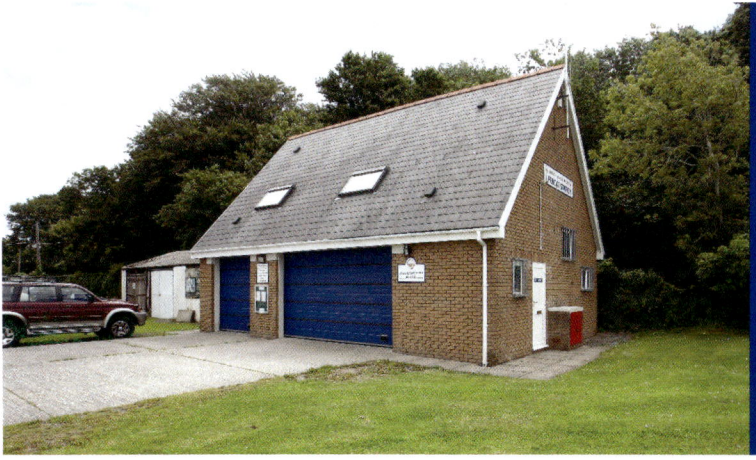

The lifeboat station at Loughor on the east bank of the River Loughor, to the north of the A484 main road. (Nicholas Leach)

LOCATION Glamorgan, South Wales
ORGANISATION Loughor Inshore Rescue
ESTABLISHED 1969
HISTORY The Loughor estuary, with a great tidal range, is notorious for its fast flowing river, shifting sandbanks and dangerous currents. In early 1969 a small boy tragically drowned near the railway bridge and local people realised that a rescue service was needed. Wilf Pitman, a member of the local St John Ambulance, called a meeting, and the outcome was the formation of the Loughor Rescue Service.

PREVIOUS ASSETS
1969 The service started with a second-hand 12ft flat-bottomed inflatable boat driven by a second-hand 25hp outboard motor, donated by neighbouring Ferryside Rescue Service.
1973 Using money raised locally and significant help from Avon Inflatables, a 4m rigid inflatable boat with a 40hp outboard was purchased. This was much faster than the original boat, and safer for the crew.
1977 A 5.4m Sea Rider rigid inflatable was purchased with a centre console and 70hp

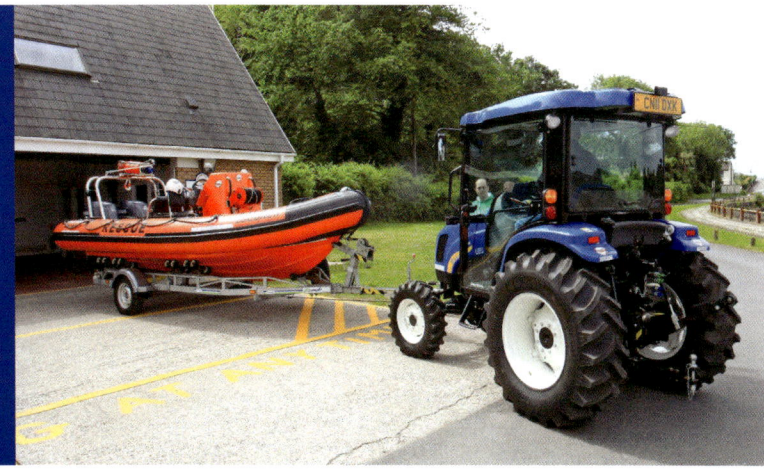

The inshore lifeboat outside the lifeboat house on its trailer, with the launch vehicle, in May 2011. (Nicholas Leach)

Independent lifeboats of Britain

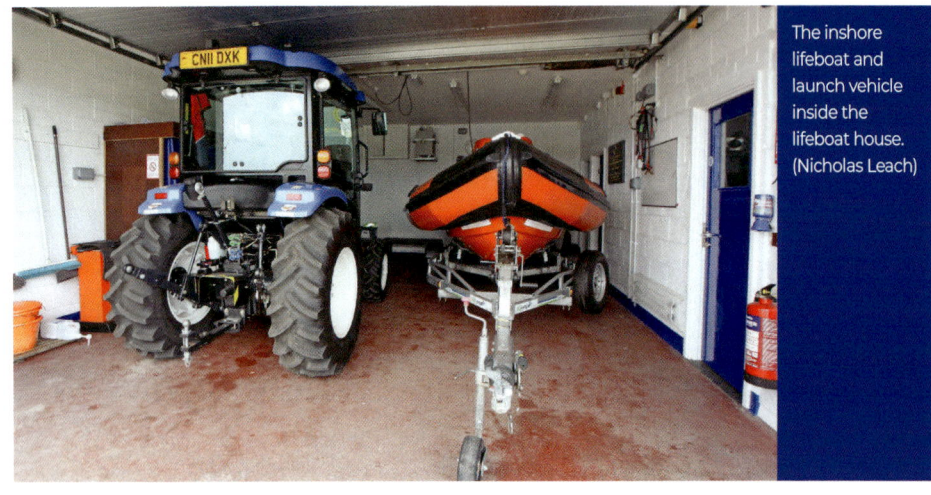

The inshore lifeboat and launch vehicle inside the lifeboat house. (Nicholas Leach)

outboard. The new boat was much bigger and faster than the boat replaced, and increased the operational capability of the service.
1988 After considerable fund-raising, and again with help from Avon Inflatables, a purpose-built 5.4m twin-engined lifeboat was purchased, and was named Community Spirit (18-01).
1998 In August Community Spirit was replaced by Community Spirit II (18-02), another 5.4m Avon Searider, made with orange fabric. The communication and navigation equipment were updated and the centre console modified.
2009 A new 5.85m rigid inflatable was built by Ribcraft, Yeovil. Powered by twin 60hp outboard engines, it had a top speed of 40 knots and carried the latest communication and satellite navigation equipment.

2020 In addition to the main ILB, a Zodiac Emergency Response Boat powered by a Yamaha 25hp outboard engine is used for shallow water response.
2022 A new inshore rescue hovercraft came into service. Initial evaluations started in 2018 when manufacturer BBV Hovercraft brought a demonstration craft to the estuary for trials. The Service subsequently purchased a new craft from BBV which was designated LH01. Following a period of crew training after the craft arrived in 2021, the hovercraft was formally launched at a ceremony in June 2022.
CURRENT ASSETS Ribcraft 5.85m Professional, launched by New Holland 3040 tractor and trailer, on station 2009; Zodiac ERB; hovercraft, on station 2020.

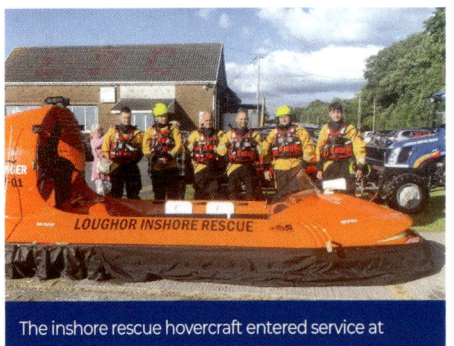

The inshore rescue hovercraft entered service at Loughor in 2022. (By courtesy of Loughor IR)

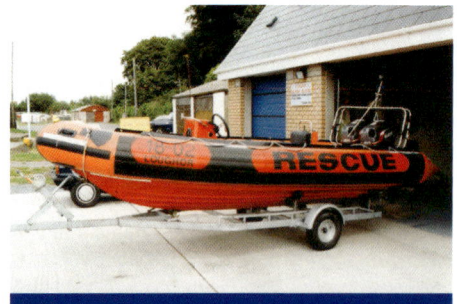

The 1998-built Avon Searider Community Spirit II (18-02) outside the boathouse. (Martin Fish)

FERRYSIDE   Glamorgan

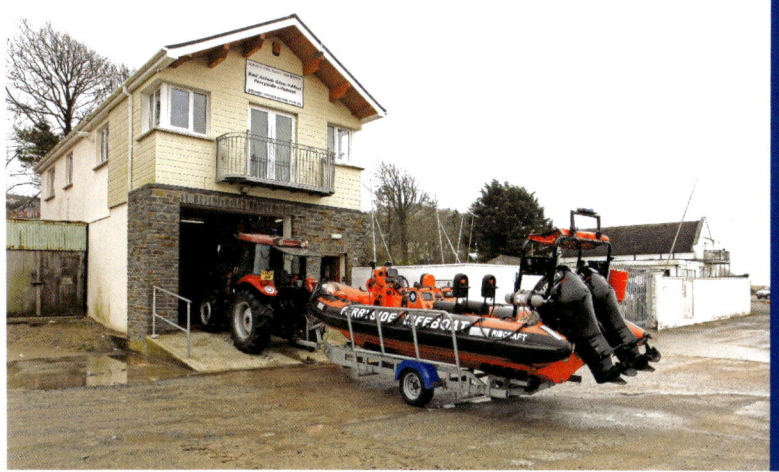

The boathouse on Ferryside foreshore, built in 2009-10, pictured in 2013 with The Freemason outside on her trailer. The old lifeboat house used by the RNLI can be seen in the background at the right. (Nicholas Leach)

LOCATION Carmarthenshire, South Wales
ORGANISATION Ferryside Lifeboat
ESTABLISHED 1966
HISTORY The RNLI operated a lifeboat at Ferryside from 1860 to 1960, with a motor lifeboat in service from 1941. With the demise of commercial shipping in the river Towy, however, the need for a lifeboat diminished and the station was closed. However, an increase in leisure activity during the 1960s resulted in the beach patrol expanding to form a lifeboat service, organised by members of the Llanelli division of St John Ambulance, Cymru. In 1966 a number of cadets began to provide a beach patrol service. This was soon extended to providing assistance on the water using a small inflatable boat, donated by Avon Inflatables Ltd from their recently opened Llanelli factory. Operations began in a small building, but a new boathouse was built on the foreshore at Ferryside in 2009-10 with improved facilities. This was opened by HRH The Duchess of Gloucester at a ceremony on 30 March 2010.

PREVIOUS ASSETS
1998 A new Narwhal rigid inflatable boat, powered by twin Mariner 50hp engines, was purchased; it was named Blundell after the benefactor of the service. A Nuffield tractor was used for launching and recovery.
2001 A Ribcraft-built 5.85m Professional Series rigid inflatable, with twin 60hp Mariner outboards and a righting airbag on a roll

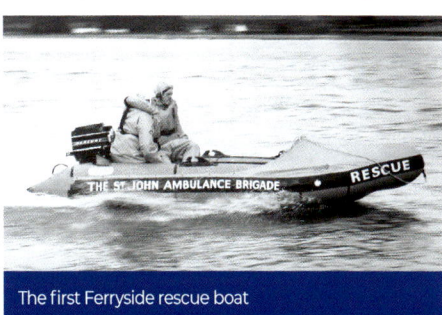
The first Ferryside rescue boat

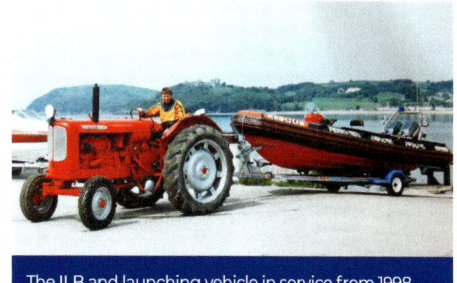
The ILB and launching vehicle in service from 1998.

Independent lifeboats of Britain   103

bar, was acquired. The lifeboat was named Blundell, being officially dedicated at a naming ceremony on 1 September 2012.
2011 A new lifeboat built by Ribcraft Ltd was delivered. It was equipped with a righting system and was powered by two Suzuki 90hp outboard engines. The £80,000 cost was largely met by a donation of £50,000 from the Freemasons.
2017 A UK government grant was used to purchase a small Vortex Services twin-engined Mistral inshore rescue hovercraft, modified for search and rescue. The hovercraft is kept on a launching trailer in a small building next to the lifeboat station. The former RNLI Talus MB-H launching tractor T112 was also acquired.
2019 A new Zodiac Milpro ZMSR 380 inshore rescue boat was obtained to replace an earlier Avon inflatable. The smaller Zodiac complements the main lifeboat and provides capabilities for shallow water rescues.
CURRENT ASSETS Ribcraft 6.4m Professional, named The Freemason, launched by Talus MBH (T112) tractor, on station 2011; Vortex Services Mistrel R hovercraft, launched by trailer, on station 2017; Zodiac Milpro ZMSR 380, launched by trailer, on station 2019.

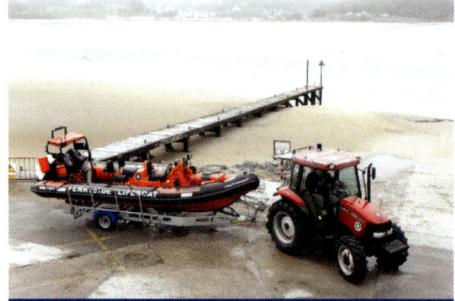

The Ribcraft rigid inflatable The Freemason on her trailer outside the lifeboat house. The boat covers the River Towy estuary and, as with all lifeboats operating in the Bristol Channel, the volunteer crew have to cope with a large tidal range. (Nicholas Leach)

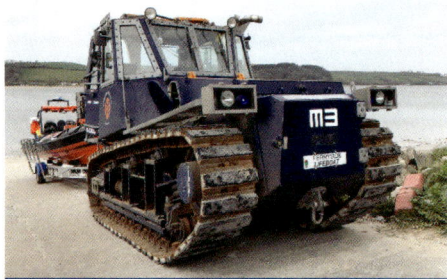

Talus MB-H tractor (ex-T112) served at Anstruther during her RNLI career before coming to Ferryside.

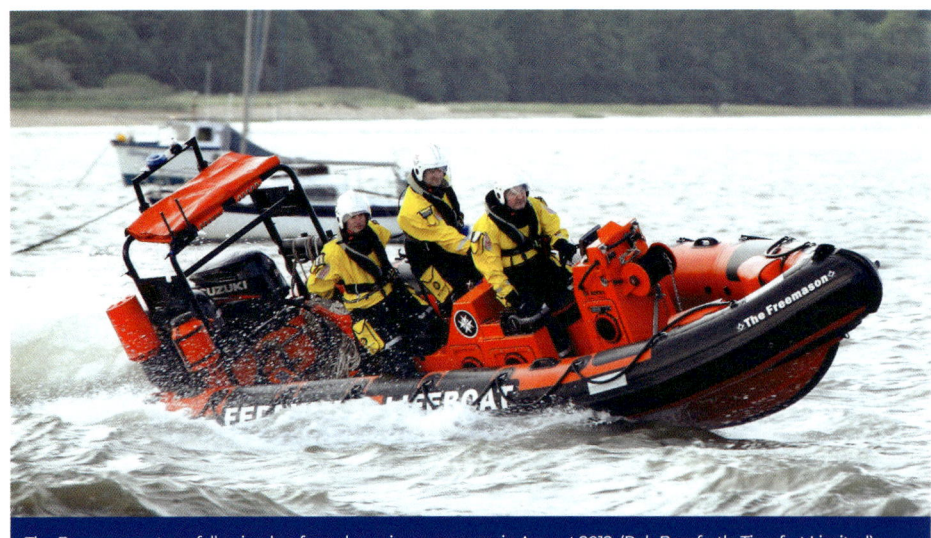

The Freemason at sea following her formal naming ceremony in August 2012. (Rob Bamforth, Timefort Limited)

ENGLAND NORTH WEST

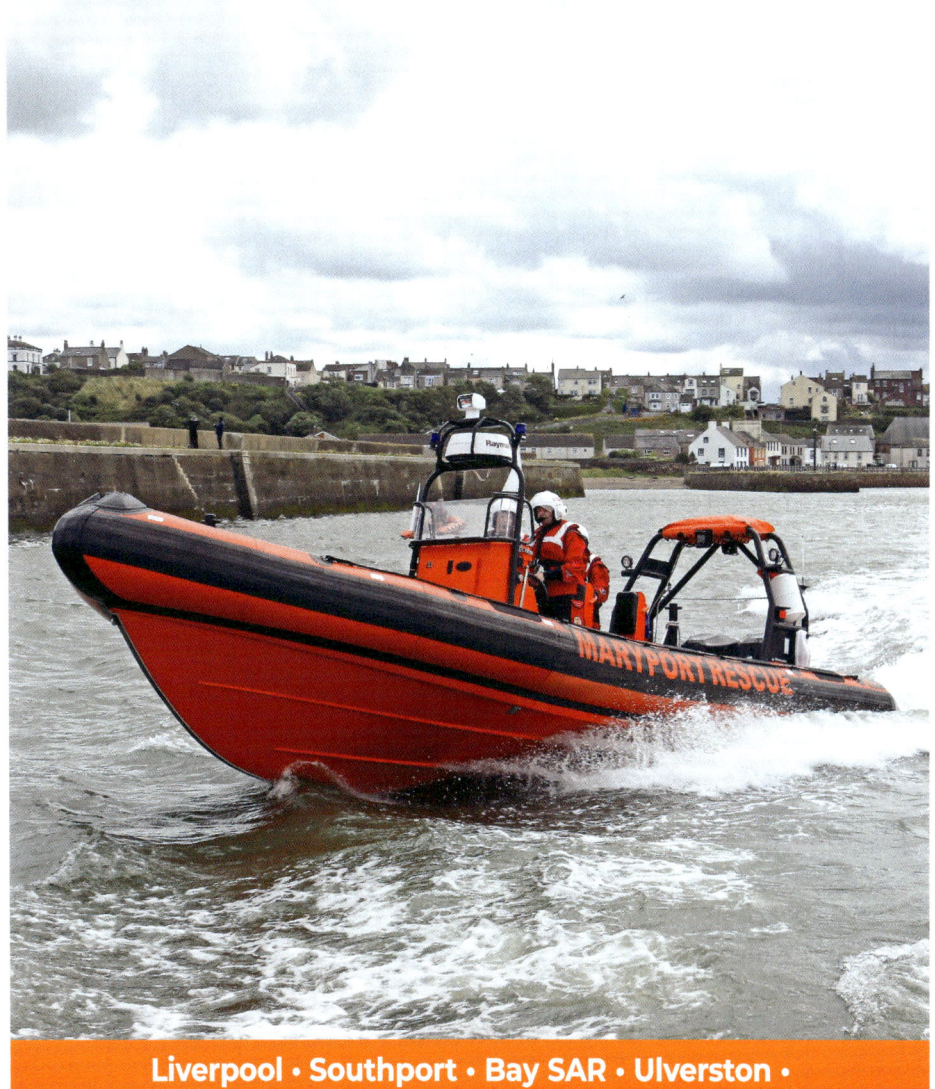

Liverpool • Southport • Bay SAR • Ulverston • Duddon • Haverigg • Maryport

LIVERPOOL — Merseyside

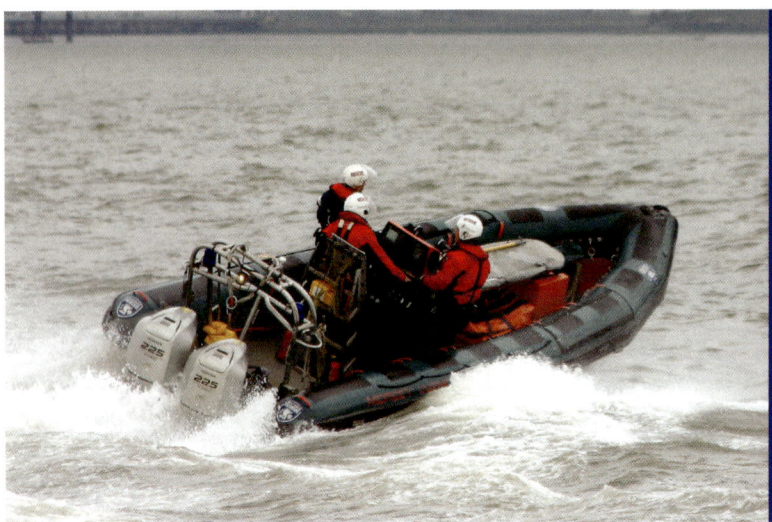

The Avon rescue boat on exercise in 2005. Introduced in 1986 this boat was modified during its years in service and is seen here in its final configuration with Honda outboard engines and the console near the stern of the craft. (Martin Fish)

LOCATION Liverpool
ORGANISATION Merseyside Fire & Rescue Service Marine Rescue Unit (MFRS MRU)
ESTABLISHED 1984
HISTORY The rescue service at Liverpool can trace its roots back to 1984, when the city hosted the International Garden Festival. As the event bordered the banks of the Mersey, organisers established a temporary rescue boat for the duration of the festival. The boat carried out many rescues, so it was decided it should become a permanent service. Established as the Mersey Inshore Rescue Service, it was the only full-time unit working on a river in the UK at the time. In addition to assisting vessels and people in the river, the charity was ready to respond to any aviation incidents arising at the adjacent Liverpool Airport.

The base for the Marine Rescue Unit Service is Pier Head on the Liverpool

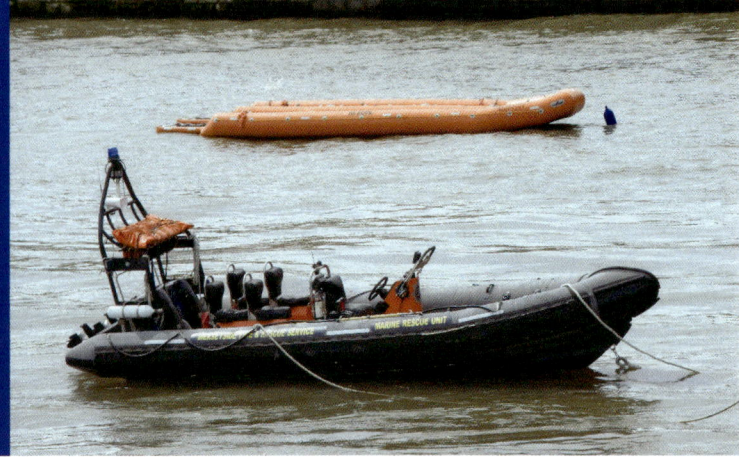

The lifeboat moored off Woodside ferry terminal in 2007 following the sinking of the Pier Head landing stage. In the background is one of the slide raft inflatables to be used in the event of a mass casualty evacuation with an aircraft ditching in the Mersey. (Martin Fish)

Independent lifeboats of Britain

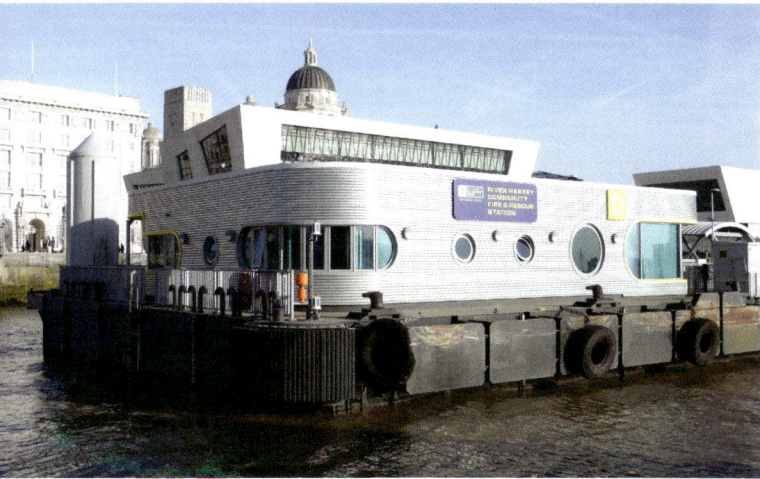

Situated at the Pier Head, the River Mersey Community Fire & Rescue Station has accommodation for duty crew on call throughout the year. (Martin Fish)

waterfront. A crew is always on call, with crew facilities on the pier. The MFRS MRU has an operational area that covers sixty miles of coastline. Funding the service as a charity proved challenging; part of the operating costs were met by grants from Liverpool Airport, local councils and other emergency services. Jaguar Cars in Halewood also offered financial support and in return the boat was branded with the company logo and renamed Mersey Jaguar.

PREVIOUS ASSETS

1986 A 7.5m Avon Searider rigid inflatable was custom-built for the Service. It had seven safety chambers in the sponsons, a carrying capacity of 20 people and, powered by twin 175hp outboards, was able reach speeds up to 52 knots, with a range of 130 nautical miles.

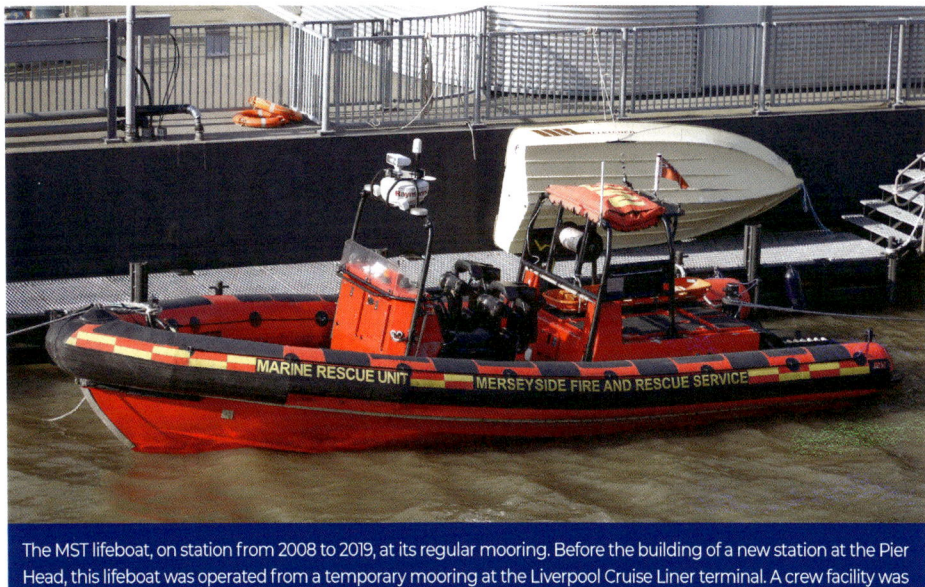

The MST lifeboat, on station from 2008 to 2019, at its regular mooring. Before the building of a new station at the Pier Head, this lifeboat was operated from a temporary mooring at the Liverpool Cruise Liner terminal. A crew facility was located in a nearby building. (Martin Fish)

Independent lifeboats of Britain

The lifeboat was subsequently upgraded with twin 225hp Honda outboards.

2005 Merseyside Fire and Rescue Authority invested in a new and improved rescue craft to cope with the unique environment of the Mersey estuary. This saw the charity cease and operations transferred to Merseyside Fire & Rescue Service. The Avon boat was replaced by a smaller RIB while a new boat was under construction.

2006 In March the Pier Head landing stage sank, along with the crew facilities for the lifeboat. The Service was temporarily relocated to the opposite side of the river, at Woodside Ferry terminal.

2008 In September a 10.5m MST Rescue 1000 craft, Marine Fire One, capable of forty knots and built by Marine Specialised Technology Ltd (MST) of Liverpool, entered service. This 10.5m boat was powered by twin 370hp Volvo diesel engines driving twin waterjets, and had a self righting capability provided by an airbag mounted on the roll-bar. A second MST rigid inflatable, Marine Fire Two, was used as a reserve boat. Powered by twin Evinrude outboards, it featured seating for four crew.

2012 In June the Unit moved to a station on the Mersey ferry terminal at Liverpool's Pier Head. The new building provided a pontoon mooring for the lifeboat and better crew facilities, including standby bedrooms for the duty crew.

2019 Two former RNLI Atlantic 75s were purchased for service on the Mersey at a cost of approximately £75,000 and replaced the waterjet-powered MST Rescue 1000 boat. One boat is kept at the Pier Head and the spare boat is usually kept in the Marina at Coburg Dock, although trailers are available to move the boats by road if necessary. The two former Atlantics, B-780 and B-791, were renamed Mersey Grace and Mersey Brave.

2022 In May Marine Fire 2 – Mersey Grace was severely damaged and capsized when a tugboat collided with the Pier Head landing stage and the lifeboat at its mooring alongside River Mersey Community Fire and Rescue Station. The second Atlantic was continued operations from a temporary mooring alongside the landing stage.

CURRENT ASSETS Two Atlantic 75 lifeboats: Marine Fire 1 – Mersey Brave (ex-RNLI B-780) and Marine Fire 2 – Mersey Grace (ex-RNLI B-791), moored afloat, on station 2019.

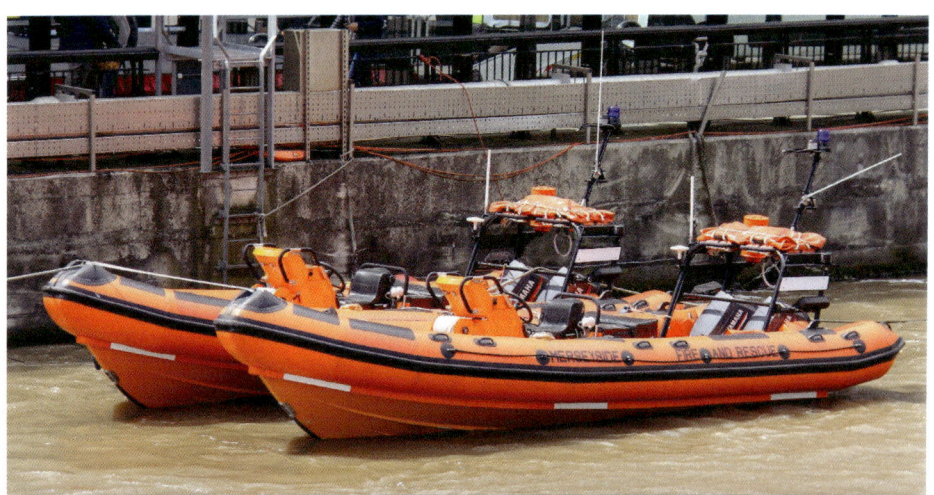

Atlantic 75 lifeboats Marine Fire 1 – Mersey Brave and Marine Fire 2 – Mersey Grace moored at the Liverpool Cruise Liner terminal in 2019 while crew training on the new boats was being carried out before they entered service. (Martin Fish)

SOUTHPORT
Merseyside

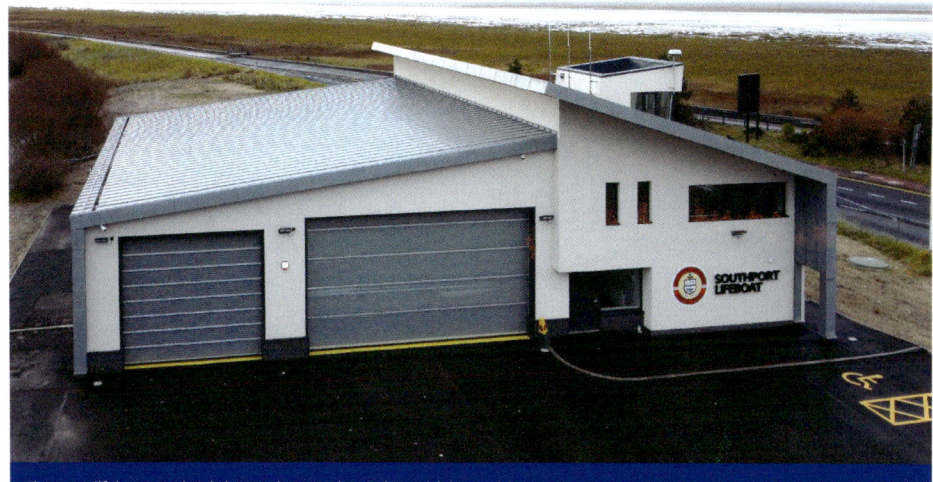

The new lifeboat station is located on Marine Drive, which provides easy access to the slipway onto the beach. Work on the building started in July 2018, with the building being completed in late 2021 after an extended build period. The delay in construction was partly caused by the lockdowns during the Covid pandemic. A look out tower on the seaward side gives views of the coast and acts as an operations control room.

LOCATION Southport, Merseyside
ORGANISATION Southport Offshore Rescue Trust
ESTABLISHED 1988
HISTORY Run by the Southport Offshore Rescue Trust, Southport Lifeboat provides a lifeboat rescue service around the Sefton coastline. The organisation builds on Southport's proud history of life-saving, which dates back to the first half of the 19th century and saw several RNLI-funded and -maintained pulling and sailing lifeboats operated until silting in the river Ribble and changes in shipping led to the eventual closure of the RNLI station in 1925. However, after a series of drownings off Southport in the 1980s, it was decided to establish an independent lifeboat. The lifeboat house of 1887 on the seafront was acquired as a base for the service, with the first lifeboat coming on station in December 1988.

The Trust's first lifeboat was a 6m Carson rigid inflatable, named Geoff Clements and powered

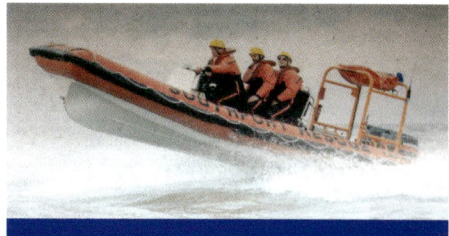

The 6m Carson RIB Geoff Clements was the first lifeboat used at Southport after the station opened.

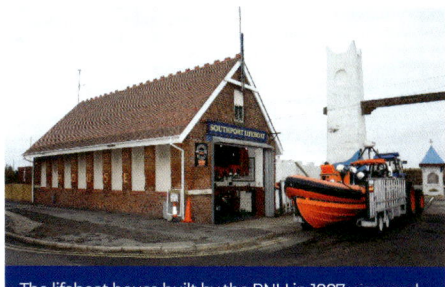

The lifeboat house built by the RNLI in 1887 was used until the pulling and sailing lifeboats were withdrawn in 1925 and the station was closed. The Southport Offshore Rescue Trust used the building from 1988.

Independent lifeboats of Britain

by twin 40hp Mariner outboards, with integral fuel tanks in the hull and a top speed of thirty knots. She had a self-righting airbag on a frame over the engines. During a refit in 1995 a single 85hp Suzuki outboard was fitted with a 10hp auxiliary engine. A modified Case agricultural tractor was used for launching and recovery.

PREVIOUS ASSETS

1995 A new 6.6m rigid inflatable, built by Delta Power Services in Stockport, was placed on station. Named Bessie Worthington, the boat was originally powered by twin 90hp Suzuki outboards. These were changed to 90hp Mariners in 1998. The lifeboat featured a console with seating for four crew, and housing a radio, GPS and echo sounder.

2000 A purpose-built launch vehicle was brought into use to launch the lifeboat across the sands. It was based on a commercial Benford dumper truck powered by a Cummins diesel engine. A second launch vehicle, a modified Muir Hill 121 tractor, was adapted for lifeboat launching.

2004 Quad bikes were introduced for searches along the shoreline and to carry mud rescue equipment for incidents in the Ribble Estuary. The first came into use in 2004, and in 2006 two Honda Foreman quad bikes were acquired. They are replaced on a three-yearly cycle.

2005 The service acquired former RNLI EA16 D class inflatable D-437 Jill Gatti. The ILB was initially used as a training boat, but following

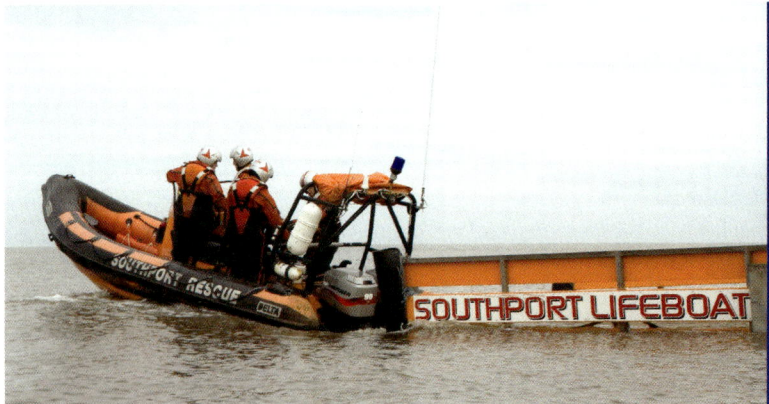

The lifeboat Bessie Worthington being launched from the beach at Southport using the bow launching trailer. (Martin Fish)

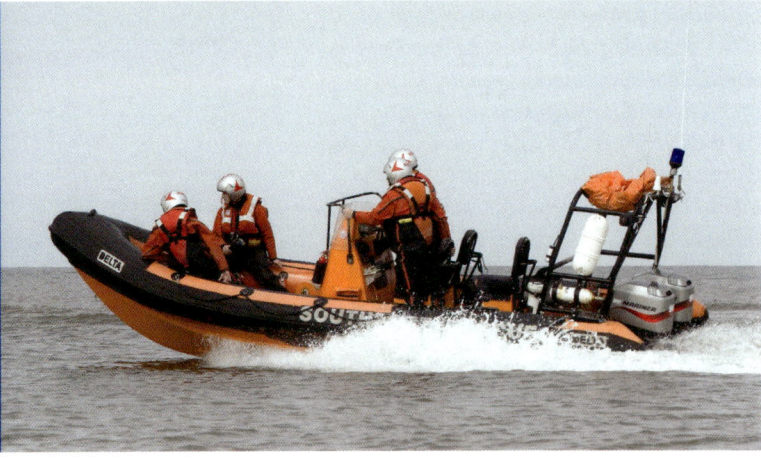

Built in 1995 by Delta Power Services in Stockport, the 6.6m Bessie Worthington served for more than a decade and is pictured on a training exercise in 2007. (Martin Fish)

Independent lifeboats of Britain

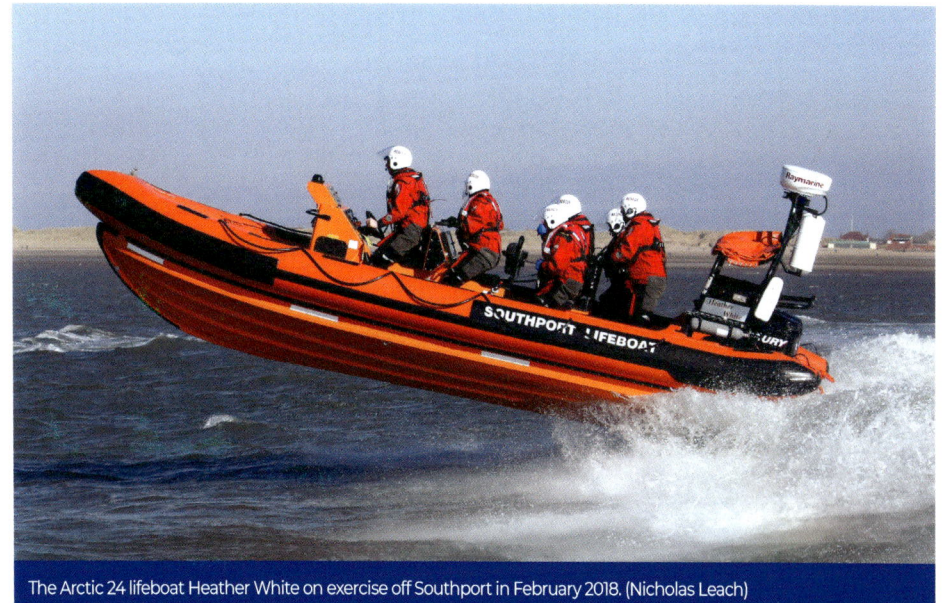

The Arctic 24 lifeboat Heather White on exercise off Southport in February 2018. (Nicholas Leach)

the arrival of a new Arctic 24 rigid inflatable in 2007 it was used in the shallow waters north of Southport Pier. The D class was powered by a single 40hp Mercury outboard.

2007 A new Arctic 24 rigid inflatable, named Heather White, came into service in May. The boat was powered by 135hp Mercury engines, which, in early 2011, were upgraded to 150hp outboards to give the boat a top speed of forty-four knots with an endurance of approximately four hours at maximum speed. The boat features a comprehensive electronic suite, including depth sounder, GPS, chart plotter, Raymarine radar, VHF radio and an intercom system. A manually activated righting airbag is fitted to a roll bar over the engines. After eleven years in service, the boat was given a major refit, being taken to the Habbeké Shipyard in the Netherlands in February 2018 for a full strip down and rebuild. This included fitting new Mariner 150hp outboards.

2014 A converted Caterpillar Challenger 65 tracked vehicle, which had previously been used by the KNRM, the Dutch lifeboat service, was purchased, arriving for trials in December before having an overhaul and entering service.

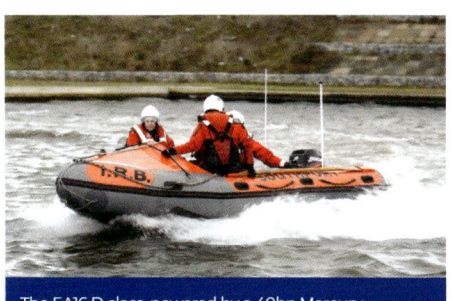

The EA16 D class, powered by a 40hp Mercury outboard, on exercise in the Marine Lake in 2009. She was on station until 2017. (Nicholas Leach)

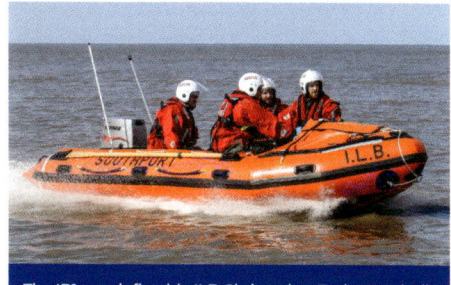

The IB1 type inflatable ILB Christopher Taylor was built for Southport Offshore Rescue Trust at the RNLI's Inshore Lifeboat Centre, Cowes in 2016. (Martin Fish)

Independent lifeboats of Britain

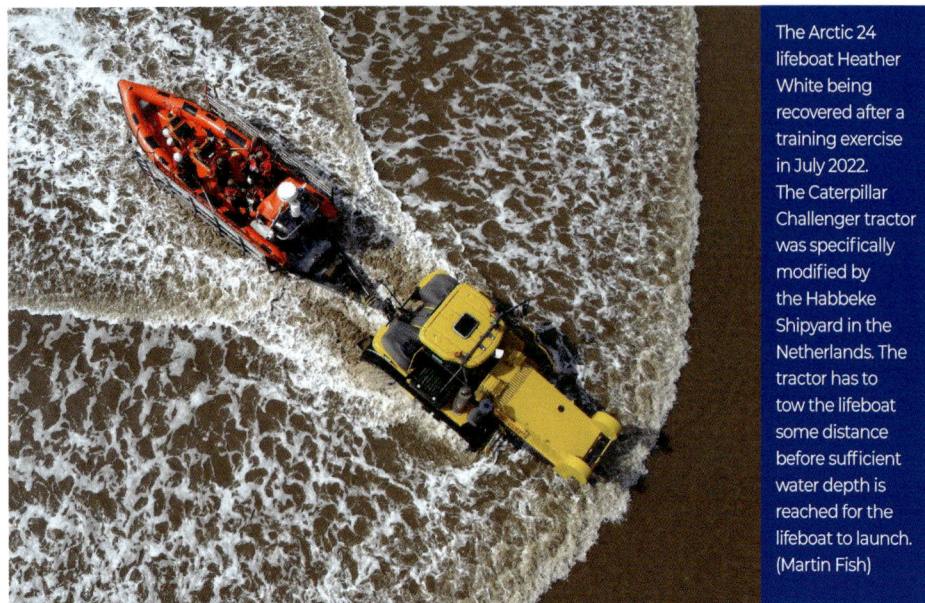

The Arctic 24 lifeboat Heather White being recovered after a training exercise in July 2022. The Caterpillar Challenger tractor was specifically modified by the Habbeke Shipyard in the Netherlands. The tractor has to tow the lifeboat some distance before sufficient water depth is reached for the lifeboat to launch. (Martin Fish)

2015 In August the Trust was granted planning approval for construction of a new boathouse on a site next to the Esplanade park and ride car park, after agreement with Sefton Council.
2016 At the beginning of March the Trust received funding from the Department of Transport's Inland and Inshore Rescue Boat Fund campaign for a new D class ILB. The latest version of the D class, the IB1, was built for the Trust by the RNLI at the ILC in Cowes and arrived in early December, becoming operational in 2017. The boat was named Christopher Taylor at a ceremony in April 2018.
2018 Following the success of the former KNRM tractor on the beach at Southport, a new tractor was obtained by the Trust. A second Caterpillar Challenger tracked tractor was converted at Habbeké Shipyard to the latest specifications as used by the KNRM. The tracks provide low ground pressure for easily crossing the soft sand and mud of Southport Beach, with full marinisation including an engine bay which can be completely sealed.
2019 A New Holland TD5 tractor was purchased as a second launch vehicle, primarily for use with the D class ILB, and the Benford launch vehicle was withdrawn. Another development was the introduction of an SAR Drone capability using two drones, both with HD and thermal imaging cameras.
2022 A new lifeboat station building became operational. Work started on the first phase of construction in July 2018, and took until late 2021 to be completed. Problems with the coating system applied to the structural steelwork required rectification works to be carried out and the build was further delayed by the Covid-19 pandemic. The trust moved into the new building on New Years Day and responded to the first call out from the new base the next day. A main boathall houses the two lifeboats and the quad bikes. The station has rooms for training and maintenance, as well as a workshop, kitchen and changing facilities.
CURRENT ASSETS Halmatic Arctic 24 built by VT Halmatic, named Heather White, launched by Caterpillar Challenger tractor and carriage, on station 2007; RNLI IB1 type D class inflatable, named Christopher Taylor, launched by New Holland TD5 tractor and trailer, on station 2017.

FLOOKBURGH/BAY Cumbria

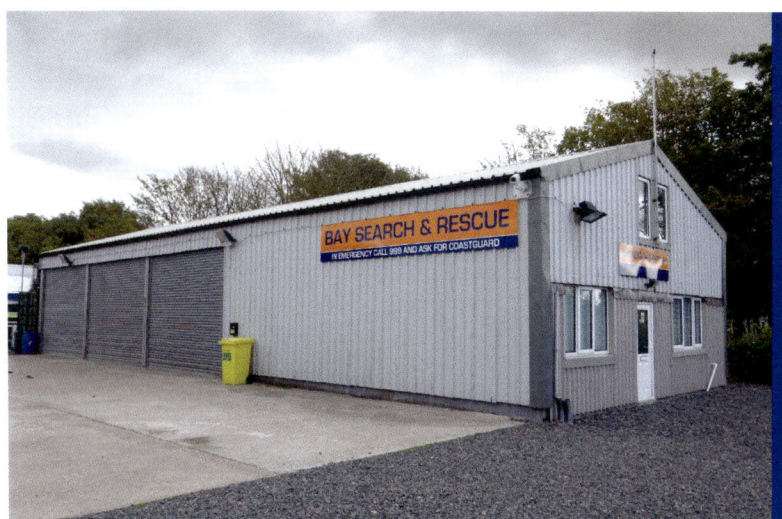

Bay SAR Headquarters building in Flookburgh. It was built on land provided by Lord Cavendish of Holker Hall. Rescue equipment is also based at a number of locations around Morecambe Bay. (Martin Fish)

LOCATION Flookburgh, Cumbria
ORGANISATION Bay Search & Rescue
ESTABLISHED 2001
HISTORY Bay Search and Rescue is a unique organisation, covering the treacherous Morecambe Bay. The service was founded in 2001 as Bay Hovercraft Rescue, being the first SAR team in the UK to use a hovercraft as a rescue vehicle. The Osprey 5 hovercraft was funded by local benefactor Ada Hillard, and carried the name Lady Ada. Supporting the hovercraft were two Argocat all-terrain vehicles, which were able to operate where conventional search and rescue craft could not. The service was originally based in an old wartime fire station in the grounds of Abbot Hall Hotel in Kents Bank. A purpose-built station was erected by team members at Moor Lane in Flookburgh on land provided by Lord Cavendish of Holker Hall. Originally specialising in quicksand rescue, the role of the team has expanded to flood and water rescue, with team members being trained as swift water rescue technicians.

PREVIOUS ASSETS
2005 The hovercraft and Argocats were

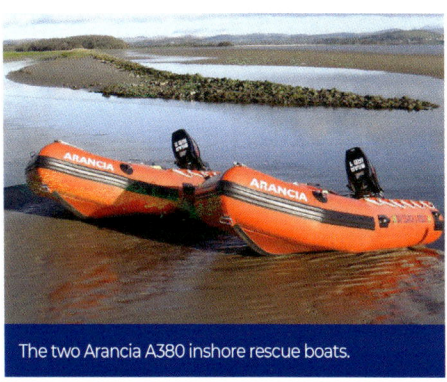

The two Arancia A380 inshore rescue boats.

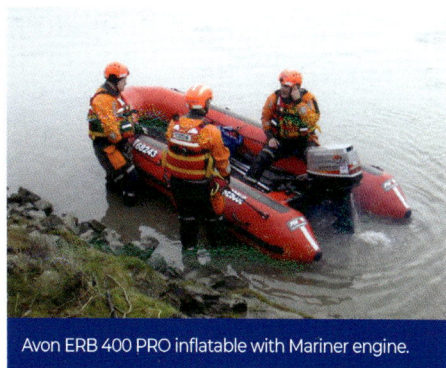

Avon ERB 400 PRO inflatable with Mariner engine.

Independent lifeboats of Britain

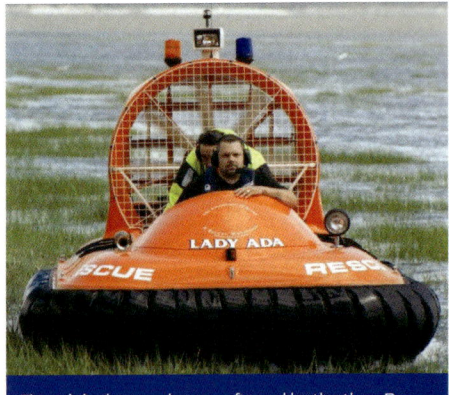

The original rescue hovercraft used by the then Bay Hovercraft Rescue, which was named Lady Ada.

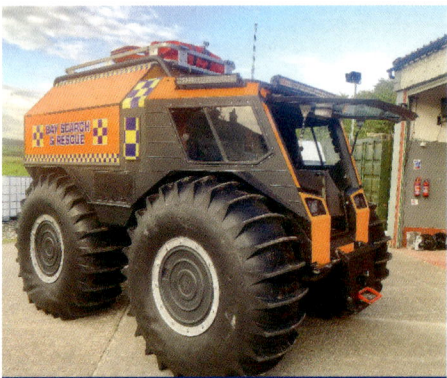

The SHERP all-terrain vehicle which came into service during 2020.

replaced by Hägglunds Bv206 articulated tracked all-terrain vehicles. The hovercraft, although better than boats for operating in the Bay, could not carry enough equipment or personnel. The Hägglunds was originally designed for military use in snow but it has proved to be versatile in many other situations for rescue work. A range of support vehicles is also used by the service, including Volvo and DAF transporter trucks and Toyota Hilux 4x4 response vehicles. The 18-tonne DAF CF transporter is fitted with tail ramps to transport a Hägglunds vehicle and rescue equipment to incidents in Cumbria or Lancashire.

2016 Prior to 2016, an Avon ERB 400 PRO inflatable boat with a 30hp Mariner two-stroke outboard was purchased with a grant from the Big Lottery Fund, primarily to be

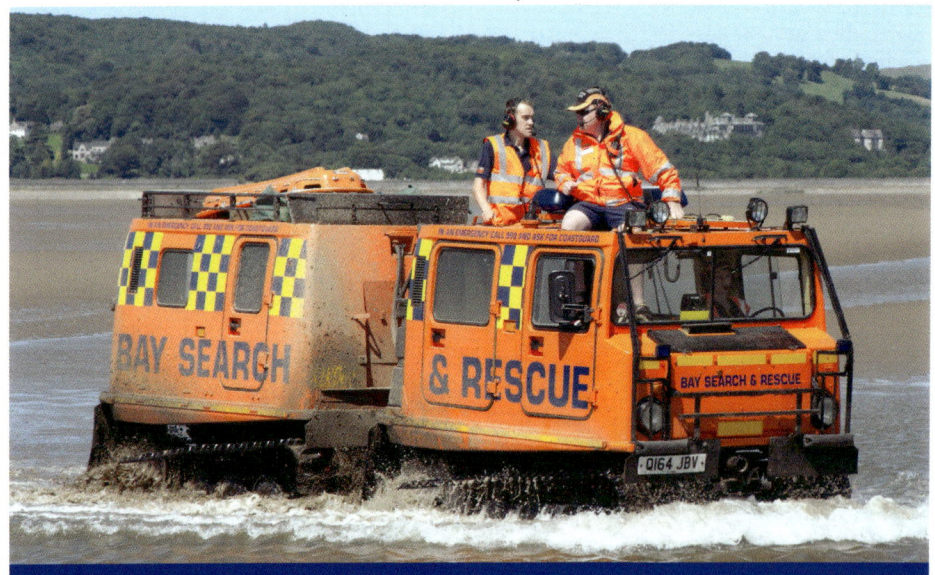

The Hägglunds Bv206, call sign BAY2, on exercise in Morecambe Bay. The Bv206 consists of two rubber-tracked units linked together by a hydraulic steering unit. The Bv206 is fully amphibious, being propelled in the water by its tracks. The vehicle features a rear load-carrying area, and a basket stretcher can be seen on the roof. (Martin Fish)

Independent lifeboats of Britain

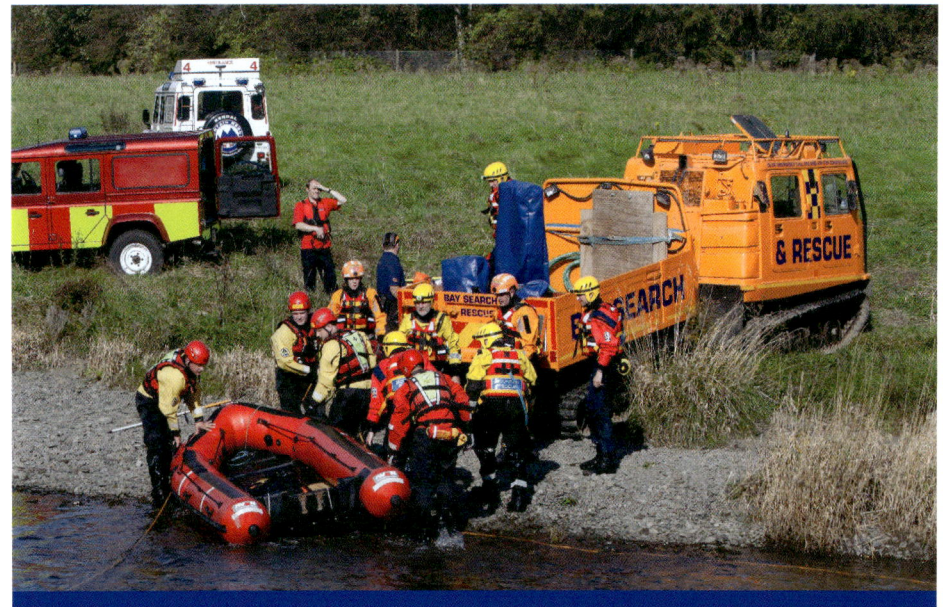

The Hägglunds Bv206 during a multi-agency training exercise on the River Kent, practising swift-water rescue techniques. (Martin Fish)

used for flood work. A 3.8m Zodiac inflatable rescue boat was also in service. The Hägglunds vehicles and Toyota 4x4s carry inflatable rescue paths, specialist inflatable water rescue stretchers and other quicksand rescue equipment. In August 2016 the rescue boats were replaced, thanks to further funding from the Big Lottery Fund, with two Arancia A380 flood rescue boats, powered by Tohatsu 30hp outboard engines, being acquired.

2020 The latest unique vehicle to go into service arrived in early 2020 with the purchase of a SHERP all-terrain vehicle. Manufactured in the Ukraine, the SHERP is a skid-steer vehicle capable of speeds of up to 25mph, powered by a Kubota diesel engine and has the ability to adjust its tyre pressures when operating on more challenging terrain.

CURRENT ASSETS Arancia A380 inshore rescue boats, on station 2016, launched by trailer and 4x4 vehicle; Diamondback SAR Airboat, launched by trailer; Hägglunds Bv206 and SHERP all-terrain vehicles.

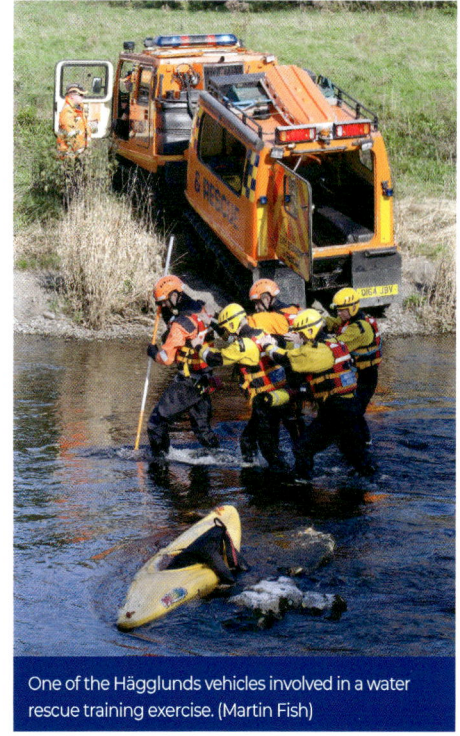

One of the Hägglunds vehicles involved in a water rescue training exercise. (Martin Fish)

Independent lifeboats of Britain

ULVERSTON
Cumbria

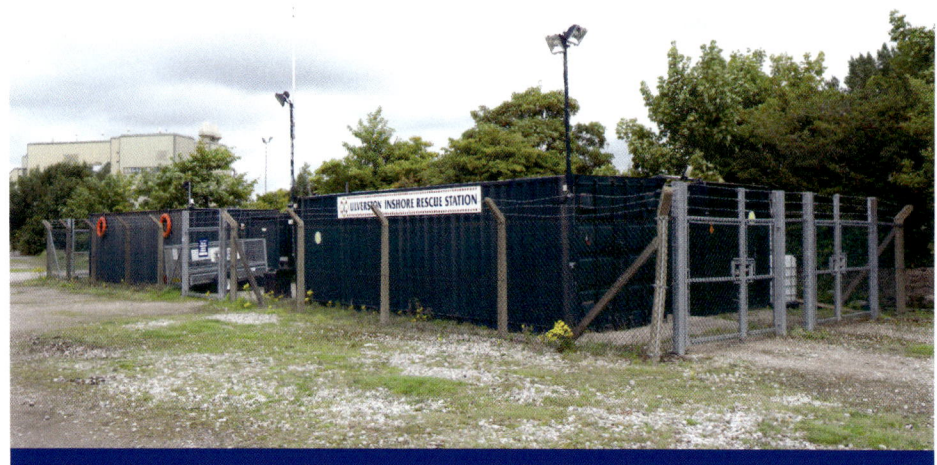

The shore facility housing lifeboats and vehicles on land provided by GlaxoSmithKline at Ulverston. (Martin Fish)

LOCATION Ulverston, Cumbria
ORGANISATION Ulverston Inshore Rescue
ESTABLISHED 2002
HISTORY Following the tragic drowning of Stewart Rushton and his nine-year-old son Adam in January 2002, members of the Ulverston Town Council established a working group to look at measures to prevent such events, including the creation of a local rescue facility. By October 2002 a land-based rescue team had been established and was meeting regularly. An enclosure, containing a crew room and three steel storage containers, was agreed with GlaxoSmithKline, who provided a site near to Canal Foot in Ulverston.

In March 2003 planning permission was granted, and the landowner repaired the access ramp to the beach and constructed a fenced enclosure. Equipment purchased for a crew of fourteen included high visibility personal protective clothing, lifebelts and shore rescue equipment, high power torches for night operations, two Quad Bikes and VHF marine radios. The Quad Bikes are capable of road use and are used for beach patrols.

PREVIOUS ASSETS
2005 A small surf rescue boat with a shallow draught, produced by Arancia Industries Ltd of New Zealand, was purchased. It was delivered in July and named Fisher 1 in recognition of funding from the Sir John Fisher Foundation. Powered by a 30hp outboard engine, the boat proved useful for shallow water operations. A Kubota 4x4 RTV Utility vehicle, for launching the boat, was funded from a donation by the Centrica Helicopter Memorial Fund.
2006 The Service obtained a second, larger lifeboat, a rescue version of the Humber 5.9m Assault rigid inflatable manufactured by Humber Fabrications (Hull) Ltd. The boat was fitted with VHF radio, GPS, depth sounder and navigation lights, and is capable of carrying up to eleven. Originally powered by a 60hp Mariner outboard, it has a seating console for the helm and a second crew member. The boat was named Lady Maria at the request of the donors, the Sir John Fisher Foundation, who have funded a number of lifeboats in Cumbria. The boat was collected from Hull in August and went into service soon

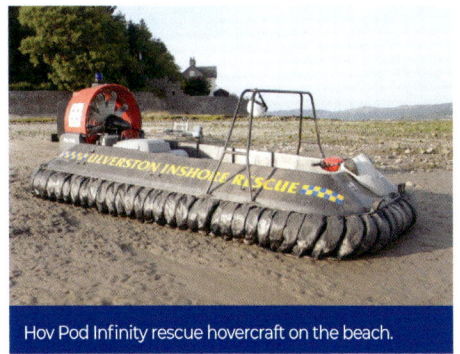
Hov Pod Infinity rescue hovercraft on the beach.

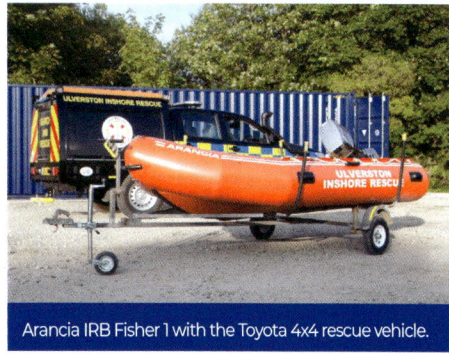
Arancia IRB Fisher 1 with the Toyota 4x4 rescue vehicle.

afterwards. In September a Ford Ranger 4x4 vehicle was purchased for towing Lady Maria to the various launching sites and to act as a mobile base during rescue operations. The boat's engine was subsequently upgraded to a 100hp Honda outboard, and a 5hp Mariner was carried in case of engine failure.

2015 In July the service took delivery of a rescue hovercraft. Manufactured by Hov Pod, the Infinity Hovercraft was funded by the Big Lottery Fund with additional funding from the Sir John Fisher Foundation and was named Patricia. A road-going launching trailer enables the hovercraft to be launched at a range of sites. The hovercraft was upgraded in 2018 with the fitting of a second lift engine to provide extra lift and give enhanced performance.

2016 A second 4x4 rescue vehicle came into service in February in the shape of a specialist Toyota Hilux rescue vehicle converted by Pickup Systems. This carries a range of rescue equipment in the rear body and acts as towing vehicle for the lifeboats and hovercraft.

CURRENT ASSETS Humber 5.9m Assault RIB, Lady Maria, on station 2006, launched by trailer and 4x4 vehicle; Arancia IRB, Fisher 1, on station 2005, launched by trailer and 4x4 vehicle or quad bike; Hov Pod Infinity Hovercraft, named Patricia, on station 2015, launched from a road-going trailer.

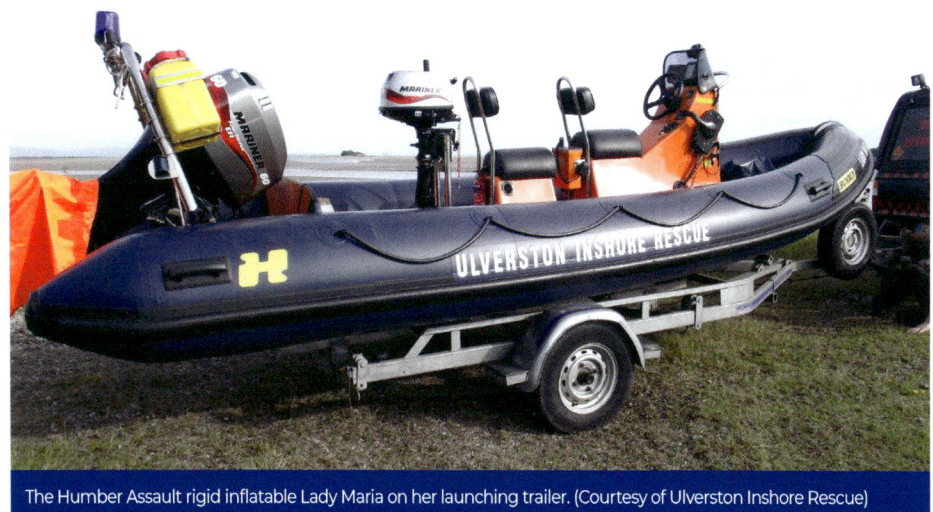
The Humber Assault rigid inflatable Lady Maria on her launching trailer. (Courtesy of Ulverston Inshore Rescue)

Independent lifeboats of Britain

DUDDON Cumbria

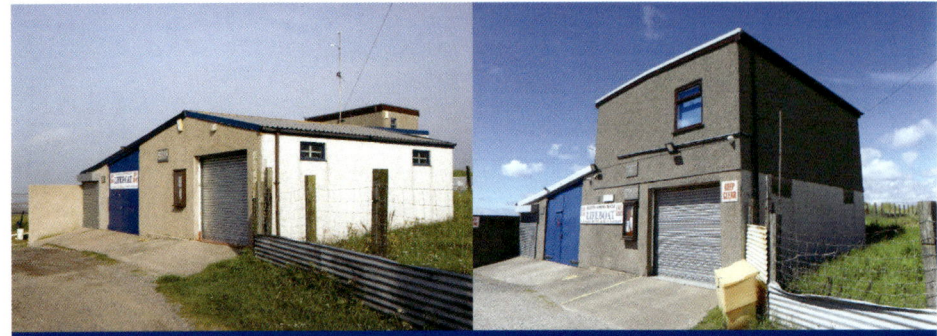

The lifeboat station built on the beach at Askam in 1969. The building has been extended several times, most recently in 2017 when a training room was added. (Martin Fish)

LOCATION Askam in Furness, Cumbria
ORGANISATION Duddon Inshore Rescue
ESTABLISHED 1969
HISTORY The catalyst for setting up a lifesaving service was the tragic drowning of two Askam brothers and a Dalton man who lost his life while holding his thirteen-year-old daughter out of the water on an incoming tide. A local committee was established and, led by Bernard McNamee, set about acquiring a rescue boat for the area. Land was found on the foreshore at Askam and construction of a boathouse began in 1969, with an official opening by Albert Booth MP in 1970. The first lifeboat on the station was a 16ft RFD inflatable, powered by a Yamaha outboard, which cost £750. Duddon's first service took place in August 1970 when two children were rescued after becoming stuck on a sandbank.

PREVIOUS ASSETS
1989 RFD inflatables were used until 1989, when a new EA16 type inflatable built by Avon Inflatables at Llanelli in Wales and powered by a Yamaha outboard engine, was introduced. The new lifeboat was to the same design as the latest generation of RNLI D class ILBs,

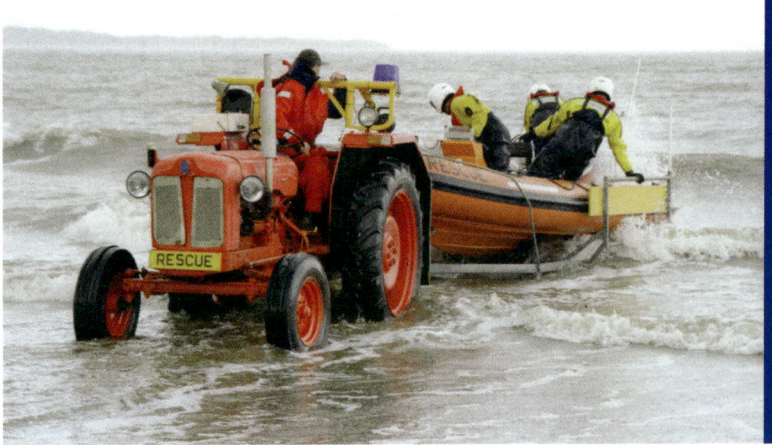

The inshore lifeboats are launched from the beach at Askam using an agricultural tractor modified for the service. (Martin Fish)

Independent lifeboats of Britain

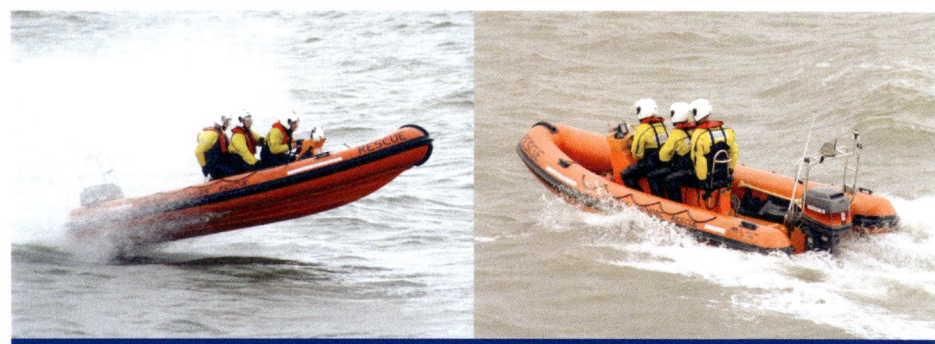

The BWM DiveRib 575 inshore lifeboat on exercise off Askham pier; she served at Duddon until 2006. (Martin Fish)

which were being built by Avon Inflatables. A stern-first launching trailer was used in conjunction an agricultural tractor. In 1990, to supplement the lifeboat, a quad bike was added to the station equipment, providing a quick response to incidents on the shoreline.

1995 An upgrade to the EA16 took place when a new BWM DiveRib 575 rigid inflatable was purchased. Powered by a single Mariner 55hp outboard engine it featured a centre console with seating for the crew and a steel frame at the stern for lights and aerials. The Reverend Danny Sanderson, vicar of Askam and Ireleth, conducted a service to bless the new £9,000 rigid inflatable.

2006 A new lifeboat, named Duddon Guardian, was placed on station following a ceremony attended by Lord Lieutenant of Cumbria James Cropper. Manufactured by Ribcraft of Yeovil, the new £35,000 boat was a 5.8m Professional rigid inflatable with a console seating three crew and powered by twin Mariner 60hp outboards. A roll bar over the engines carried a righting airbag activated by the crew in the event of a capsize. A Case 895 Tractor was used with a trailer to launch the lifeboat stern first across the beach.

2010 Changes in the Duddon estuary meant the effectiveness of the rigid inflatable lifeboats was being limited due to lack of water at low tide. This led to a change in lifeboats, with the EA16 inflatable again being the boat of choice. The service obtained lifeboat D-567 from the RNLI, which had previously served at Barrow and was refitted and modified for use at Duddon.

2015 The trailer was updated to a bow-first launch to improve launching arrangements.

2016 The RNLI agreed to supply a new IB1 inflatable. Built at the RNLI Inshore Lifeboat Centre in Cowes, the ILB is powered by a 50hp Mariner outboard and has a bow pod which contains the electronic equipment. The IB1 was delivered in February and on 19 June a naming

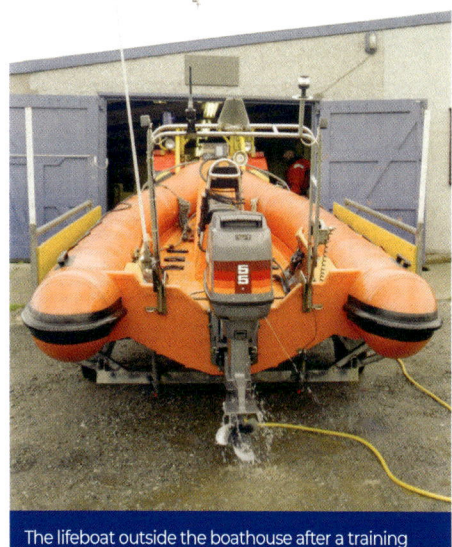

The lifeboat outside the boathouse after a training launch in 2001. (Martin Fish)

Independent lifeboats of Britain

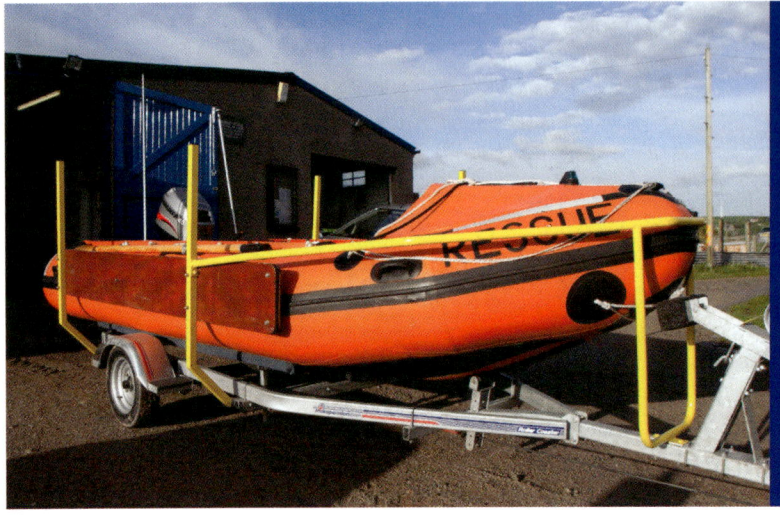

The former RNLI EA16 D class inflatable on her launching trolley in May 2011. Originally D-567 Spirit of Tamworth, the boat served the RNLI station at Barrow until 2010. (Martin Fish)

ceremony took place for the boat, which had been donated in memory of Anyon Arthur Kay. A second EA16 inflatable, powered by a 40hp Mariner outboard, is used as a reserve and training boat, and housed in a storage container.
2017 A two-storey extension to the lifeboat station was completed and officially opened in October 2017 to provide a bespoke training and meeting area for the volunteer crew. The extension was dedicated to the memory of one of the founding members of the Service, Bernard McNamee, MBE.
2018 A New Holland TD5.85 tractor was acquired in November, funded by the Ørsted's Walney Extension Community Fund. The service continues to operate the Honda quad bikes for a shore-based response, together with a 4x4 support vehicle which carries search and medical equipment.
CURRENT ASSETS IB1 type inflatable inshore lifeboat, on station 2016, launched by New Holland TD5.85 tractor and trailer.

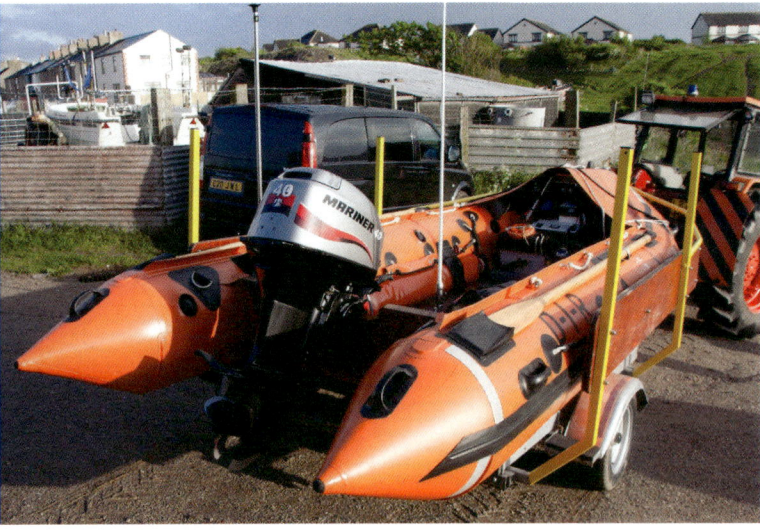

The former RNLI EA16 D class inflatable served from 2010 having been refitted and modified for use at Duddon. (Martin Fish)

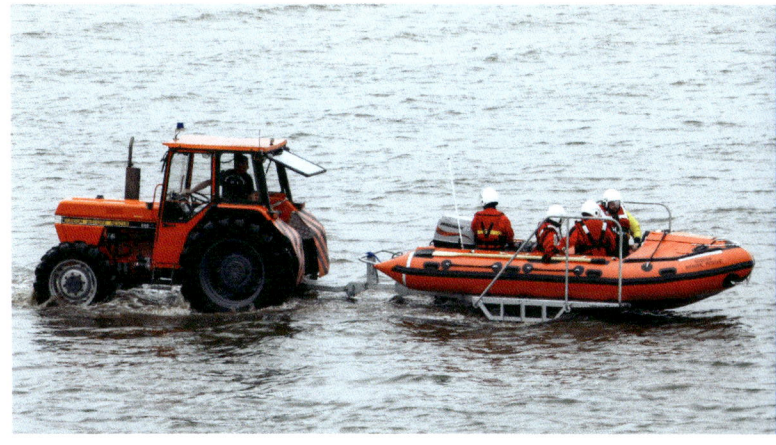

The current inshore lifeboat being launched using the Case tractor. (Martin Fish)

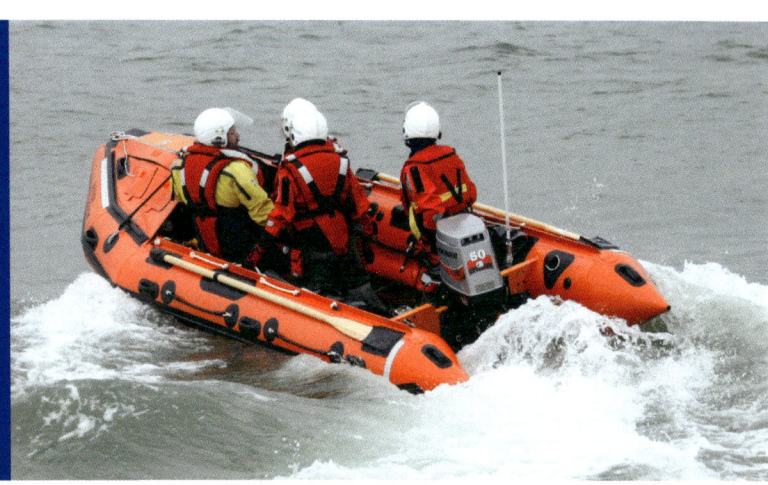

The IB1 type D class inshore lifeboat under way off Askam Pier following the boat's formal dedication in June 2016. (Martin Fish)

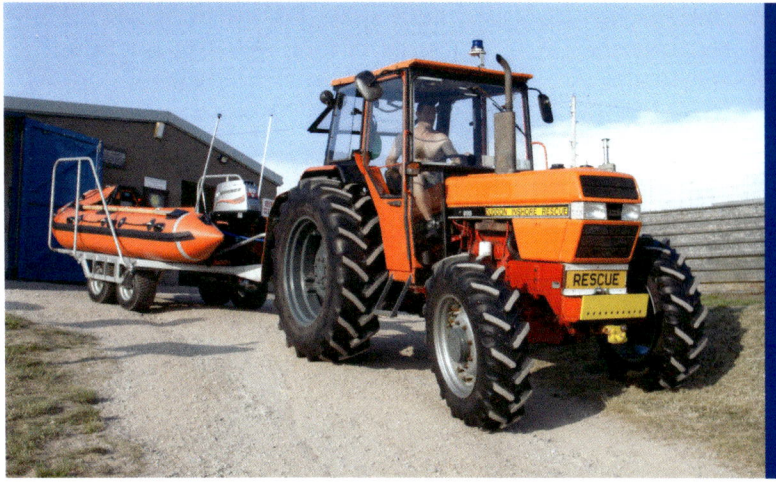

The D class inshore lifeboat on her launching trolley outside the boathouse in June 2016, soon after arriving on station. (Martin Fish)

Independent lifeboats of Britain

HAVERIGG

Cumbria

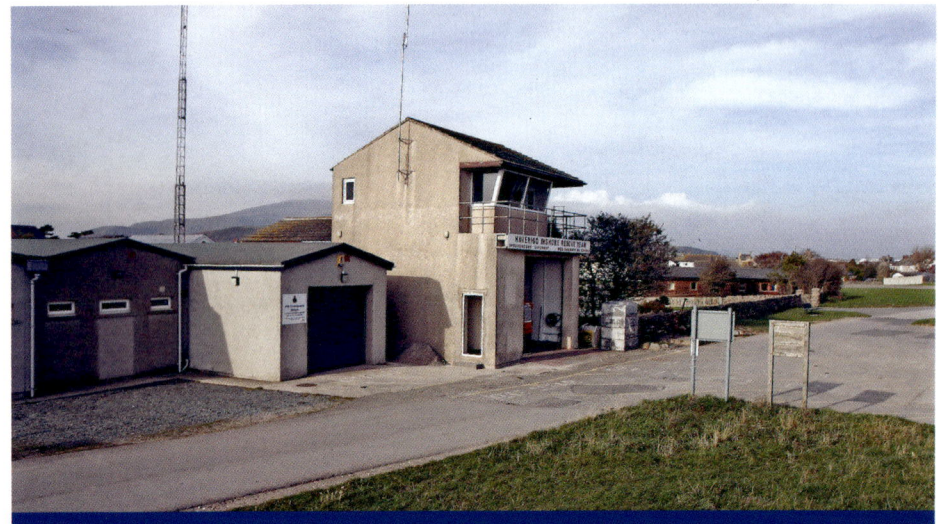

The two-storey lifeboat station is situated on the seafront at Haverigg at the southern end of the Sea View road, opposite the beach across which the lifeboat is usually launched.

LOCATION Haverigg, Millom, Cumbria
ORGANISATION Haverigg Inshore Rescue Team
ESTABLISHED 1973
HISTORY Haverigg Inshore Rescue Team was formed in 1973 following the tragic drowning of a local boy in a boating accident. Based in the village of Haverigg, the team is crewed by volunteers from Haverigg and Millom. The service's first lifeboat was an Avon S650 Inflatable Sports Boat powered by a 40hp outboard. An old Nuffield two-wheel-drive agricultural tractor was obtained and the volunteers built a launch trailer. This equipment was stored in a shed at a local caravan site while negotiations for a suitable permanent site for a boathouse were ongoing with the local council.

In 1976 a boathouse was built, and this has been gradually modified by the crew to provide improved facilities. The two-storey building has a boat hall for the lifeboat and tractor, as well as a workshop area, crew changing area and a lookout/operations room on the first floor.

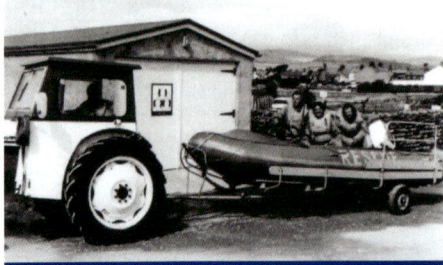

The station's first lifeboat, an Avon Sports Boat, on her trailer outside the station's first boathouse.

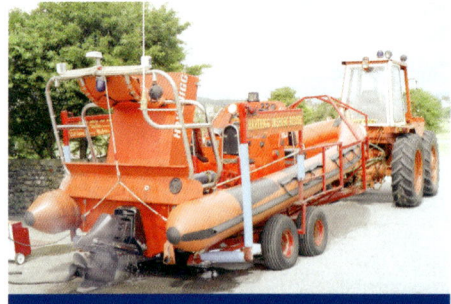

The 1991 Osprey RIB on the stern first launch trailer.

Independent lifeboats of Britain

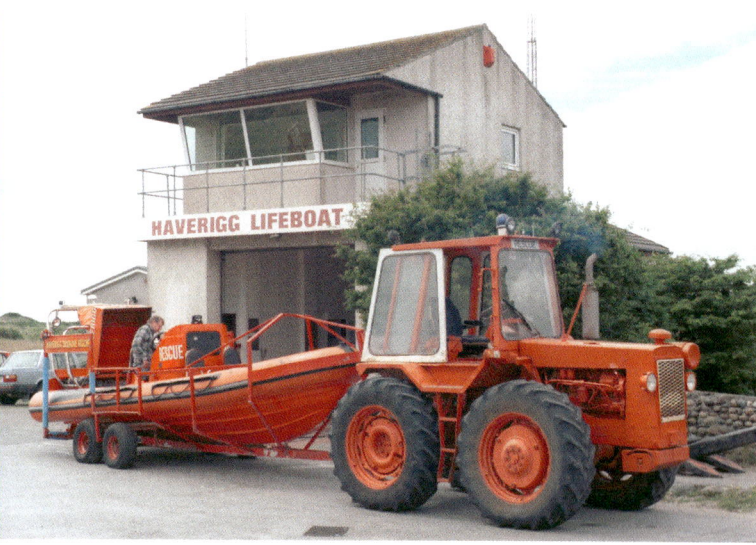

The lifeboat station with the boat hall on the ground floor and the lookout/operations room on the first floor. (Martin Fish)

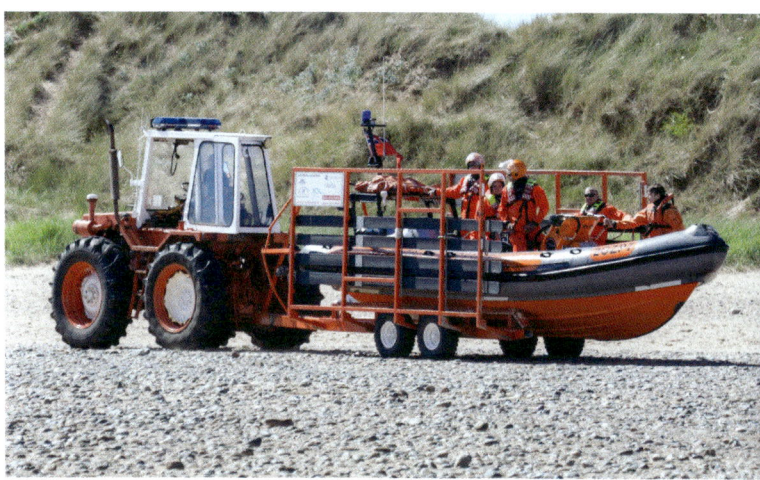

The Muir Hill launching tractor has high ground clearance and is modified to allow it to enter the water when launching the lifeboat. (Martin Fish)

PREVIOUS ASSETS
1979 Following a number of rescues undertaken in heavy seas it was apparent that the sponsons on the Avon Sports boat were suffering from stretching so a replacement was needed. A more robust 4.5m Gordon inflatable with a Johnson 40hp outboard and a seating console for the helm was purchased. The boat was slightly larger than the Avon and had an aluminium floor, which was more durable. Later during the boat's service, a righting airbag was fitted with a roll bar frame.

1985 A new 7m Flatacraft rigid inflatable boat was acquired. Powered by a 140hp Johnson outboard, it had righting airbag fitted to a frame over the rear engines; the frame also carried the navigation lights and VHF radio aerial. Crew members designed and built a trailer for stern-first launching, and modified an old four-wheel drive loading shovel to serve as a launch vehicle, replacing a David Brown tractor, which was no longer suitable.
1991 A new 7m Osprey Viper rigid inflatable, powered by an inboard engine driving a single

Independent lifeboats of Britain

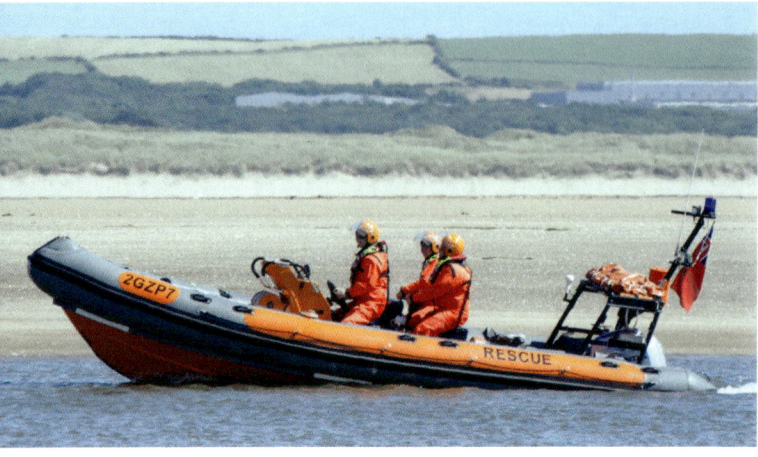

The first former RNLI Atlantic 75 to serve at Haverigg, ex-B-734, was operational from 2013 to 2017, and is pictured in July 2014 after her formal blessing ceremony. (Martin Fish)

sterndrive unit, was purchased. Originally installed with a 236hp OMC petrol engine, the boat was able to achieve a top speed of about thirty-five knots. A centre console featured a dedicated helm position with seating for four crew and containing the communications and navigation equipment. A roll bar was installed over the engine casing with aerials, lights and the righting airbag, activated by the crew in the event of a capsize. During a mid-life refit, the OMC engine was replaced by a Steyr diesel unit. The lifeboat was launched using a Muir Hill Tractor, which was modified to work in salt water. Originally the boat was launched stern first, but this was changed to bow first launching using a bespoke carriage built by crew members. Towards the end of 2006 the lifeboat was re-engined again, this time with a new Mercruiser 360 petrol engine which had greater power and reliability.

2013 With the Osprey RIB approaching the end of its life, a former RNLI Atlantic 75 was purchased. Originally built in 1997 as B-734, it had served as a relief lifeboat and at RNLI stations on the Thames. It was refitted with new 90hp Honda outboards. A blessing ceremony for the new boat was held outside the lifeboat station at Haverigg in July 2014.

2017 In February the service obtained a newer Atlantic 75 from the RNLI, B-766, formerly at Hartlepool having been built in 2000. The main difference from the earlier boat was the orange-coloured sponsons. The 90hp Honda engines were transferred to the new boat with ex B-734 being sold, becoming a dive boat in southern Ireland.

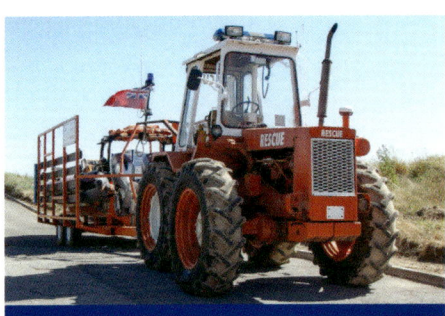

The Muir Hill Tractor, modified to work in salt water, is used to launch the Atlantic 75. (Martin Fish)

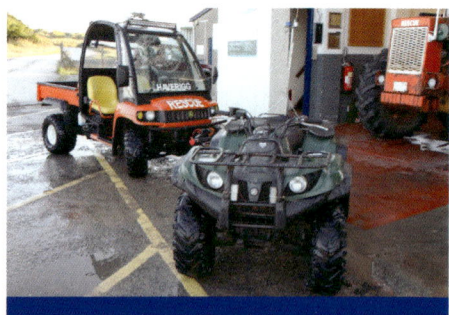

The John Deer Gator utility vehicle and Yamaha Grizzly quadbike used for shoreline rescue.

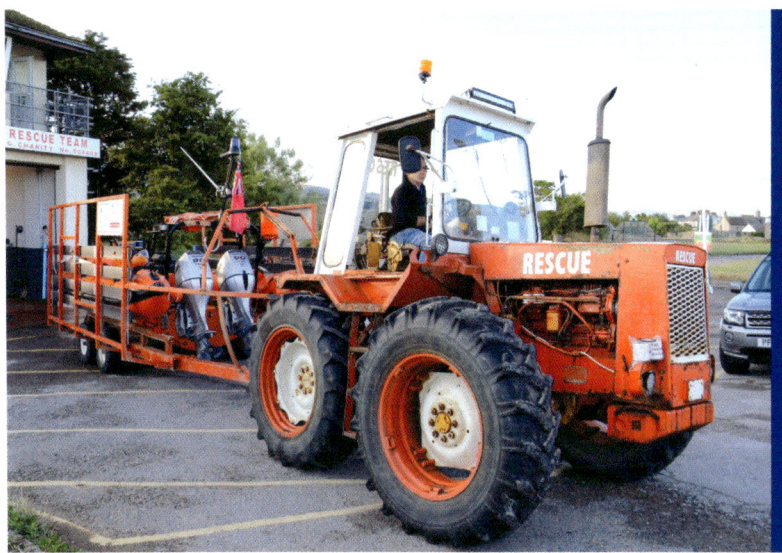

The Atlantic 75 is launched across the beach at Haverigg by the Muir Hill launch tractor from a bow first launch trailer, specially manufactured for the service. (Martin Fish)

2018 To improve response to incidents in shallow water, the service placed a Sea-Doo personal watercraft (PWC) into service as a quick response asset to support the main lifeboat. In addition to the PWC, the service operates a Yamaha Grizzly quad bike and John Deere 4x4 utility vehicle for incidents on the shoreline. To house these additional assets, storage containers have been placed adjacent to the lifeboat station.

CURRENT ASSETS Atlantic 75 Rigid Inflatable (Ex-RNLI B-766), on station 2017, launched by Muir Hill tractor and carriage; Sea-Doo PWC, on station 2018, launched by trailer with John Deere Gator Utility Vehicle or using the Yamaha Grizzly quadbike.

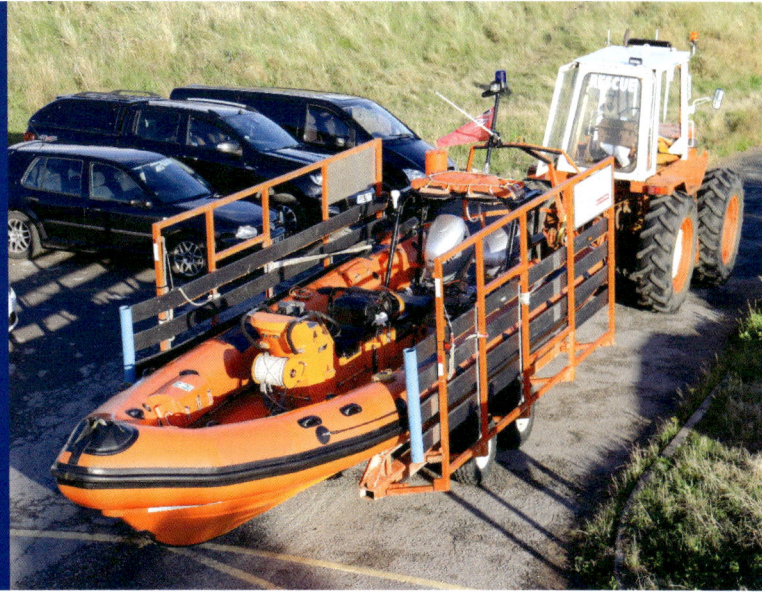

The former Hartlepool Atlantic 75 B-766 at Haverigg in her launching carriage. (Martin Fish)

Independent lifeboats of Britain

MARYPORT   Cumbria

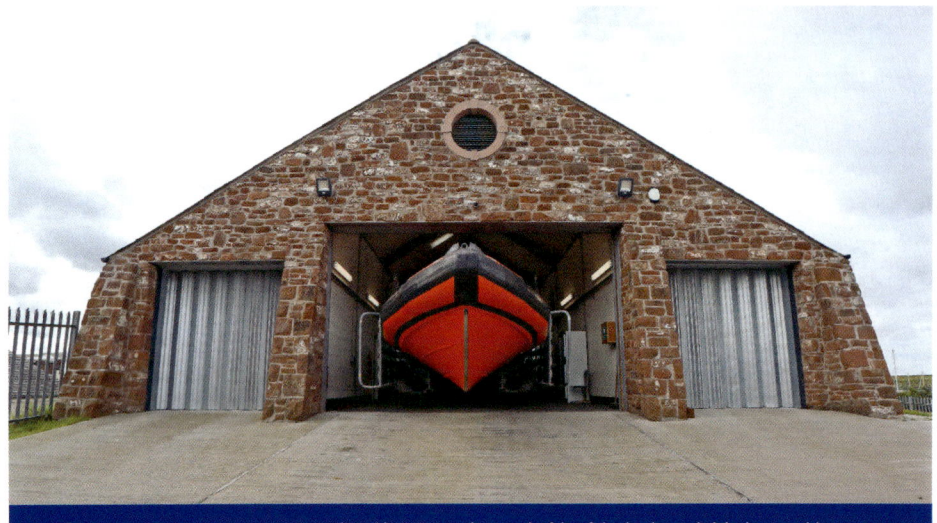

The lifeboat house at Maryport was completed in 2014 on the south side of the harbour. (Nicholas Leach)

LOCATION Maryport, Cumbria
ORGANISATION Maryport Inshore Rescue
ESTABLISHED 1978
HISTORY Lifeboat provision in Maryport dates back to 1865, when the RNLI opened the station operating a 32ft self-righting pulling and sailing lifeboat. A lifeboat house was built in the harbour, and in 1931 the station was supplied with a motor lifeboat. However, in 1949, with silting in the harbour hindering operations, the RNLI decided to close the station and reopen the station at neighbouring Workington. As a result Maryport was without a lifeboat, until the 1970s. Then, in 1978, an independent lifeboat service was founded by six local people after an accident at sea when three crew on the local fishing boat Osprey lost their lives.

PREVIOUS ASSETS
1978 A basic rigid inflatable boat, powered by a single outboard, was acquired, operating out of the old RNLI lifeboat house, built in 1908,

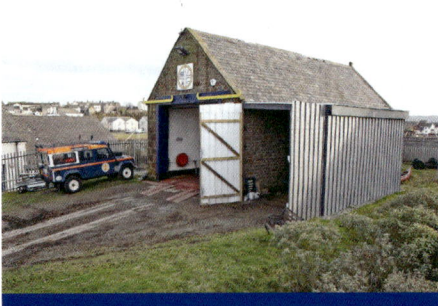

The lifeboat house, built by the RNLI in 1908, was used by Maryport lifeboat from 1978 until 2013, when it was demolished. (Nicholas Leach)

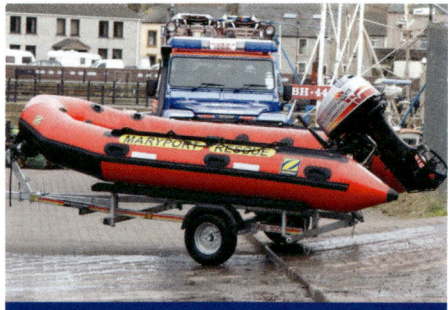

The Zodiac Milpro ERB inflatable used primarily for flood response work and is towed by one of the station's two Land Rovers. (Martin Fish)

Independent lifeboats of Britain

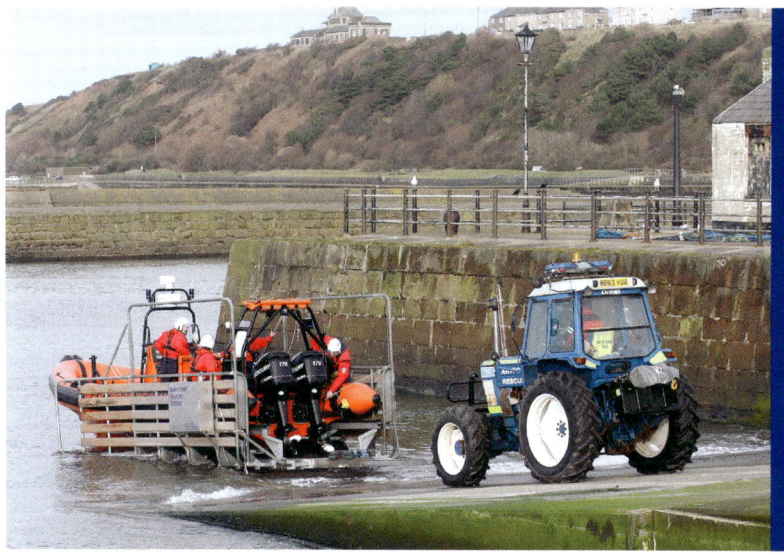

The MST rigid inflatable E.ON Spirit of Maryport being launched down the concrete slipway into the harbour at high tide, February 2009. At low tide, the boat is launched across the beach. (Nicholas Leach)

in the harbour. The next ILB was a Humber rigid inflatable, named Ronnie Farish after a local fundraiser. Powered by a single Evinrude outboard, she had a seating console for three, a VHF aerial and radar reflector. A second Humber rigid inflatable, named Symon Grant, upgraded the station. Powered by twin outboard engines, she had a centre seating console for a helm and two crew members and a manually activated self-righting airbag fitted to a roll bar.

2008 In May a new lifeboat arrived, built by Liverpool-based Marine Specialist Technology, costing £104,000. E.ON, the electricity generating company operating wind farms off the Cumbrian coast, contributed £50,000 to a local appeal and the lifeboat was named E.ON Spirit of Maryport. The 9m boat was initially powered by twin 175hp Mercury outboards, but in 2018 these were changed for new 150hp Mercury outboards. A console provides seating for four crew, a collapsible mast at the front of the console carries radar, blue beacons and a searchlight, and a righting airbag is fitted on a roll bar A Ford 7710 tractor was used for

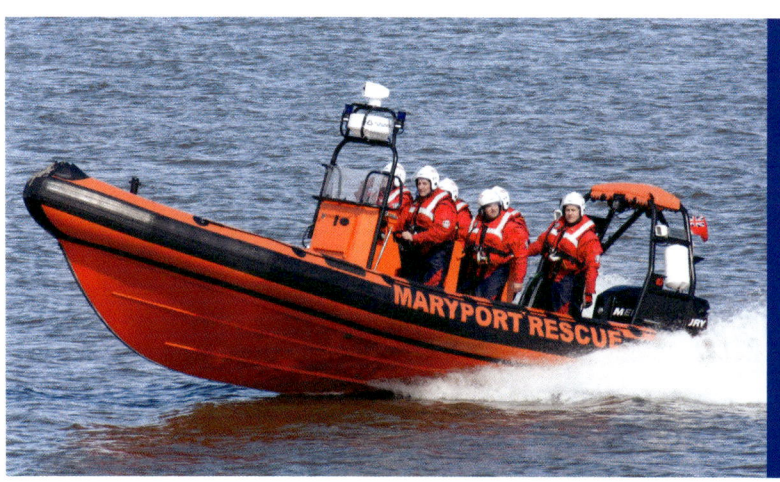

Maryport lifeboat E.ON Spirit of Maryport taking part in a multi-agency exercise simulating an aircraft crash into the Solway Firth, 2012. (Martin Fish)

Independent lifeboats of Britain

launching from a bow first launching carriage.
2009 In March seven members of the crew became qualified Rescue 3 Swift Water Technicians, enabling the service to provide cover for inland flood rescue incidents. Maryport volunteers helped during severe flooding in Cockermouth and Workington in November.
2012 A new Zodiac Milpro ERB was placed on station. Powered by a 40hp Mariner outboard engine, this boat was primarily to support flood rescue operations. It was funded through charitable grants, including funds from the Sir John Fisher Foundation.
2012 A new lifeboat station was built to replace the old boathouse, which was demolished. The new building has a boathall for the lifeboat and tractor, with garages for the Land Rover and flood rescue boat, and improved crew facilities. It was opened in June 2014 by Sir Tony Cunningham.
2021 A new IB1 inshore lifeboat was purchased from the RNLI, built for Maryport at the Inshore Lifeboat Centre, Cowes. Powered by a 50hp Mariner outboard engine, the ILB has a bow pod housing radio and navigation equipment. The lifeboat was named Lady Anne Cunningham at a ceremony on 21 November 2021 at the lifeboat station. A

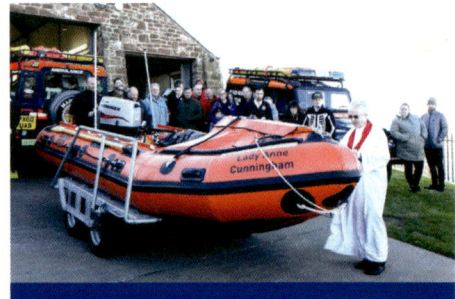

Naming and dedication ceremony of the D class inflatable Lady Anne Cunningham. (Martin Fish)

new mezzanine extension to the boathouse, funded by the Grand Lodge of Mark Master Masons, was opened at the same time.
2022 A Loglogic Tooltrak tracked vehicle was purchased from East Sutherland Rescue Association to improve launch and recovery arrangements for the D class when launching into the harbour or from the secondary launch site across the beach.

CURRENT ASSETS MST Rescue 900, named E.ON Spirit of Maryport, funded by Energy company E.ON and a local appeal, launched by Talus MB-H tractor and carriage, on station 2008; IB1 D Class named Lady Anne Cunningham, launched by Loglogic Tooltrak, on station 2021; Zodiac Milpro ERB 4.3m, launched by Land Rover and trailer, on station 2012.

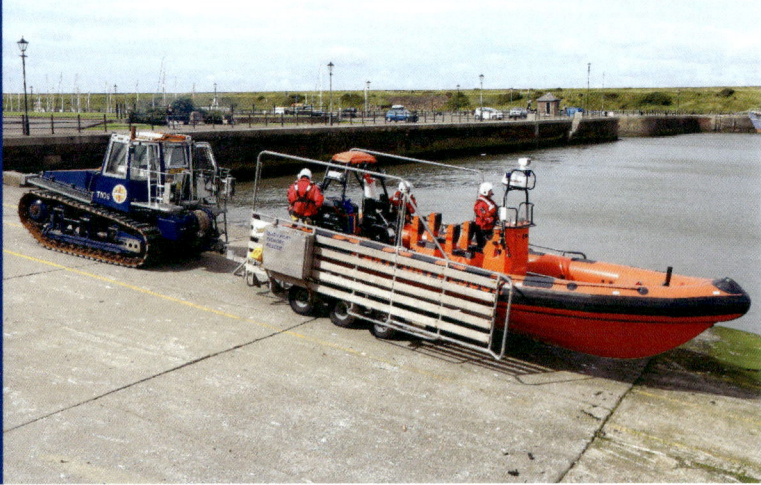

Maryport lifeboat E.ON Spirit of Maryport being launched on exercise in August 2017 by the ex-RNLI Talus MB-H tractor, numbered T106 by the RNLI, which served the RNLI stations at Scarborough and Filey. (Martin Fish)

Independent lifeboats of Britain

SCOTLAND

Nith • Port William • Fleet Bay • Glasgow • Loch Lomond • East Sutherland • Moray • St Abbs

Independent lifeboats of Britain

NITH — Dumfries

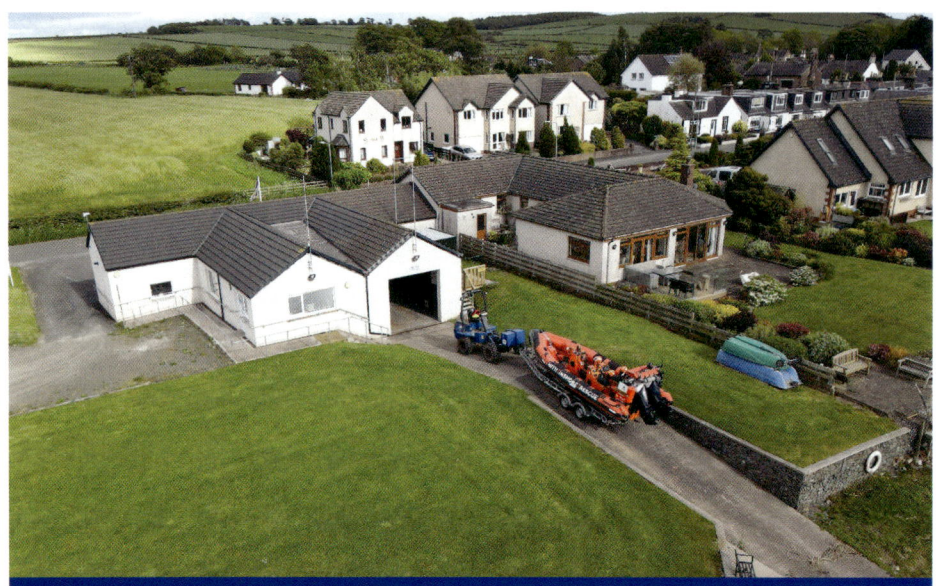

The Nith Inshore Rescue lifeboat house on the banks of the river Nith in Glencaple. The boathouse, which has been extended since the service was founded, is situated on land leased from the Caerlaverock Estate. (Nicholas Leach)

LOCATION Glencaple, south of Dumfries
ORGANISATION Nith Inshore Rescue
ESTABLISHED 1981
HISTORY Nith Inshore Rescue, based in Glencaple, five miles south of Dumfries, covers the estuary of the River Nith where it joins the Solway Firth, together with other rivers and lochs in the area. The service was established in the winter of 1981-82 following a series of tragedies in the tidal waters of the Nith, which were covered by the RNLI station at Silloth, across the Solway in Cumbria, the nearest lifeboat. Local people decided the Glencaple area needed its own rescue boat, to be based in the village. Following extensive fundraising, donations from private individuals and local businesses the first boat was purchased. The lifeboat was a 12.5ft Zodiac inflatable fitted

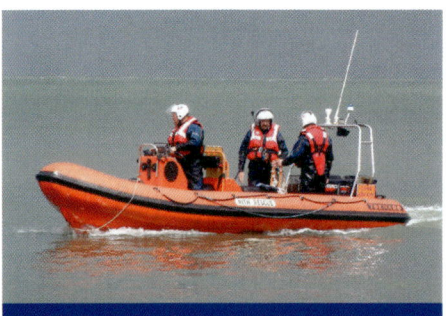

The 6.5m Tornado rigid inflatable Lena Burton served at Nith from 1997 to 2010. (Nicholas Leach)

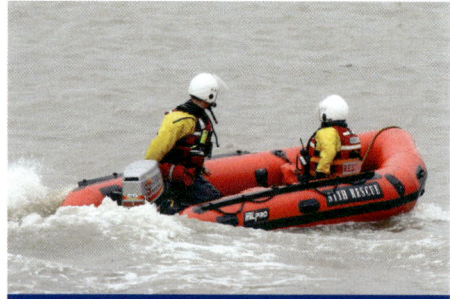

Nith Inshore Rescue's Zodiac Milpro ERB 380, named Cauley, at Kippford in July 2019. (Martin Fish)

Independent lifeboats of Britain

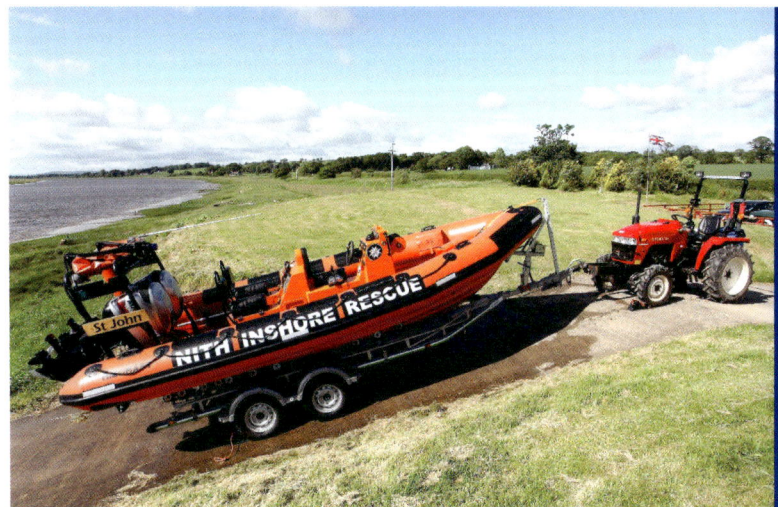

The twin-engined 6.8m Ribcraft rigid inflatable St John, acquired in 2010, pictured in June 2012 with the small launch tractor. (Nicholas Leach)

with a 35hp outboard engine and a VHF radio.
PREVIOUS ASSETS
1989 The first boat served until 1989 when, due to its age and the increased area the Service was being required to cover, a new lifeboat was deemed necessary. The Service managed to raise enough money to buy the second boat, a 5.1m rigid inflatable lifeboat fitted with a 60hp outboard.
1997 The lifeboat was again upgraded with a 6.5m Tornado rigid inflatable. Named Lena Burton, it was powered by twin 60hp Mercury outboards and a seating console for the helm and two crew. A stainless steel roll bar over the engines provides mounting for the VHF radio aerials, lighting and GPS navigation equipment. The lifeboat could operate in as little as two feet of water and carried fuel for six hours of running up to speeds of 30 knots. The lifeboat was launched stern first down a

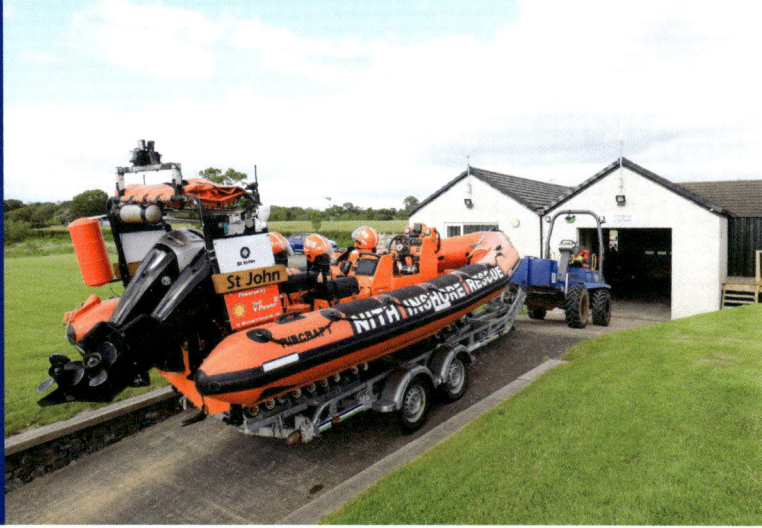

The main lifeboat in service at Nith is the 6.8m Ribcraft St John, which was funded by the St John The Priory of Scotland organisation. The Benford 4x4 launch vehicle is specially adapted for launching the lifeboat into the tidal estuary. (Nicholas Leach)

Independent lifeboats of Britain

slipway by tractor at Glencaple.

2010 In preparation for the new Rescue Boat Code of Practice, the service upgraded the main lifeboat to a Ribcraft 6.8m Professional rigid inflatable powered by twin Mariner 90hp outboards. A roll bar provides mounting for a righting airbag and electronic equipment. A grant of £25,000 towards the new boat was received from St John The Priory of Scotland, and the new boat was named St John in recognition of their support. The new lifeboat became operational in February 2010.

2015 The Service also operates a second smaller Avon ERB inflatable, which is towed by a Land Rover on a trailer to access incidents inland from Glencaple and on lochs if required. In 2015 a new 3.8m Zodiac Milpro inflatable, powered by a 25hp Mariner outboard, was acquired. Dedicated to the memory of Dumfries teenager Macauley McQueen, who tragically died in the River Nith, the boat was named Cauley in a ceremony performed by the charity's patron, Lady Herries of Terregles.

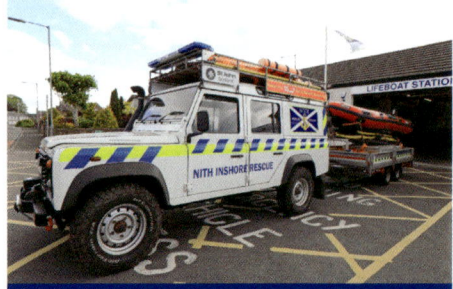

Land Rover 110 used for launch and recovery of the smaller Zodiac Milpro boat, which can be taken to different launch sites. (Nicholas Leach)

2017 In May an extension to the lifeboat station at Glencaple was completed following an extensive refurbishment of the building to include a training room and enhanced crew facilities. The building houses both lifeboats and launch vehicles with a dedicated access slipway into the River Nith.

CURRENT ASSETS 6.8m Ribcraft Professional, St John, on station 2010; Benford 4x4 vehicle and trailer; Zodiac Milpro ERB 380, named Cauley, on station 2015; Land Rover and trailer.

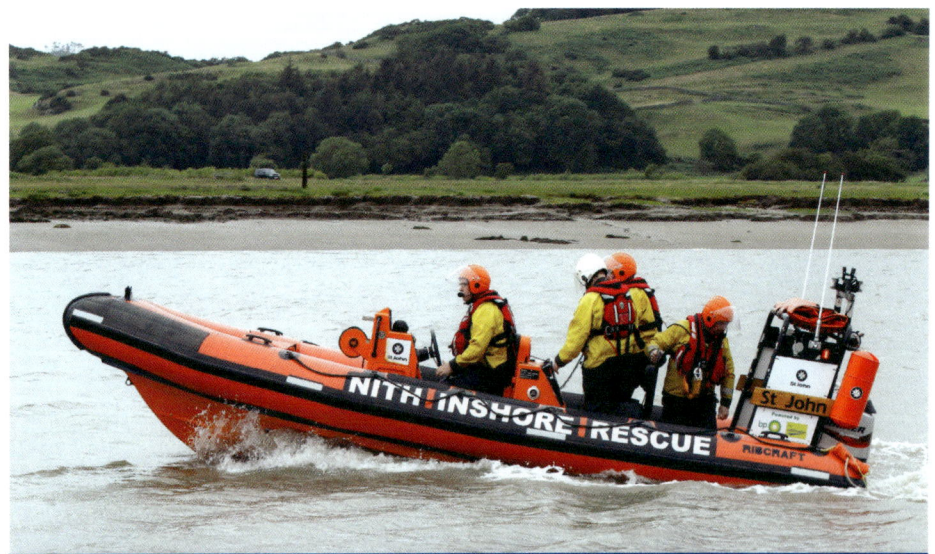

The Ribcraft rigid inflatable St John at Kippford RNLI's annual open day, July 2019, at which various neighbouring lifeboats were in attendance, including Workington RNLI and Kirkcudbright RNLI. (Martin Fish)

PORT WILLIAM
Dumfries and Galloway

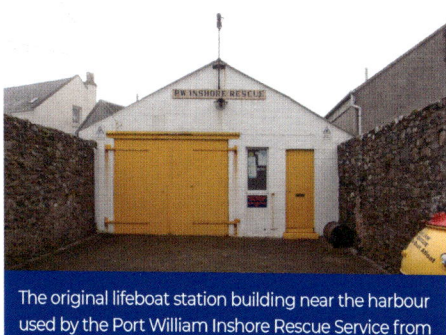

The original lifeboat station building near the harbour used by the Port William Inshore Rescue Service from its establishment in 1979 until 2015. (Martin Fish)

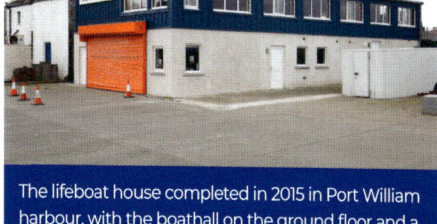

The lifeboat house completed in 2015 in Port William harbour, with the boathall on the ground floor and a shop and cafe on the first storey. (Martin Fish)

LOCATION Dumfries and Galloway
ORGANISATION Port William Inshore Rescue Service
ESTABLISHED 1979
HISTORY Port William Inshore Rescue Service was formed in 1979 after a fisherman got into difficulty and the nearest lifeboats were some distance away in Kirkcudbright and Portpatrick. An initial approach was made to the RNLI, who declined to establish a station at Port William, so a local committee was established and an independent service was set up to cover the Luce Bay and surrounding areas. After local fund-raising a semi-rigid inflatable boat was purchased and put into service, crewed by local volunteers. The 5m Avon Searider was powered by a single 50hp Yamaha outboard engine and the crew were seated at a console, which also contained the helm controls and radio. The first lifeboat was known as PIRSAC I (Port William Inshore Rescue Service Action Committee) and went

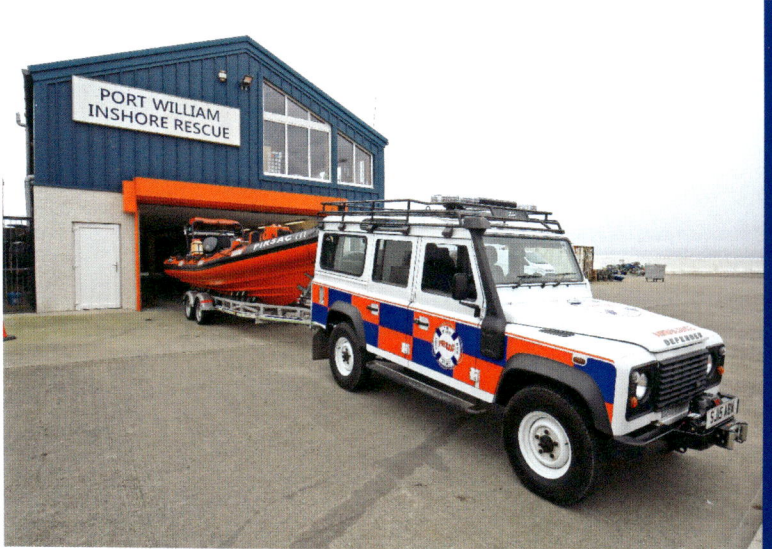

Following significant funding received from the Dumfries and Galloway European Fisheries Fund, the Service acquired a new Ribcraft lifeboat and new shore facilities in 2015. (Martin Fish)

Independent lifeboats of Britain

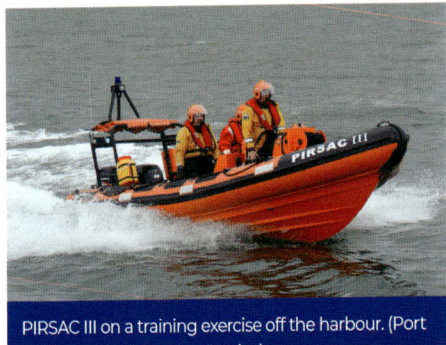

PIRSAC III on a training exercise off the harbour. (Port William Inshore Rescue Service)

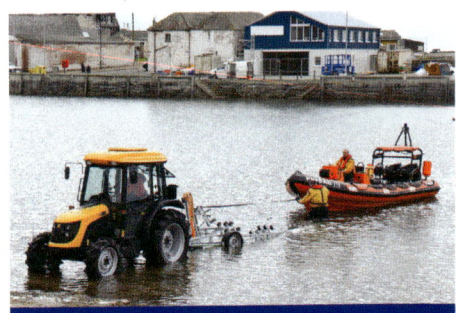

JCB 360 tractor used for launching the lifeboat in the harbour. (Port William Inshore Rescue Service)

into service in June 1979. The Service operated from a small boathouse in the harbour at Port William, which housed the lifeboat and launch vehicle, with basic crew facilities.

PREVIOUS ASSETS

1998 A new 5.5m rigid inflatable with a GRP hull and inflatable sponsons, initially powered by twin 40hp Yamaha engines, was acquired. Named PIRSAC II, it was built by Tornado RIBs of Hull. The outboard engines were subsequently upgraded to 60hp to improve the boat's performance. The boat featured a centre console in a delta configuration with jockey seats for the helm and the crew. A roll bar was fitted at the stern as a mounting for the VHF aerial and navigation lights. For launching and recovery, the boat was towed on a road trailer by a Land Rover Defender 110.

2013 In December Dumfries and Galloway European Fisheries Fund awarded the Service more than £240,000 towards the cost of both a new fully-equipped rigid inflatable rescue boat and the construction of a new lifeboat station building.

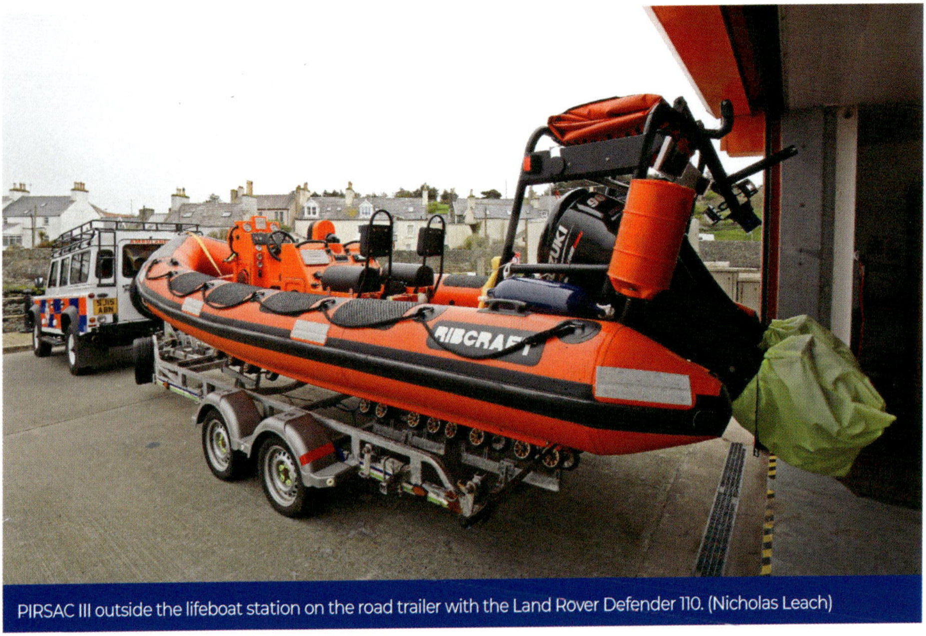

PIRSAC III outside the lifeboat station on the road trailer with the Land Rover Defender 110. (Nicholas Leach)

Independent lifeboats of Britain

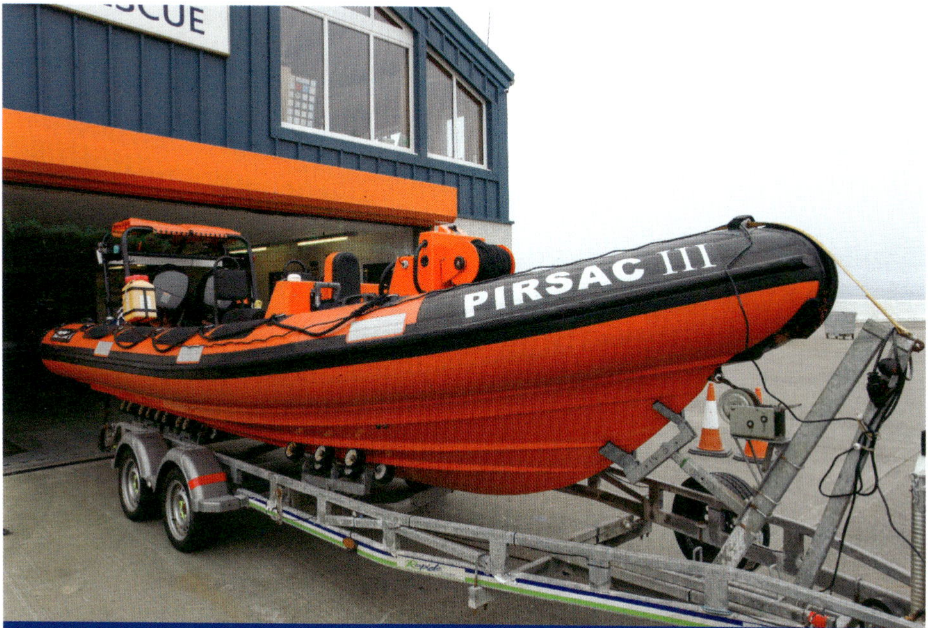

The 6.4m Ribcraft Professional lifeboat PIRSAC III placed on station in 2015. The Ribcraft design is used by a large number of UK independent lifeboats. (Nicholas Leach)

2015 The Service's third new boat arrived in August. The 6.4m Ribcraft Professional rigid inflatable was built by Ribcraft at Yeovil, with orange Hypalon inflatable sponsons and anti-slip decking. A crew console has three seats, for helm and two crew. The fuel system has twin 20 gallon stainless steel under deck fuel tanks feeding twin 90hp Suzuki four-stroke outboard motors. An aluminium roll bar frame for a self-righting airbag is fitted over the engines. The roll bar also provides mounting for the navigation lights, aerials and radar reflector. In addition to the new boat, the funding award also enabled a replacement Land Rover launching vehicle to be acquired.

The new two-storey boathouse was completed in November 2015. The ground floor features a large boathall to house lifeboat and launching vehicles, a crew changing area and office. A community hub, including a coffee and gift shop, on the upper level provides income for the charity. The move into the new building allowed a JCB tractor to be purchased as an additional option for launching into the harbour at Port William, with the Land Rover being used to take the lifeboat by road to alternative launch sites as required. An opening ceremony for the new building took place in June 2017.

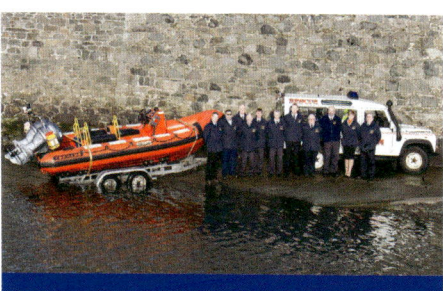

The Tornado RIB PIRSAC II with the Land Rover and crew at the harbour in Port William. (Port William Inshore Rescue Service)

CURRENT ASSETS Ribcraft 6.4m Professional, named PIRSAC III, on station 2015; Benford 4x4 vehicle for launch and recovery, on station 2021.

Independent lifeboats of Britain

FLEET BAY (MOSSYARD)
Dumfries and Galloway

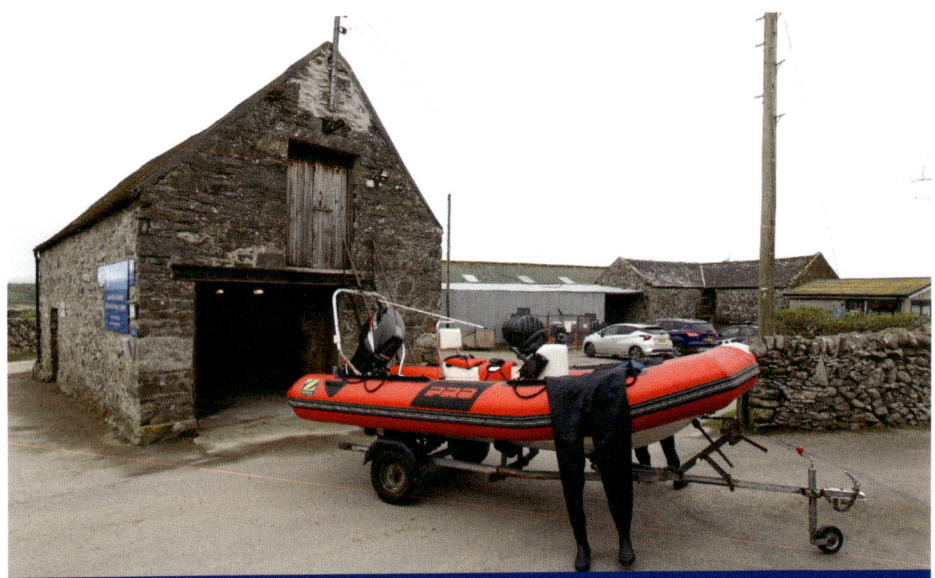

The Fleet Bay Inshore Rescue Boat outside the boathouse at Mossyard Caravan Park. (Martin Fish)

LOCATION Gatehouse of Fleet, Dumfries
ORGANISATION Fleet Bay Inshore Rescue Boat
ESTABLISHED 1974
HISTORY The Fleet Bay Inshore Rescue Boat operates from a small boathouse at Mossyard Caravan Park, where water sports and sea-based activities are undertaken all year round. The Rescue Boat Committee ensures the service provides a quick response to any incidents and emergencies in Fleet Bay. The service is financed by public donations and annual contributions from holiday park owners around the Fleet Bay area.
PREVIOUS ASSETS
1974 The first lifeboat was funded by donations made by the caravan park owners and cost £858. The boat was kept on a trailer in a small boathouse on the Mossyard Caravan Park site, being towed by a 4x4 vehicle to the beach to launch when required.
2003 In October 2003 a new lifeboat was provided. After eight years of fundraising and a successful application to the National Lottery a more modern version of the original boat was acquired. A £5,000 lottery grant was used as a contribution towards the cost of the new Zodiac Pro 3 rigid inflatable. A central console has a seated helm position with seating for two crew members.
CURRENT ASSETS Zodiac Pro 3 RIB, on station 2003; launched by trailer.

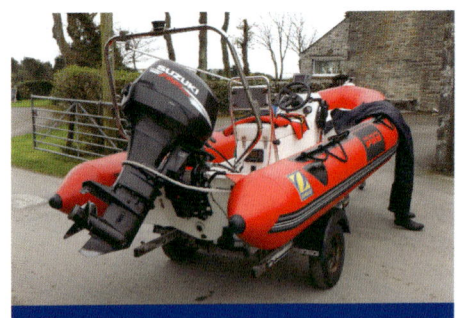

The Fleet Bay IRB is a small Zodiac Pro 3 fitted with a Suzuki four-stroke outboard engine. (Martin Fish)

Independent lifeboats of Britain

GLASGOW

Glasgow

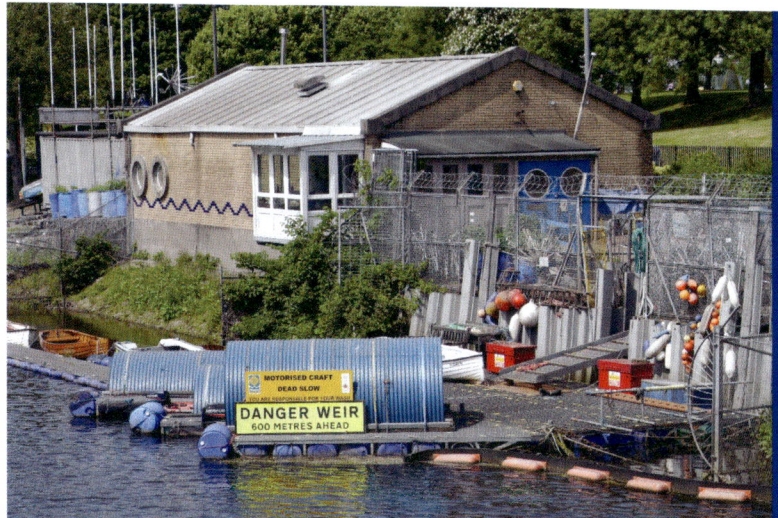

The boathouse at Glasgow Green, on the north bank of the River Clyde, with pontoon berths for a range of motor and rowing rescue boats. (Martin Fish)

LOCATION Glasgow Green, Glasgow
ORGANISATION Glasgow Humane Society
ESTABLISHED 1790
HISTORY Glasgow Humane Society has been saving lives on and around Glasgow's waterways for over 230 years. It is the oldest practical lifesaving organisation in the world, and has been based at Glasgow Green since 1790. The Society is a registered charity and relies on donations from the public and support from Glasgow City Council. It was established by members of the Royal College of Physicians and Surgeons of Glasgow, who were concerned with the high loss of life on the River Clyde, and so appointed a full-time Officer to provide a dedicated rescue and recovery service.

In 1795 the Lord Provost and Magistrates attended a meeting of directors, and suggested that a house should be built to accommodate the Society's boat and provide a residence for a Society Officer. This was subsequently built on Glasgow Green. Since then, a full-time Society Officer has managed the service, supported by volunteers, who patrol the waterways of Glasgow and undertake rescues, primarily using a range of small rowing lifeboats and bankside rescue equipment.

Today, the Society carries out a variety of water safety and rescue work for several different groups, including the local rowing clubs and emergency services, as well as private businesses for specific event related safety provision. The Society is contracted by Glasgow City Council to maintain the public rescue equipment along the River Clyde and works with community groups along to promote water safety, education and drowning prevention.

KEY EVENTS
1934 The first motorised lifeboat went into service, when the Society received permission to use a motor boat on the river in an area under the jurisdiction of the Clyde Navigation Trustees.
1935 The Humane Society boathouse, in need of replacement, was demolished in 1935, to be replaced by a new building on Glasgow Green.
1991 A new riverside boathouse was opened which is the current base for operation and maintenance of the rescue boats.
2005 The immediate response to water rescue

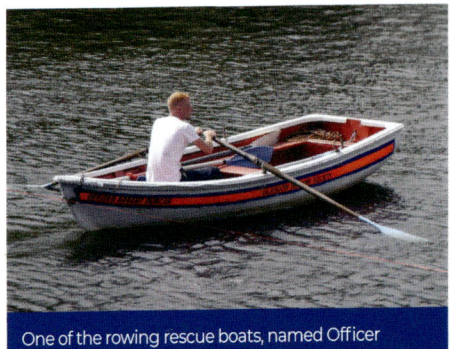

One of the rowing rescue boats, named Officer Robert Duncan, on patrol on the Clyde. (Martin Fish)

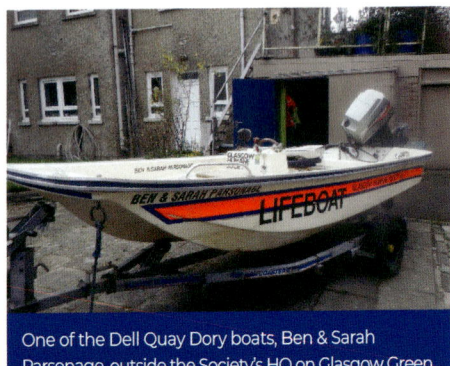

One of the Dell Quay Dory boats, Ben & Sarah Parsonage, outside the Society's HQ on Glasgow Green.

incidents passed to Strathclyde Fire and Rescue Service, then to the national Scottish Fire & Rescue Service. The Humane Society went from being the dedicated resource for waterway rescue in the Greater Glasgow area to being an additional resource, enabling the Society to concentrate on accident prevention but still being available for rescue and recovery tasks in the immediate area around Glasgow Green.

2021 In May a new rescue boat was acquired with the purchase of a Whaly 500 rigid boat, powered by a 50hp Yamaha outboard; named Lede, it is based at Kelvin Harbour.

CURRENT ASSETS The Humane Society operates a range of rescue boats from its boathouse at Glasgow Green. The small rowing lifeboats are built to a design refined by the Society with great inherent stability to allow casualties to be pulled out of the water without swamping the boat. In addition to the rowing lifeboats, a number of motorised small rescue boats are used, including a Dell Quay Dory, named Ben & Sarah Parsonage, which is powered by a Mercury outboard engine.

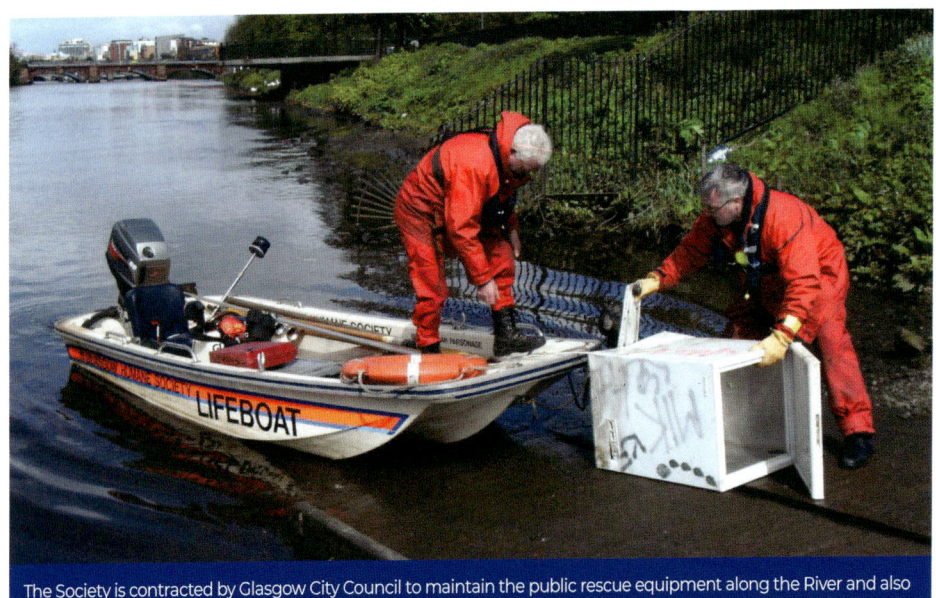

The Society is contracted by Glasgow City Council to maintain the public rescue equipment along the River and also undertake a wide range of work to ensure the safety of waterways in the City. (Courtesy Glasgow Humane Society)

LOCH LOMOND
Argyll and Bute

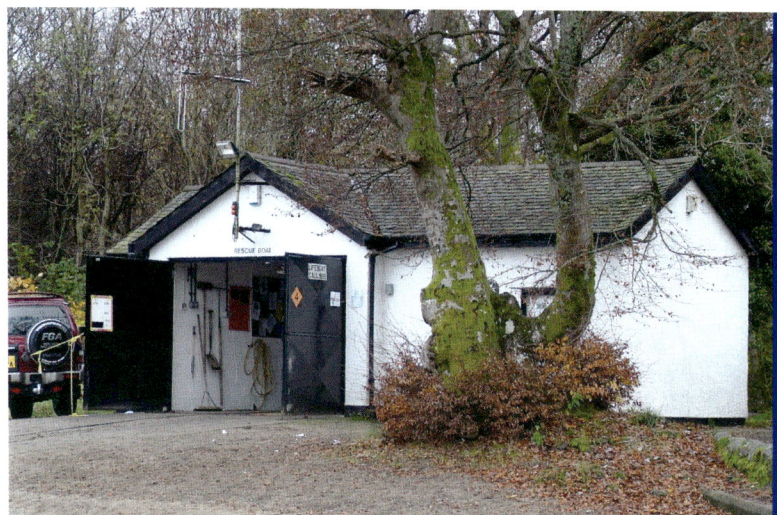

The boathouse used by the Loch Lomond Rescue Boat on the launch trolley built at a site on the Western shore of the Loch at Luss. St John Scotland funded an £18,000 extension to the boathouse.

LOCATION Luss, western shore of the Loch
ORGANISATION Loch Lomond Rescue Boat
ESTABLISHED 1977
HISTORY The Loch Lomond Rescue Boat organisation was founded in 1977 when an anonymous sailor donated £10,000 to provide a rescue service to cover the 27 square miles of the picturesque Loch. The Royal Society for the Prevention of Accidents (ROSPA) supported the new venture and have it operated under their umbrella. The first lifeboat, obtained in 1978, was a rigid inflatable powered by a 55hp Evinrude outboard engine with a central seated console for the helm and a second crew member. The boat was named Luss Younger by HRH Prince Charles.

Governance of the rescue boat charity changed when the Loch Lomond Association took over from ROSPA, and in the 1990s a standalone committee was formed for overseeing the running the rescue boat.

BOATHOUSE The boat is kept on a trolley in a boathouse at Luss. A winch cable is used to get the launch trolley in and out of the water. The station was extended during 1992-93 and fully rebuilt in 2000, funded largely by the Order of St John in Scotland.

PREVIOUS ASSETS
1992 A new lifeboat was obtained to replace the original boat. The Avon Searider rigid inflatable boat, powered by twin Mariner outboard engines, was purchased after the Hugh Fraser Foundation provided funding for the new boat, which cost £25,000. The craft was formally named Sir Hugh Fraser at a ceremony by Mrs Elma Mills, wife of Vale of Leven Councillor Duncan Mills. A folding roll bar over the engines provided a mounting for VHF and GPS aerials, and lights.

The first Loch Lomond rescue boat, named Luss Younger, was placed in service in 1978.

2006 The service purchased a VT Halmatic Arctic 22 rigid inflatable boat, which can reach speeds of around 40 knots, enabling it to reach the furthest ends of the Loch within 20 minutes. The main contributor to the £105,000 cost was St John Scotland, who gave £32,000. The boat was formally named St John in 2006 by HRH Princess Royal at a ceremony attended by crew, families, committee members and local dignitaries.

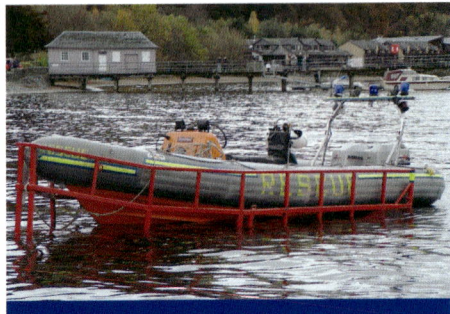

The Avon RIB Sir Hugh Fraser on the launching trolley.

2022 A planning application was submitted for a new station building at Balloch, on a new site near Balloch Pier, close to the mouth of the River Leven. The popularity of the wider Loch Lomond area has been delaying crew members from reaching the existing station at Luss. For a trial period the lifeboat had been kept afloat at Duncan Mills Memorial Slipway, close to the new site, and crew response times greatly improved. Funding in the region of £300,000 is needed.

CURRENT ASSETS VT Halmatic Arctic 22 6.5m rigid inflatable, named St John, powered by two 115hp Mercury four-stroke outboard engines, launched with trolley and winch.

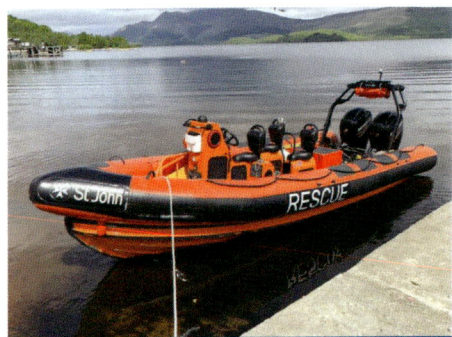

The current Loch Lomond lifeboat St John has a Halmatic Arctic hull, a design used by a number of independent lifeboats around the UK.

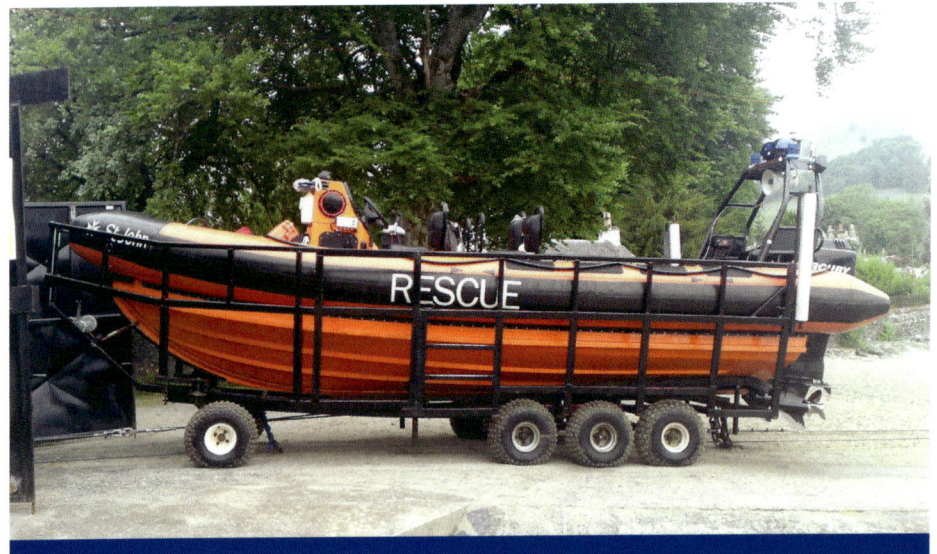

The current Loch Lomond lifeboat Sir Hugh Fraser outside the boathouse.

Independent lifeboats of Britain

EAST SUTHERLAND

Sutherland

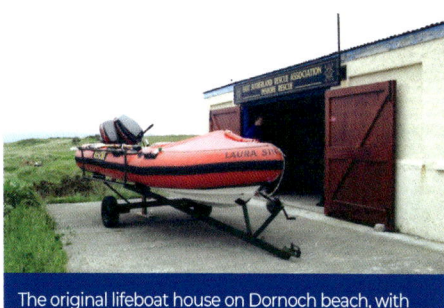

The original lifeboat house on Dornoch beach, with the Association's second ILB outside.

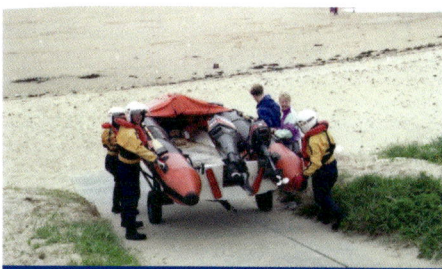

The small open rigid inflatable Laura Sinclair served as the Association's first lifeboat from 1982 to 1987.

LOCATION Dornoch, Sutherland
ORGANISATION East Sutherland Rescue Association (ESRA)
ESTABLISHED 1981
HISTORY East Sutherland Rescue Association, also known as Dornoch Inshore Rescue, is located on Dornoch beach. The Service was formed in 1981 following concerns about the level of emergency response in the area, particularly around popular beaches at Dornoch and Embo. Local people established a committee to fund an inshore lifeboat and train a crew. A boathouse on the beach was obtained in 1982 and fitted out, but lacked mains water and electricity. Training was undertaken using borrowed equipment. The first lifeboat, an open rigid inflatable with a tiller-controlled outboard engine, arrived in 1982 and was named Laura Sinclair after the first casualty rescued. The young girl from Thurso had been swept out to sea on an inflatable dinghy. The Service covers the east coast of Sutherland and Easter Ross, bordering the Dornoch Firth.

In March 2021 construction started on a new lifeboat station building to provide much improved facilities. The new building was completed during the summer of 2022, and was formally opened at a ceremony on

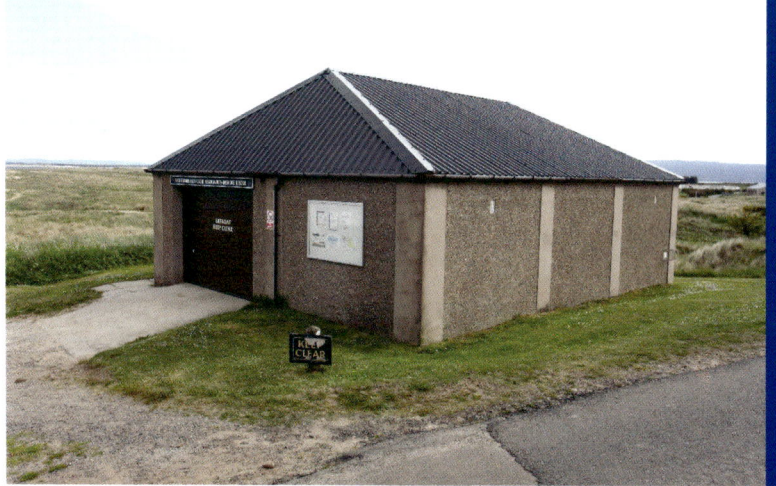

The lifeboat house used by the East Sutherland Rescue Association, situated at Dornoch beach car park, pictured in June 2013. The building was replaced in 2022. (Nicholas Leach)

Independent lifeboats of Britain

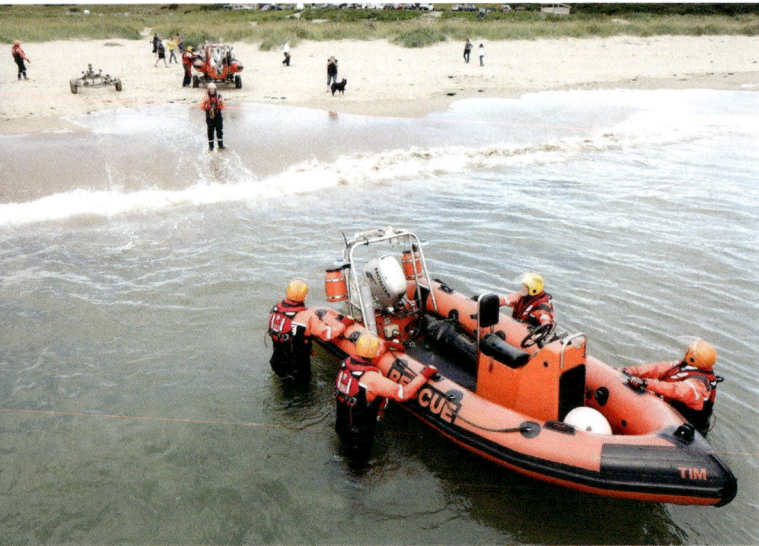

The 4.8m Ribcraft lifeboat Tim Jarvis off the beach at Dornoch with the second lifeboat Glen Cassley and lifeboat station in the background. (Photo by courtesy of East Sutherland Rescue Association)

14 August 2022. The Highland Council provided the site for the new building, adjacent to the original boathouse. The new £550,000 building was formally opened by main benefactor Charles Cadogan, 8th Earl Cadogan, who contributed more than £400,000 towards the cost of the spacious boathouse. Rev John Chambers conducted the service of dedication. The two-storey building has an enlarged boathall for two rescue boats and launch vehicle, together with toilets, showers, changing and drying rooms, kitchen, training room and first aid facilities.

PREVIOUS ASSETS
1988 A larger rigid inflatable, named Laura Sinclair II, was acquired. It had a seated helm position, a roll bar at the stern for navigation lights and aerials, and a single outboard engine.
1997 A new 4.8m Ribcraft rigid inflatable was obtained and named William B. Ashplant; it was powered by a 50hp Yamaha.
2005 A new 4.8m Ribcraft, powered by a 50hp Honda outboard, was purchased. The lifeboat was named Tim Jarvis after a founder member of the service who collapsed following a heart attack during a training session in October 2004.
2015 A Loglogic Tooltrak tracked vehicle was purchased for launching and recovery.
2016 An updated version of the Ribcraft boat,

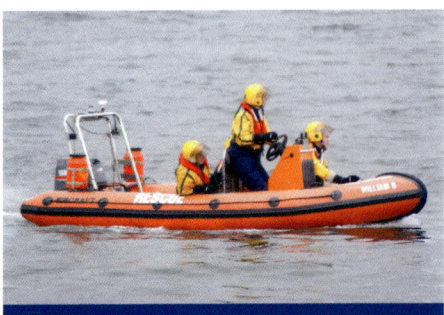

The 4.8m Ribcraft rigid inflatable William B. Ashplant was acquired by the Association in 1997.

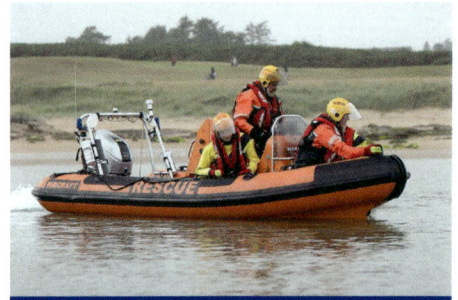

The 4.8m rigid inflatable Glen Cassley was funded by Lord Cadogan and built by Ribcraft of Yeovil.

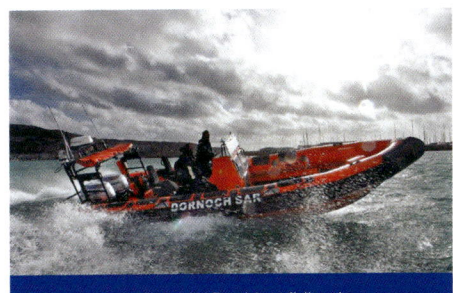
The new Ribcraft rigid inflatable Wildlands.

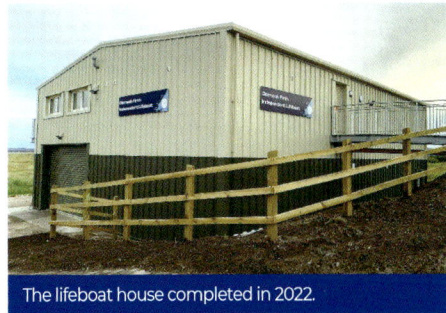
The lifeboat house completed in 2022.

with a 60hp Honda outboard, was obtained. Named Glen Cassley, she featured enhanced electrical equipment with a console behind the helm position for the radio and GPS equipment.
2022 A new 7.8m Ribcraft rigid inflatable, named Wildlands, was built, as well as a Loglogic Softrak launch and recovery vehicle, funded by Highland-based land conservation and tourism business Wildland Limited owned by Danish billionaire Anders Holch Povlsen.
CURRENT ASSETS Two 4.8m Ribcraft rigid inflatable lifeboats: Glen Cassley (in service 2016) and Tim Jarvis (in service 2007); latter

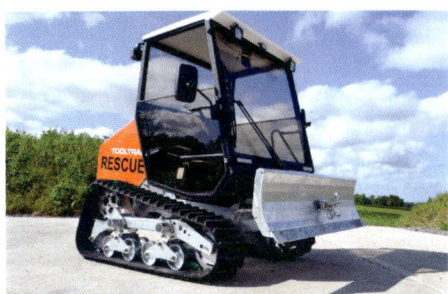
The Loglogic Tooltrak vehicle used by the ESRA.

used as a reserve. Loglogic Softrak tracked vehicle used for launch and recovery.

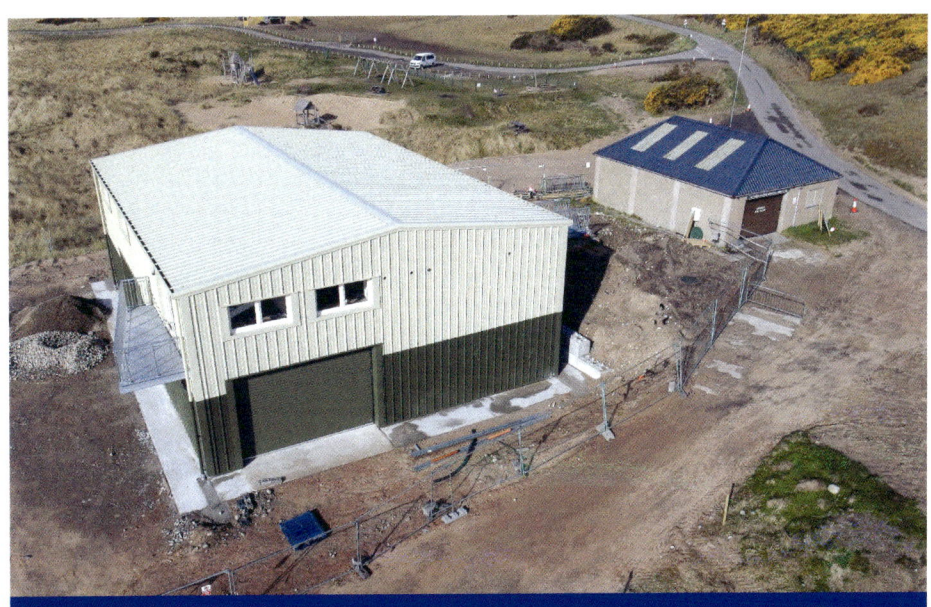
The new lifeboat house at Dornoch under construction in April 2022. Situated adjacent to the original boathouse, the new building provides greatly improved crew facilities. (Martin Fish)

Independent lifeboats of Britain

MORAY

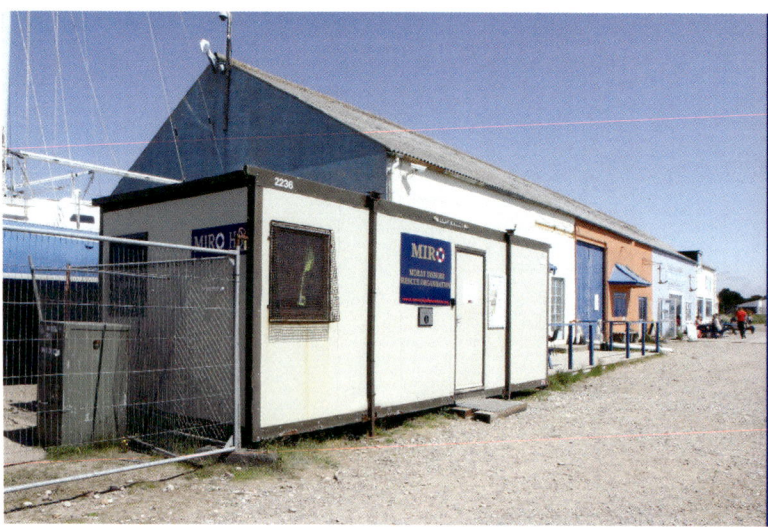

The shore facility used by MIRO volunteers is located in Findhorn Marina at the mouth of the River Findhorn. (Nicholas Leach)

LOCATION Findhorn, Moray
ORGANISATION Moray Inshore Rescue Organisation (MIRO)
ESTABLISHED 2005
HISTORY The Moray Inshore Rescue Organisation (MIRO) was established in July 2005 as a rescue service covering Findhorn Bay and its approaches. The Maritime Coastguard Agency agreed that a dedicated rescue service was required and tasked MIRO to cover Findhorn Bay as well as the inshore waters of the Moray Firth between Burghead and Nairn.

In August 2005 MIRO launched its first boat, a 5.8m Humber Destroyer rigid inflatable powered by twin Mercury 60hp outboards, with a seated helm position. The boat was named Glyn Whitehead after a Findhorn sailor who tragically lost his life at sea in 2003. In August 2007 MIRO became an MCA declared facility with volunteers on call 24 hours a day. The Service operates from a base at Findhorn Marina, with the lifeboat being kept afloat during the summer and ashore on a trailer at other times. Crew facilities are provided in a temporary building within the marina site.

PREVIOUS ASSETS
2013 Supported by funding from the Budge Trust, MIRO purchased a new boat. Slightly larger than the first boat, the 6.5m Humber Ocean Pro rigid inflatable was powered by twin 90hp Mariner outboard engines and had seating for the helm and two crew. A roll bar over the engines carried a righting airbag. After delivery from the Humber factory, the boat was fitted with engines and ancillary kit by Findhorn Marina prior to undergoing sea trials. The boat was officially launched in June 2013 by Mrs Lorraine Budge at Findhorn Marina and named Glyn Whitehead II.
2016 In April a Barrus SeaSearch inflatable powered by a 20hp Honda outboard engine was acquired. This additional lifeboat was for use as a shallow water rescue boat to supplement the Humber RIB. The boat was named Graham Millar in memory of one of the organisation's crew members.
2019 A Humber Ocean Pro boat was purchased, funded after MIRO undertook a £68,000 campaign for a new boat to improve capabilities, helped by a Department of

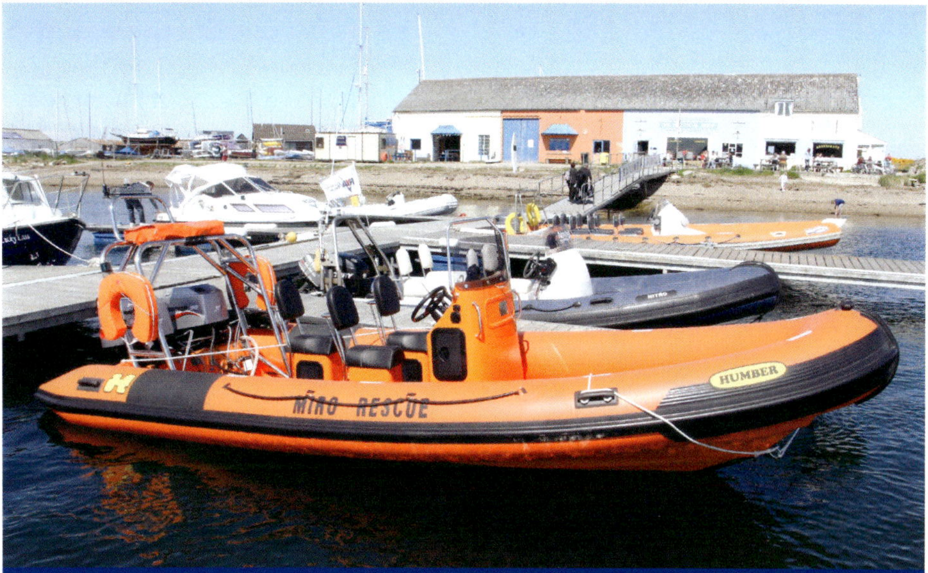

Glynn Whitehead II afloat in Findhorn Marina, pictured in June 2013. (Nicholas Leach)

Transport funding grant. The new boat had a larger console with seating for four crew, and, for the first time on a MIRO boat, radar was fitted to the rear roll bar. In November 2019 Grenville Johnston, Lord Lieutenant of Moray, named the boat Glyn Whitehead III.

2020 To improve the launch and recovery procedure, a £15,500 contribution from the UK Government's Department for Transport's rescue boat grant fund enabled the purchase of a Kubota tractor, removing the need to utilise other marina vehicles. A further improvement to launch and recovery was made when funding from the Gordon and Ena Baxter Foundation enabled MIRO to purchase a floating drive-on docking system for use when the lifeboat is afloat in the Marina, to keep it out of the water.

CURRENT ASSETS Humber Ocean Pro, named Glyn Whitehead III, launched from a floating VersaDock or Kubota L1421 tractor and trailer, on station 2019; SeaSearch SS420 HD inflatable, named Graham Millar, launched by trailer; on station 2016.

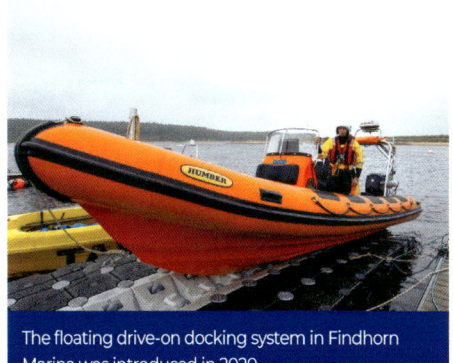

The floating drive-on docking system in Findhorn Marina was introduced in 2020.

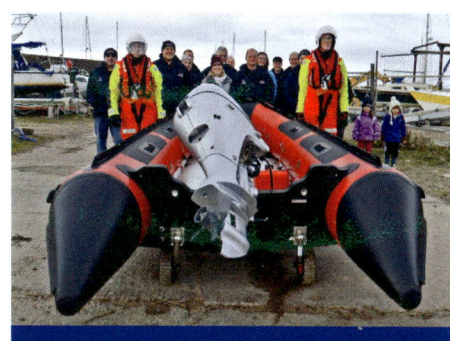

The SeaSearch SS420 HD inflatable Graham Millar is used for shallow water rescues.

Independent lifeboats of Britain   145

ST ABBS

Borders

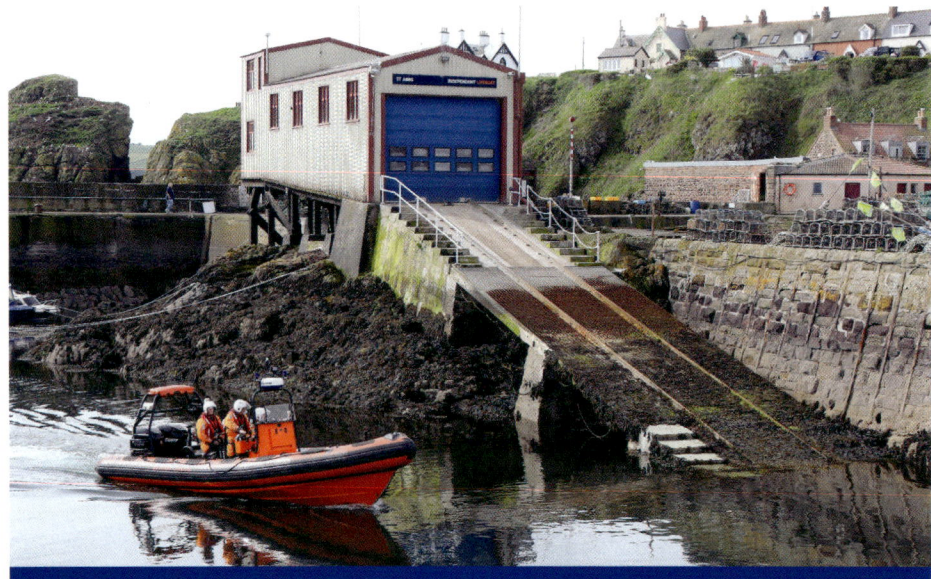

The lifeboat station in the small picturesque harbour at St Abbs. The slipway was built by the RNLI in 1911, and the lifeboat house was added in 1915; the house was adapted and extended for subsequent lifeboats. (Nicholas Leach)

LOCATION Scottish Borders
ORGANISATION St Abbs Lifeboat
ESTABLISHED 2016
HISTORY The independent lifeboat service was set up in response to the RNLI withdrawal in 2015. Following a Coast Review, the RNLI decided to close the station and their Atlantic 75 lifeboat left for the last time on 8 September 2015. Local people strongly opposed the closure, and decided to raise funds to purchase a lifeboat, which would be operated independently. Considerable fund-raising work was undertaken, and, with a generous donation from Boyd Tunnock, enabled the new organisation to purchase a new MST 900W lifeboat. This boat was officially named Thomas Tunnock by the donor in honour of his late brother and

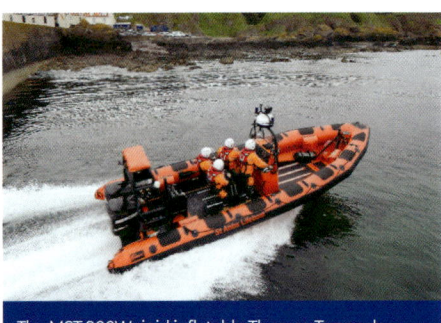

The MST 900W rigid inflatable Thomas Tunnock heading out of St Abbs harbour on exercise.

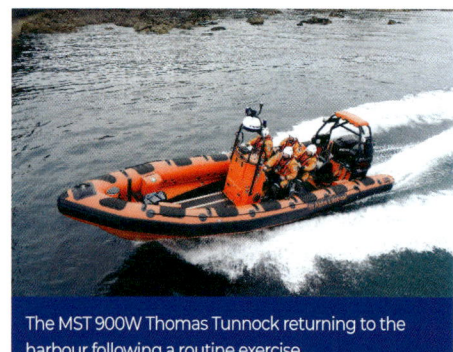

The MST 900W Thomas Tunnock returning to the harbour following a routine exercise.

Independent lifeboats of Britain

grandfather, at a ceremony on 17 September 2016, which was attended by Nicola Sturgeon, MSP, First Minister of Scotland. The lifeboat operates from the boathouse and slipway used by the RNLI; the slip, built in 1911, and the boathouse, in 1915, were subsequently modified.

CURRENT ASSETS Marine Specialised Technology 900W rigid inflatable, named Thomas Tunnock, 9m by 3.05m by 0.7m, powered by twin 200hp Mercury OptiMax outboard engines, speed in excess of 45 knots, range 150 nautical miles.

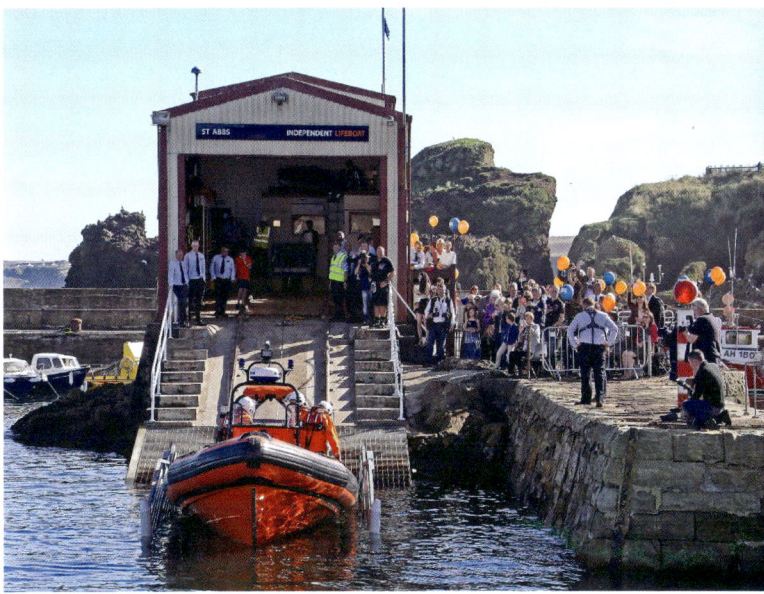

The scene during the naming ceremony of Thomas Tunnock on 17 September 2016, attended by hundreds of people, who lined the harbour to watch the proceedings. (Nicholas Leach)

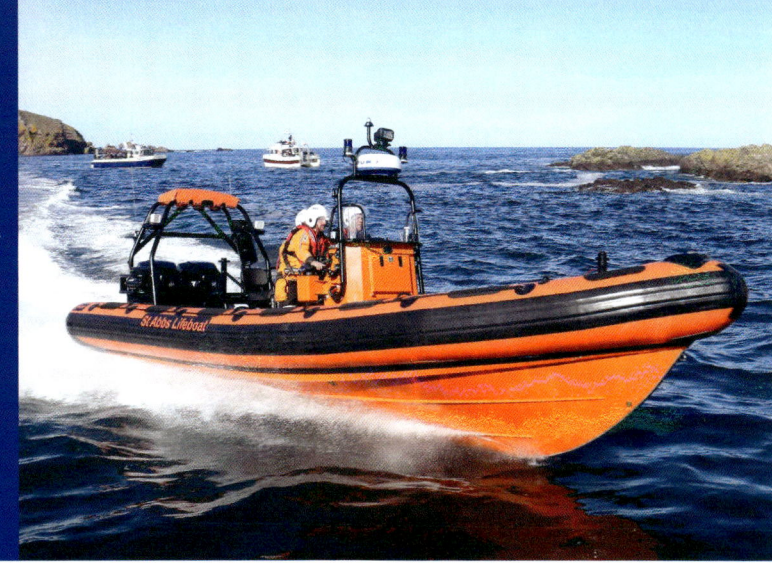

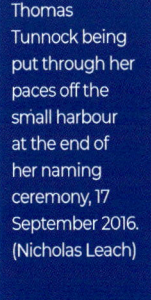

Thomas Tunnock being put through her paces off the small harbour at the end of her naming ceremony, 17 September 2016. (Nicholas Leach)

Independent lifeboats of Britain

INLAND STATIONS

YORK

HISTORY York Rescue Boat is an independent search and rescue charity based in the city of York. The charity was founded in 2014 after a series of deaths in the rivers Ouse and Foss, which run through the city. A Memorandum of Understanding with North Yorkshire Fire and Rescue Service enables the Service to call upon York Rescue Boat to assist with rescues, missing person searches and any other incidents on the water.

ASSETS The Service operated a Humber rigid inflatable boat powered by a Mercury outboard engine, with a central steering console for the helm. The lifeboat was kept moored at a pontoon on the River Ouse. The charity uses a Mitsubishi 4x4 rescue vehicle and a Ford Transit support vehicle to provide an operating base during patrols. In July 2021 the Service ordered a new lifeboat financed by extensive local fund-raising undertaken in memory of Sonny Ferry, who drowned in the River Foss. The new lifeboat, named Spirit of Sonny, was built by Highfield and is based on their Patrol 660 hull, with bespoke modifications to suit requirements at York.

FLOOD RESCUE In addition to response work on the rivers, York Rescue provides a national Flood Rescue Team as part of Surf Life Saving GB's network of flood rescue trained volunteers. For flood response York Rescue has a Bay Industrial FRB-400 inflatable rescue boat powered by a 30hp Mariner outboard engine and a specialist RescueONE Connector flood rescue boat.

WATERSAFE UK

HISTORY Watersafe UK Search & Rescue Team is a voluntary search & rescue organisation and registered charity based in the East Midlands. The Team provides operational support to the Fire Service, Police and other blue light services, operating from a base at Redhill Marina at Ratcliffe on Soar near Nottingham. The Team was established in 2009 in response to the National Flood Enhancement Project led by the Department of the Environment, Food & Rural Affairs (DEFRA). This Government project organised the water rescue assets around the UK and assessed them against national standards so that, in the event of widespread flooding these assets can be called upon, and they will operate to common standards.

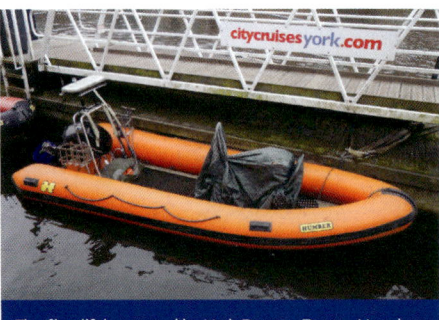

The first lifeboat used by York Rescue Boat, a Humber rigid inflatable, on the River Ouse at York. (Martin Fish)

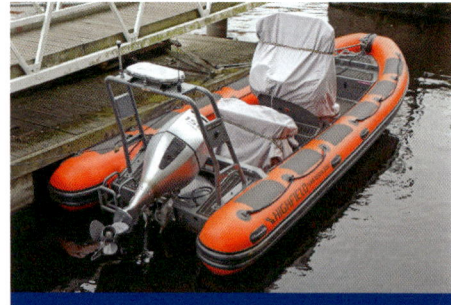

The Highfield Patrol 660 boat, formally named in July 2022, at the King's Staith Landing in York. (Martin Fish)

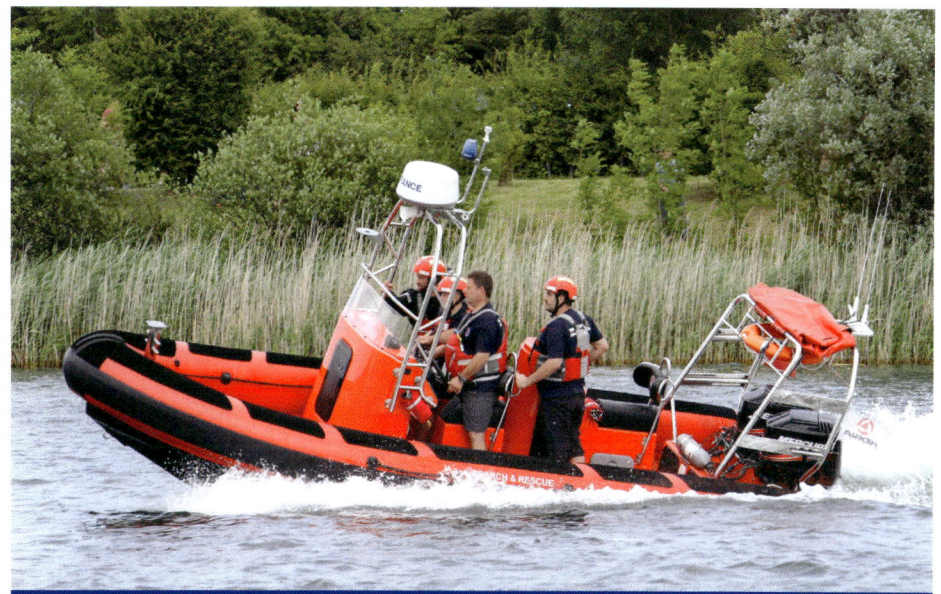

The Parker 650 rigid inflatable taking part in a Rescue Day event at Crowle in July 2015. (Martin Fish)

ASSETS For flood response work, Watersafe UK operates various SeaSearch MX390 inflatable boats powered by Mariner or Mercury outboards, and a Pioneer Multi rigid boat with a 50hp Mercury outboard. The Service continued to enhance the rescue assets available. In 2013 an AB Inflatable Profile RIB with a 50hp Mariner outboard was obtained. Two larger rigid inflatable lifeboats were obtained in 2015 and 2016. Parker RIBs of Gdynia, Poland, built a Parker 650 rigid inflatable, powered by twin Mercury 90hp outboard engines, with a comprehensive electrical fit out including radar. A Parker 510 boat, powered by a single 90hp Mercury outboard with post immersion start, was purchased in 2016. The boat's electronics included a down scan and side scan sonar.

A Nissan Navara 4x4 and van-based support vehicles and road-going trailers are used to launch the boats. The assets are based at a facility in Redhill Marina which has space for the boats and vehicles, and portacabin buildings providing training space.

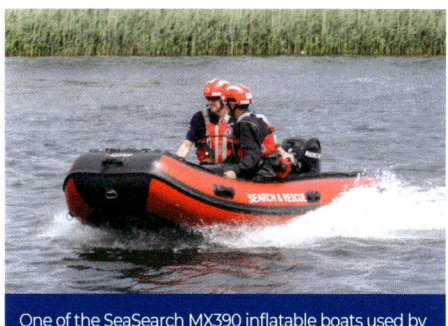

One of the SeaSearch MX390 inflatable boats used by Watersafe UK. (Martin Fish)

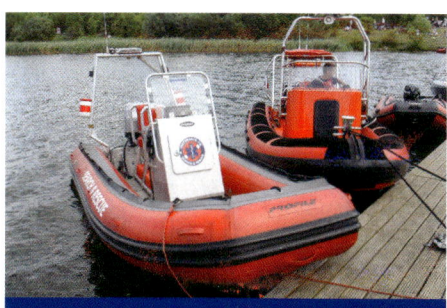

Watersafe UK Search & Rescue boats moored at Crowle. (Martin Fish)

Independent lifeboats of Britain

CLOSED STATIONS

BLYTH

YEARS OF OPERATION 2006 to 2012.
HISTORY The Blyth Volunteer Lifeboat Service (BAWLB) was formed when the RNLI withdrew its all-weather lifeboat. The volunteers of BAWLB subsequently raised £120,000 to buy the former Caister lifeboat Bernard Matthews, which was renamed Spirit of Blyth and Wansbeck. BAWLB became a declared facility with the Maritime and Coastguard agency in April 2006. However, the declared facility status was revoked in December 2012, and subsequent efforts to reinstate the operation failed, despite the acquisition in 2016 of the former RNLI 52ft Arun class lifeboat Sir William Arnold, which was named Samuel J. The boat never became

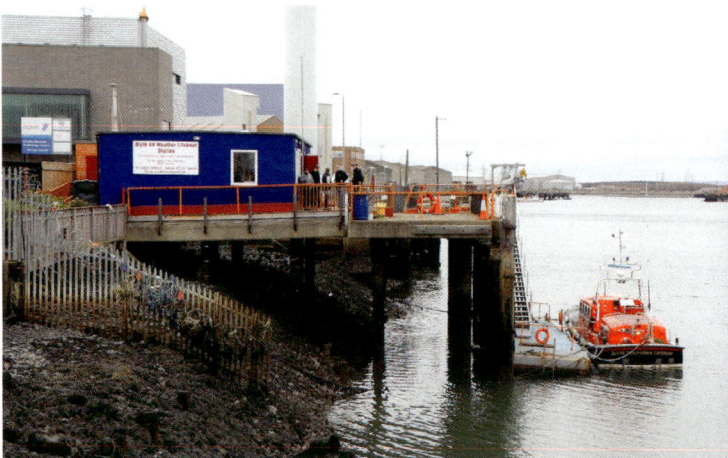

The shore facility at The Old Tugboat Jetty, on High Quay provided the crew with an operations room, meeting space and changing facilities. A mooring pontoon and access gangway were in place in front of the station buildings, with the Lochin 38 lifeboat moored in the River Blyth. (Nicholas Leach)

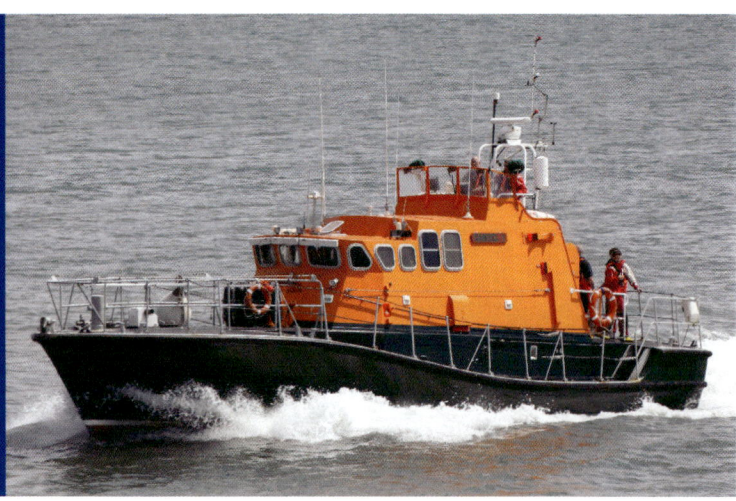

Following revocation of Blyth's declared facility status, the Service made a number of attempts to restart operations. The former RNLI 52ft Arun class lifeboat Sir William Arnold was acquired from Ireland, where it had been named Samuel J in private ownership, but this was the last lifeboat before the Service disbanded. (Martin Fish)

150 Independent lifeboats of Britain

a declared asset, and in 2019 it was sold on to a private buyer and left Blyth.
ASSETS 38ft 6in x 13ft Lochin 38 lifeboat, numbered 38-01, named Spirit of Blyth and Wansbeck, built 1991, Lochin Marine, Rye; in service at Caister 1991 to 2004.

CLEETHORPES

YEARS OF OPERATION 1969 to circa 2012.
HISTORY In November 1969 a group of parents who had tragically lost their children after a riding accident on Cleethorpes Beach formed the Cleethorpes Vigilantes Inshore Lifeboat Service. The intention was to support and assist the Coastguard, police and council and duties included beach searches, assistance with flood relief, and search and rescue at sea. Cleethorpes Rescue, as it became known, was operated by volunteers and funded by local business people, community organisations and public donations.

Funds raised equipped the service with premises, lifeboats, launch vehicles and all the safety equipment required to ensure the safety and security of the users of the Cleethorpes resort as well at the waters around the Humber Estuary. The main area covered was between Immingham Docks to North Coates, across to Spurn Point and back to Hawkins Point. During the summer months regular beach patrols were undertaken to ensure the safety of swimmers and individuals using power craft offshore. The organisation was disbanded circa 2012.

BIRLING GAP

YEARS OF OPERATION 1984 to 2016.
HISTORY The Birling Gap Safety Boat organisation was established in 1984 by Graham Collins, owner of the Birling Gap Hotel, and operated from the pebble beach set below the backdrop of the Seven Sisters cliffs, close to the village of East Dean. The service operated a number of small inflatable

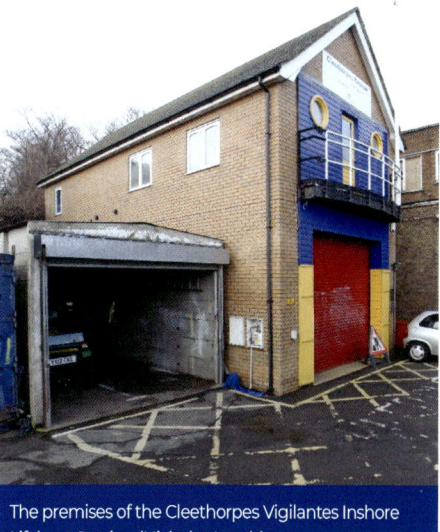

The premises of the Cleethorpes Vigilantes Inshore Lifeboat Service. (Nicholas Leach)

lifeboats, powered by outboard engines, and was operational at weekends and bank holidays. A boathouse was in place at the cliff top and a unique rail mounted crane was used to lift the lifeboat and launch trolley down onto the beach. The boat was pushed on its trolley over the beach into the water.

Coastal erosion ultimately caused the end of the service at Birling, as the chalk cliffs of were particularly vulnerable. In 2014 the boathouse had to be demolished due to erosion and loss of land. Further land loss meant that continued operation of the lifeboat became unviable and in 2016 the Birling Gap Safety Boat organisation was wound up with the boat and other rescue assets being transferred to a local volunteer lifeguard service in nearby Eastbourne.

GUERNSEY ST JOHN

YEARS OF OPERATION 1961 to 2018.
HISTORY The St John Guernsey Ambulance and Rescue Service was established in 1936, and within two years became Guernsey's only ambulance service when it took over the States Ambulance Service. Offering a

Independent lifeboats of Britain

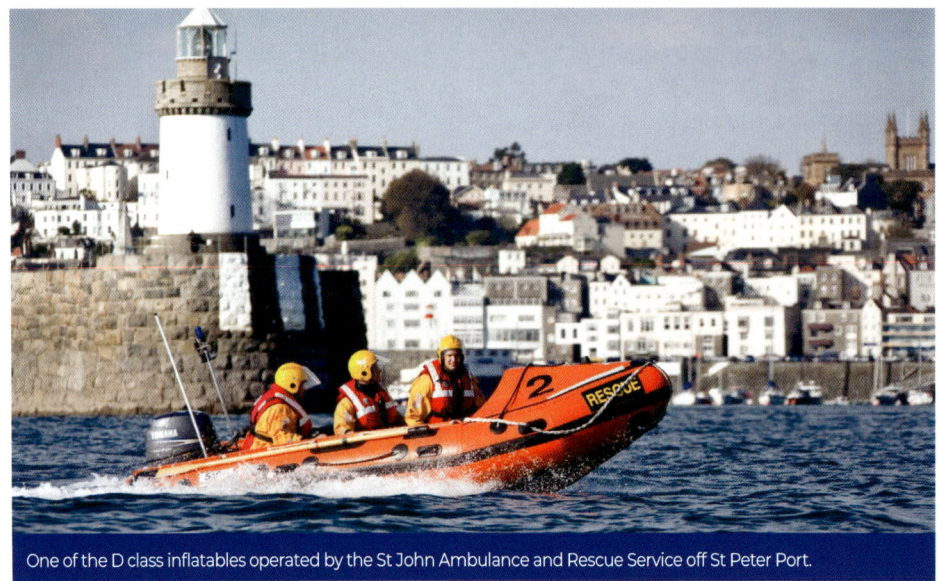

One of the D class inflatables operated by the St John Ambulance and Rescue Service off St Peter Port.

wider emergency response than traditional ambulance services, it expanded its range of activities during the 1950s and 1960s to include a marine ambulance, the operation of inshore rescue boats, a cliff rescue team and a recompression chamber.

The Service pioneered the use of inflatable boats for inshore rescue work in the late 1940s and 1950s before the RNLI adopted the craft. The early inflatable dinghies were launched from rigid boats and were paddled by oars. During the 1950s the St John Service assisted designers with research into the requirements of such craft for inshore rescue work, and in 1961 introduced Guernsey's first powered inflatable inshore rescue boat.

Experiments with rigid keels and broader boats were also conducted, and for a time the Service maintained a 17ft Beachcraft with a double-skinned fibreglass hull, operating from a mooring in St Peter Port harbour. This boat was powered by twin 40hp outboards giving a speed of 30 knots. In 1992 the Service also purchased an all-aluminium craft, as used in some parts of New Zealand, and conducted extensive trials in local waters.

The extensive experience in inshore rescue boat operations resulted in St John having a

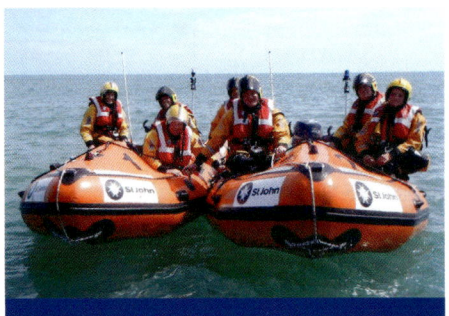

The two D class inflatables operated by the St John Guernsey Ambulance and Rescue Service.

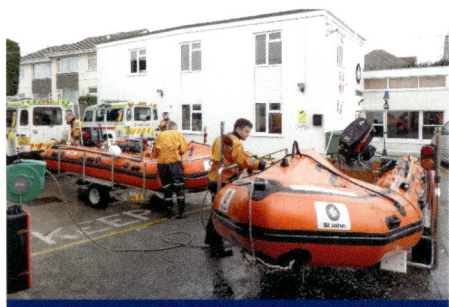

The two D class inflatables being washed down at the St John's HQ in St Peter Port after a training launch.

preference for inflatable boats, which could be placed against the rocks at the base of cliffs or driven into shallow surf in gullies. Initially using D class type inflatable boats manufactured by RFD, the Service progressed through the various generations of the D class design.

Two inshore boats, on call 24 hours a day, were housed at St John Headquarters on the outskirts of St Peter Port. They were towed overland by two Land Rovers to launch from slipways nearest to any reported incident. The boats were D class EA-16 type inflatables, manufactured by Avon Inflatables and powered by single 40hp four-stroke outboards giving a maximum speed of about 20 knots. Both boats were fitted with marine VHF radio, emergency ambulance communications and GPS satellite navigation equipment. Hand-held spotlights and illuminating flares were carried on board for night searches.

The Service was involved in may incidents, until 2017, when St John's inshore rescue capability was reviewed. Guernsey Harbour Master, Guernsey Coastguard and the RNLI were consulted as part of an independent review. The outcome of the review was announced in May 2018, with St John in Guernsey changing its focus to providing pre-hospital medical care and support in line with the changing health demands in the Island and withdrawing from the Inshore Rescue Boat (IRB) service at the end of the summer. The RNLI confirmed it would begin a two-year trial of a B Class Atlantic 85 inshore lifeboat in St Peter Port, and the Service's two D class inshore lifeboats were sold, with one going to Hornsea Inshore Rescue.

CLOVELLY

YEARS OF OPERATION 1990 to 1998.
HISTORY When the RNLI closed the lifeboat station at Clovelly in 1988, withdrawing the Clyde cruising lifeboat after a fast Tyne class lifeboat was stationed at nearby Appledore,

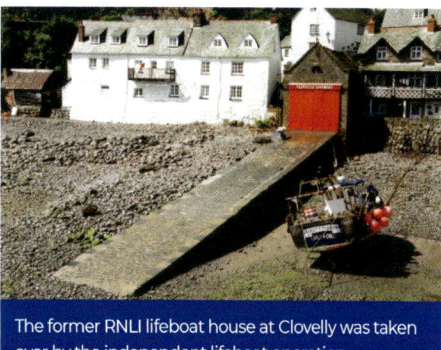

The former RNLI lifeboat house at Clovelly was taken over by the independent lifeboat operation.

the Clovelly Lifeboat Trust was established in November 1990 under the direction of the Hon John Rous of the Clovelly Estate. An 18ft Osborne Pacific rigid-inflatable named Pride of Clovelly was provided through donations raised locally and was operated our of the old RNLI lifeboat house. The lifeboat was powered by twin 40hp Mariner Magnum outboards, giving a top speed of approximately forty knots. However, after just eight years the RNLI returned and took over the station. On 14 May 1998 the station formally came under RNLI auspices after an Atlantic 21 had been sent to Clovelly the previous year for evaluation trials.

PORTISHEAD

YEARS OF OPERATION 1995 to 2015.
HISTORY The Portishead Lifeboat Trust was founded in 1995, following the closure of the Portishead Yacht & Sailing Club marine rescue service after twenty-five years. Headed by John McCorquodale as Chairman, the Board of Trustees responsible for the running of the Trust began a major fund-raising campaign and, within just over a year, a new 6.5m Ribcraft rigid-inflatable had been funded by local subscriptions and donations. On 6 October 1996 the lifeboat undertook its first rescue. A boathouse was built at Sugar Loaf Bay, adjacent to Portishead Yacht & Sailing Club, on a site two miles west of the docks, with a long slipway down to the water.

Independent lifeboats of Britain

ASSETS The first boat served until June 2003, when it was replaced by a newer rigid-inflatable of the same type, which was named Denbar Sage, having been largely funded by Barbara Palmer. Denbar Sage was in service from 2003 to 2012. On 28 August 2008, during a training exercise, she was damaged by heavy seas, and the Trust had to borrow a lifeboat from Geoff Dawe while repairs were undertaken to the boat by Ribcraft.

On 5 November 2008 the RNLI approved the adoption of PLT, a decision confirmed at a meeting of the RNLI Trustees in April 2009. However, this was just the start of a fairly long drawn out process as a new shore facility was needed for the RNLI to complete the adoption. Between 2011 and 2015, while PLT was being adopted and a suitable location for a station was being found, the RNLI leased two Atlantic 75s to the PLT. The first was B-729, which had served at Kilrush for fourteen years. She was replaced by the former Burnham-on-Crouch

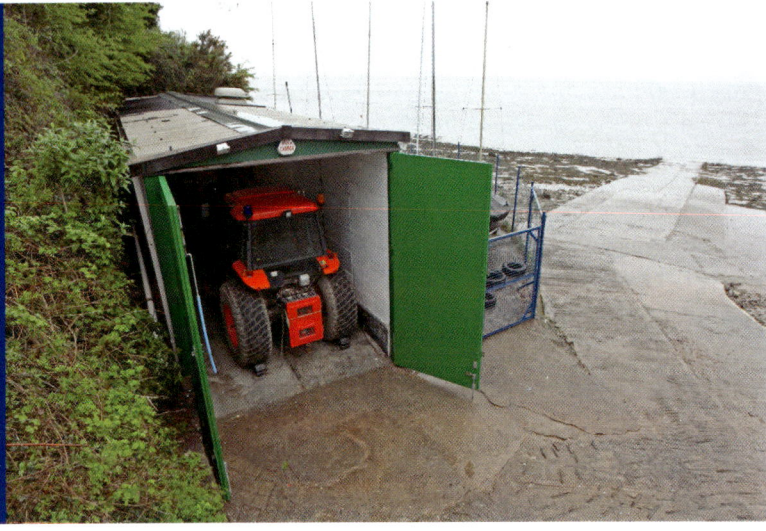

The small boathouse at Sugar Loaf Bay, Portishead, pictured in April 2010, was used by the Portishead Lifeboat Trust throughout its existence. (Nicholas Leach)

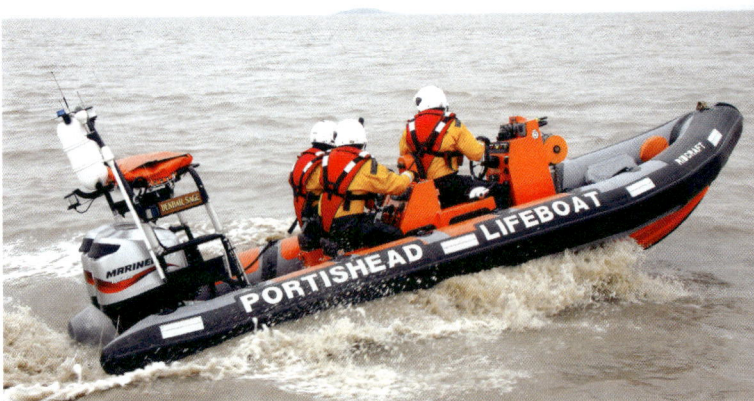

The Ribcraft type rigid-inflatable Denbar Sage on exercise off Portishead in March 2010. During her career, which ended in 2012, she launched 158 times and saved eleven lives. (Nicholas Leach)

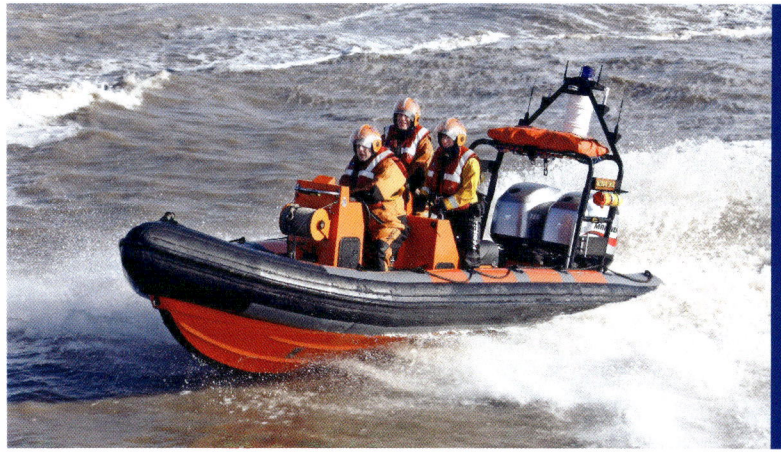

The Ribcraft type rigid-inflatable Denbar Sage on exercise off Portishead in March 2010. During her career, which ended in 2012, she launched 158 times and saved eleven lives. (Nicholas Leach)

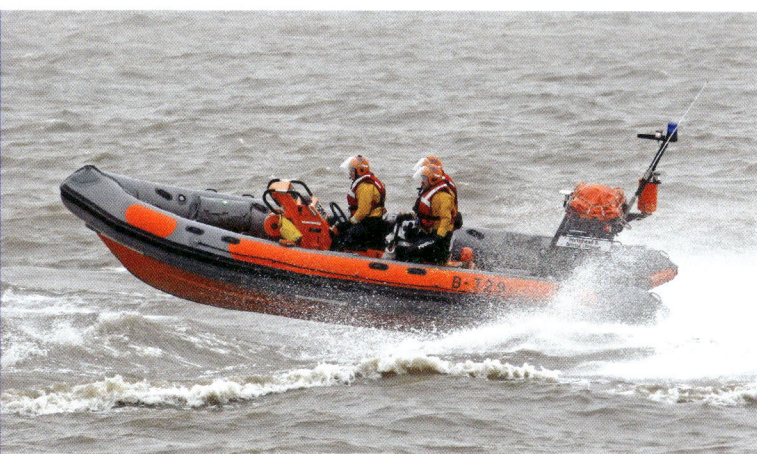

The Atlantic 75 B-729 (originally named Rose West and stationed at Kilrush) in the Bristol Channel. She was leased to the Portishead Lifeboat Trust by the RNLI from 2011 to May 2013. (Nicholas Leach)

Atlantic 75 Brandy Hole (B-733) in May 2013, which remained until 2015. In April 2015 the RNLI formally took over the station.

STONEHAVEN

YEARS OF OPERATION 1984 to 2013.
HISTORY The Maritime Rescue Institute (MRI) began as a training centre at Stonehaven. It was set up by Hamish McDonald in 1984 in response to a need for advanced specialised boat training and emergency response in a maritime environment. The commercial division provided marine safety training to the oil and gas sector and Merchant Navy. MRI Ltd employed up to 18 staff with up to 40 trainees per week. In addition to training, the training base, boats and instructors provided an independent rescue unit declared to HM Coastguard from Stonehaven. MRI took over sea rescue work from the RNLI, who had operated a D class ILB between 1967 and 1984.

The late 1990s saw an increased demand from industry for training facilities to cover a wider range of safety, survival and emergency response training. The financial investment that this would have required from MRI Ltd was not viable and so the company's commercial trade and associated assets were sold to RGIT Montrose on 1 December 2003. The funds gained from this sale were

Independent lifeboats of Britain

utilised to develop Maritime Rescue Institute as a standalone charity and allowed it to focus on the development of waterborne rescue training services throughout Europe and developing countries. The centre's work included supporting SAR response organisations, carrying out research and development programmes, and delivering specialised training to lifeboat crews from around the world. The charity also delivered education programmes to schools, focussing on environment awareness and coastal safety.

PREVIOUS ASSETS MRI operated a number of different rigid inflatable lifeboats. The main lifeboats were MRI 24, MRI 28 and MRI 42. MRI 24, named Janet Buchanan Smith, was built in 1978 as part of a joint research programme between the Robert Gordon's Institute of Technology and the Department of Trade and Industry, and was powered by twin 90hp Yamaha petrol outboards giving a speed of thirty knots. A fixed buoyancy block provided a self-righting capability, and navigational aids included a VHF, radar and GPS plotter. The boat was completely rebuilt in 2002.

MRI 28, built in-house by MRI in 2003, was based on an Avon 8.5 hull and entered service in January 2004. Powered by twin Steyr diesel inboard engines driving Alamarin waterjets, the boat had a top speed of 30 knots. The craft had an endurance of 180 nautical miles or six hours duration at full speed. An open central console was covered by a fixed roof which provided buoyancy for self-righting. A crew of five persons, two stretcher cases plus six other persons could be carried. Electronic equipment included a VHF, radar and GPS plotter with night vision.

The MRI's largest lifeboat was MRI 42 David Stogdon MBE, one of the RNLI's Medina class boats, which was built in 1984 as a trial craft. Designated official number 1091 by the RNLI, the boat was obtained by MRI in 2000 from Liverpool, totally stripped, having had a variety of uses since being disposed of by the RNLI. The boat was rebuilt by Amble Boatyard and relaunched in October 2001. David Stogdon MBE was the designer of the original RNLI Medina, and he came to Stonehaven for the naming ceremony on 31 October 2001.

Powered by twin Caterpillar engines driving Hamilton waterjets, MRI 42 had a top speed of twenty-four knots with an endurance of approximately 150 nautical miles or six hours at top speed. The enclosed wheelhouse provided seating for five crew, and a separate survivor space could hold two stretchers plus twelve other persons. Electronic equipment included VHF radios, VHF direction finder, GPS, radar and an integrated chartplotter.

The MRI's last lifeboat came into service in 2010. MRI trustee Bill Beattie donated

The MRI's boats moored in Stonehaven harbour in August 1998. (Nicholas Leach)

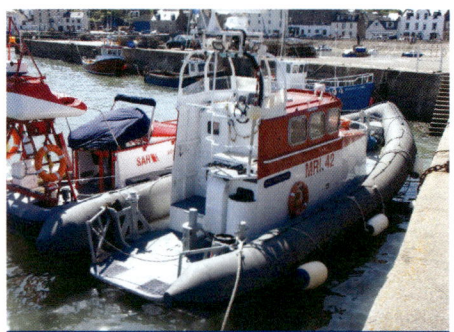

The former RNLI Medina class MRI42 (ex-ON-1091) in service at Stonehaven in 2010. (Martin Fish)

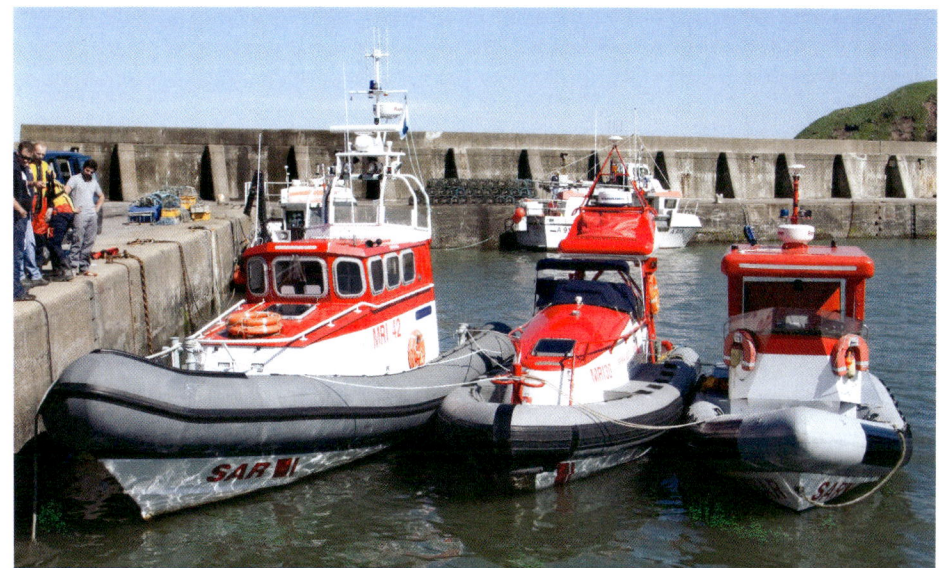

The MRI at Stonehaven operated a variety of rescue craft. Pictured in 2010 are, left to right, the former RNLI Medina class MRI42 (ex-ON-1091), named David Stogdon MBE; the former KNRM 9, Antje class rigid inflatable MRI 30, named Barbara Lesley; and MRI 24, named Janet Buchanan Smith. (Martin Fish)

funds to purchase MRI 30, which was named Barbara Lesley after his wife. The 9m Antje class lifeboat, which had a top speed of thirty-six knots and was powered by twin 230hp engines driving twin waterjets, was built by the KNRM, the Dutch lifeboat service, in 1997 and operated at Cadzand, named Jacoba Elisabeth. A substantial roll bar at the stern supported a fixed buoyancy block to give the boat a self-righting capability.

CLOSURE The MRI operation came to an end in December 2012, when Stonehaven suffered extensive storm damage. MRI's rescue boats, as well as the buildings, were damaged so badly that the organisation was put out of action. In February 2013 it was announced that MRI had been struggling with falling donations and, in the wake of the storm, the charity's board decided there was no option apart from to close the operation. In response to the closure, the RNLI established a station in 2014 with an Atlantic 75 ILB.

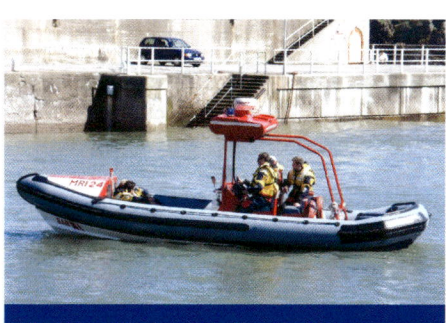

MRI 24 Janet Buchanan Smith undertaking crew training in the harbour, May 2010. (Martin Fish)

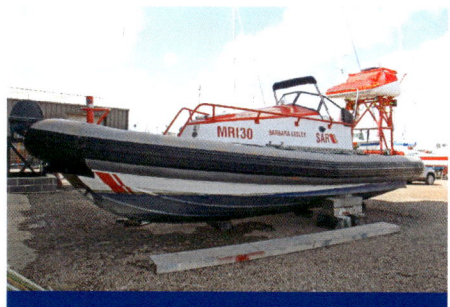

MRI 30 Barbara Lesley at Amble Boatyard after the MRI service was closed. (Martin Fish)

Independent lifeboats of Britain

SUMMARY OF INDEPENDENT LIFEBOAT ST

Location	Organisation	Founded	Page
ENGLAND – EAST COAST			
Boulmer	Boulmer Volunteer Rescue Service	1969	12
Runswick	Runswick Bay Rescue Boat	1982	14
Hornsea	Hornsea Inshore Rescue	1994	16
Hessle	Humber Rescue	1990	20
ENGLAND – EAST ANGLIA			
Mundesley	Mundesley Volunteer Inshore Lifeboat	1973	26
Sea Palling	Sea Palling Independent Lifeboat	1972	29
Hemsby	Hemsby Lifeboat	1977	32
Caister	Caister Volunteer Lifeboat Service	1969	35
Felixstowe	Felixstowe Volunteer Coast Patrol	1997	41
ENGLAND – SOUTH COAST			
Pett Level	Pett Level Independent Rescue Boat	1971	44
Southsea (Portsea Rescue)	Portsmouth and Southsea Voluntary Lifeguards	1933	47
Gosport	Gosport and Fareham Inshore Rescue Service	1969	50
Hamble	Hamble Lifeboat	1968	54
Lepe Country Park	Solent Rescue	1971	58
Sidmouth	Sidmouth Independent Lifeboat	1968	61
Hope Cove	Hope Cove Lifeboat	2010	65
ISLE OF WIGHT			
Ryde	Ryde Inshore Rescue	1969	68
Sandown	Sandown & Shanklin Independent Lifeboat	1972	72
Freshwater	Freshwater Independent Lifeboat	1972	76
CHANNEL ISLANDS			
St Helier	Jersey Fire & Rescue Service	1960	80
St Helier	Jersey Lifeboat Association	2018	82
BRISTOL CHANNEL			
Burnham-on-Sea	BARB Search & Rescue (Burnham Area Rescue Boat)	1992	85
Wyre Forest (Kidderminster)	Severn Area Rescue Association	2005	99
Tewkesbury	Severn Area Rescue Association	2007	100
Upton-upon-Severn	Severn Area Rescue Association	2019	100

...NS OF ENGLAND, WALES AND SCOTLAND

Location	Organisation	Founded	Page
Sharpness	Severn Area Rescue Association	1986	94
Beachley	Severn Area Rescue Association	1973	88
WALES			
Newport	Severn Area Rescue Association	2014	99
Loughor	Loughor Inshore Rescue	1969	101
Ferryside	Ferryside Lifeboat	1966	103
ENGLAND – NORTH WEST			
Liverpool	Merseyside Fire & Rescue – Marine Rescue Unit	1984	106
Southport	Southport Offshore Rescue Trust	1988	109
Flookburgh	Bay Search & Rescue	1999	113
Ulverston	Ulverston Inshore Rescue	2002	116
Askham	Duddon Inshore Rescue	1969	118
Haverigg	Haverigg Inshore Rescue	1973	122
Maryport	Maryport Inshore Rescue	1978	126
SCOTLAND			
Glencaple	Nith Inshore Rescue	1981	130
Port William	Port William Inshore Rescue	1979	133
Mossyard	Fleet Bay Inshore Rescue Boat	1974	136
Glasgow	Glasgow Humane Society	1790	137
Luss	Loch Lomond Rescue Boat	1977	139
Dornoch	East Sutherland Rescue Association	1981	141
Findhorn	Moray Inshore Rescue Organisation	2005	144
St Abbs	St Abbs Lifeboat	2016	146
INLAND LIFEBOATS			
York	York Rescue Boat	2014	148
Redhill Marina, Ratcliffe on Soar, Nottingham	Watersafe UK Search & Rescue Team	2009	148

ACKNOWLEDGEMENTS
The authors are extremely grateful to the very many volunteers at the independent lifeboat stations for their assistance in the compilation of this book; without their input we could not have completed our researches. We also wish to thank all those who have allowed their photographs to be used, and, while we have made every effort to accurately credit the images, we apologise in advance if this has not been possible. Finally, many thanks to Ian Moignard for proofing the book with his usual thoroughness.

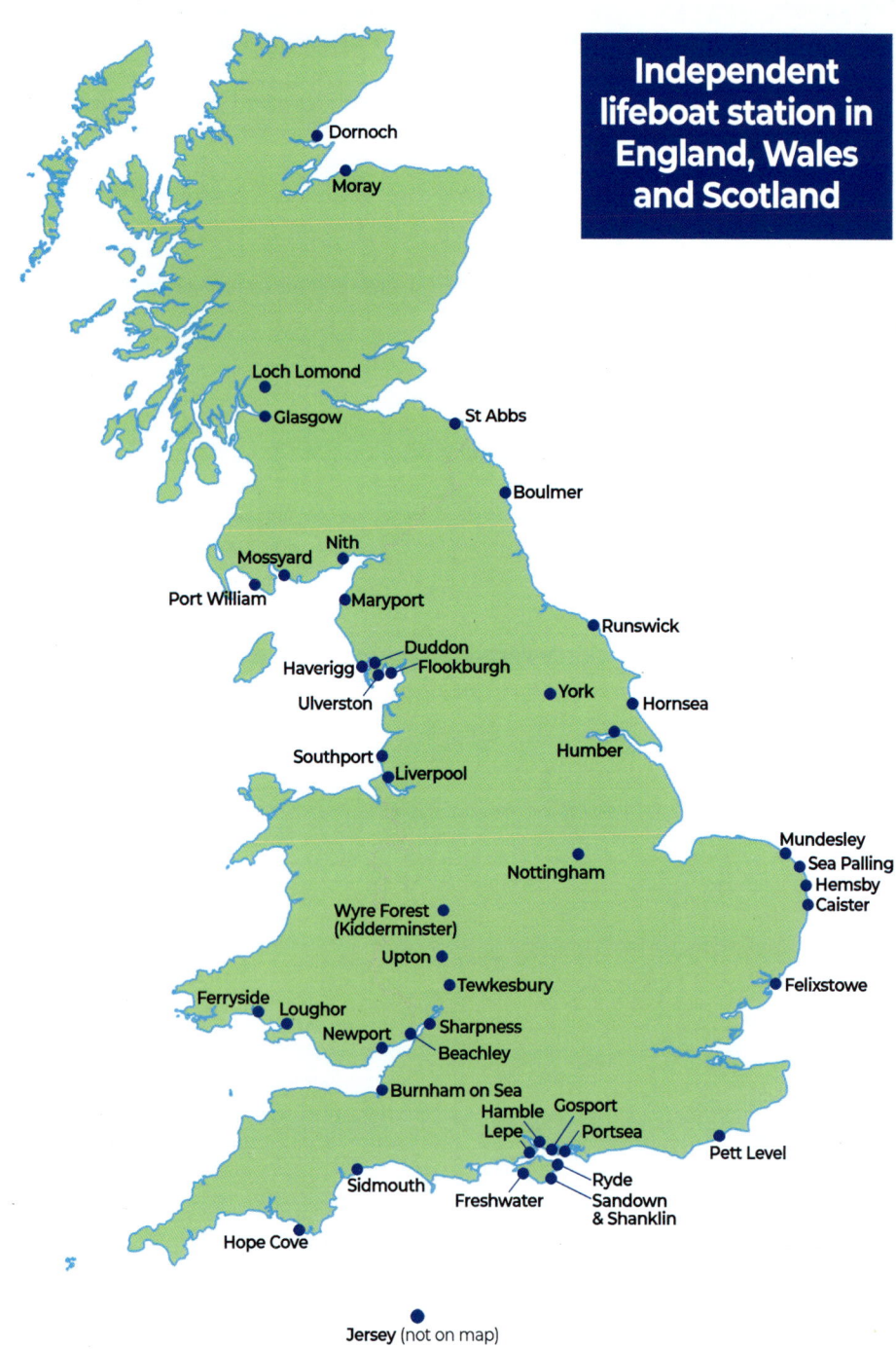